# Introduction to Surgical Trials

Stephen Lyman • Olufemi R. Ayeni
Jason L. Koh • Norimasa Nakamura
Jón Karlsson
Editors

# Introduction to Surgical Trials

Springer

ISAKOS
International Society of Arthroscopy, Knee Surgery and Orthopaedic Sports Medicine

*Editors*
Stephen Lyman
Hospital for Special Surgery
New York, NY, USA

Medical Education
Kyushu University School of Medicine
Fukuoka, Japan

Jason L. Koh
Mark R. Neaman Family Chair
of Orthopaedic Surgery
Orthopaedic & Spine Institute
Endeavor Health
Evanston, IL, USA

Clinical Professor, University of
Chicago Pritzker School of Medicine
Chicago, IL, USA

Adjunct Professor, Northwestern
University McCormick School of
Engineering
Evanston, IL, USA

Jón Karlsson
Department of Orthopaedics
Sahlgrenska University Hospital
Sahlgrenska Academy
Gothenburg University
Göteborg, Sweden

Olufemi R. Ayeni
Division of Orthopaedic Surgery
Department of Surgery
McMaster University
Hamilton, ON, Canada

Department of Health Research
Methods, Evidence, and Impact
McMaster University
Hamilton, ON, Canada

Norimasa Nakamura
Institute for Medical Science in Sports
Osaka Health Science University
Osaka, Osaka, Japan

ISBN 978-3-031-92304-3 ISBN 978-3-031-77563-5 (eBook)
https://doi.org/10.1007/978-3-031-77563-5



This Springer imprint is published by the registered company Springer Nature Switzerland AG
The registered company address is: Gewerbestrasse 11, 6330 Cham, Switzerland

# Foreword

This *Introduction to Surgical Trials* is a welcome and much-needed addition to the body of knowledge in both sports medicine and orthopedic surgery, more broadly. As a specialty society, ISAKOS has demonstrated its global objective of advancing the field of sports medicine by commissioning this work, thereby providing a vital resource to the much broader surgical research community.

While there have been well-conducted randomized controlled trials (RCTs) in sports medicine over the past two decades, many more collaborative networks to plan, design, and conduct trials are needed to further advance patient care. Lyman, Ayeni, Koh, Nakamura, and Karlsson are to be commended for recruiting the most experienced clinician scientists and researchers in the field to provide this comprehensive collection of resources for investigators in this field. The title includes the word "Introduction"; however, this resource is far more than an introduction. The text provides details that can indeed educate investigators just starting their careers, but it will also serve as a resource for mid-career and even senior clinical investigators.

The first chapter broadly introduces the topic, pointing out salient issues in each chapter. This is useful for the trainee or early-career researcher before moving on to subsequent chapters with greater detail. The final chapter on the future of trials provides a valuable summary of the importance of trials and the benefits of various trial designs, making it particularly useful for experienced researcher.

The midsection (Chaps. 2–18) is authored by experienced investigators, covering the details required for the appropriate trial design, conduct, and monitoring. The final section on alternative designs to the gold-standard RCTs is particularly useful in guiding both early-career and experienced investigators. The entire text will educate the reader not only on the details of optimum trial design but also on the limitations of RCTs. These alternative study designs each have a place in the researcher's toolbox.

All trial designs are useful for some research questions, but not for all. The involvement of senior, experienced clinician researchers in trial design cannot be underestimated. This text can fulfill that role to a great degree.

The field of sports medicine and surgery will be advanced by the authors' efforts in providing this cutting-edge information, and I am hopeful that it will be widely used to advance this goal.

Department of Orthopaedic Surgery
University of Minnesota
Minneapolis, MN, USA

Marc F. Swiontkowski

# Preface

As with any modern textbook, this *Introduction to Surgical Trials* is a collaborative effort. When we decided to undertake this project at the 2019 ISAKOS World Congress in Cancun, Mexico, we did not appreciate the time or effort this would require. Between a global pandemic, the loss of colleagues, and the ever-shifting landscape of clinical research best practices, what we initially anticipated would take 18 months has taken more than 60.

Nevertheless, we are proud to provide the orthopedic sports medicine community with this comprehensive guide to the conduct of surgical trials. Our field has long been considered behind many other fields of medicine, largely due to the challenges of studying therapeutic efficacy and safety in surgery. With a pharmaceutical intervention, the drug can always be stopped if the patient is having an adverse reaction. In surgery, there are no do-overs. As such, studying these procedures using drug trial methods is suboptimal. This text provides a road map to success in conducting surgical trials, rather than dressing drug trials up as surgical trials.

I owe a debt of gratitude to my co-editors, Drs. Ayeni, Koh, Nakamura, and Karlsson, who represent mentors, colleagues, trainees, and friends from across my own orthopedic research career. Their personal introductions to many of the chapter authors were vital in securing the best possible team of contributors. Further, when the burden became too much for me to handle alone, they were there to communicate with the authors or take a fresh look at chapters. Finally, they were there to hold me accountable when something languished in my inbox for too long.

Fortunately, due to the global professional relationships developed over decades, my co-editors and I were able to put together a team of accomplished clinical investigators from across the globe (nine countries on three continents) to write each chapter in this textbook. These authors graciously provided insights into their own fields of expertise. This was not a work for their enrichment, but for yours.

Finally, I would like to extend sincere thanks to Madison Thompson, MD, who has been a mentee of mine since she was a precocious undergraduate, introduced to me by Todd Albert, MD, former Chief of Surgery at Hospital for Special Surgery. Those personal mentorship requests from higher-ups do not always work out. In this case, it has been a tremendous success. Without her assistance, *Introduction to Surgical Trials* may not have happened.

We sincerely hope that this textbook will help continue to improve the quality of orthopedic sports medicine research and advance the field as we endeavor to provide the best evidence-based care possible to those in need.

Warm Regards,

Fukuoka, Japan Stephen Lyman

# Contents

# Part I

# Trial Design

# Why Do We Need Surgical Trials?

1

Stephen Lyman

## 1.1 Introduction

At its foundation, surgical innovation should be safe, effective, and cost-effective. Randomized controlled trials remain the gold standard in human subjects research to evaluate these surgical innovations. The limitations of surgical trials will be documented throughout this text with every effort made to mitigate the challenges through current best practices based on both previous research and the extensive experience of the individual chapter co-authors.

Orthopedic surgery is littered with failed innovations that were at best costly and ineffective and at worst catastrophic. The classic example is the use of Gore-Tex as a synthetic anterior cruciate ligament (ACL) in the 1980s. Despite preliminary evidence of successful knee stabilization, complications and graft failure occurred at alarming rates [1]. Severe osteolysis was discovered in some patients, destroying the integrity of the knees of these otherwise healthy patients. The product was pulled from the market in 1993.

You'd think we would have learned from this disaster, but in the early 2000s, the metal-on-metal hip-bearing surface was introduced broadly. In attempting to resolve osteolysis from polyethylene wear, innovators created metal particulate debris that led to devastating soft tissue destruction and permanent disability in thousands of patients worldwide [2]. Failure rates as high as 50% were seen in some cohorts, particularly among patients receiving smaller diameter femoral heads. Blood serum levels of cobalt, chromium, and molybdenum levels were seen to rise by 10–10,000% in patients with metal-on-metal implants [3]. The long-term effects of these high metal ion levels are at present unknown.

In both of these illustrative examples, a well-designed, well-controlled, adequately powered surgical trial could have identified the unacceptably high risk these implants posed to patients prior to broad clinical use. Of course, that would also require the Food and Drug Administration (FDA) and similar agencies globally to competently review premarket approval applications for implantable medical devices. In the US, the FDA's 510(k) premarket notification approval process is offered as a fast track to market for substantially equivalent implanted medical devices considered to be of minimal or medium risk [4]. Most orthopedic implants fall into these two classes because they are not considered life-sustaining or at unreasonable risk of causing serious injury or illness. In most cases, this is true, though in the case of both the Gore-Tex ACL and metal-on-metal hip implants, there was an unreasonable risk of serious injury or illness.

S. Lyman (✉)
Hospital for Special Surgery, New York, NY, USA

Medical Education, Kyushu University School of Medicine, Fukuoka, Japan
e-mail: LymanS@hss.edu


S. Lyman et al. (eds.), *Introduction to Surgical Trials*,
https://doi.org/10.1007/978-3-031-77563-5_1

The balance of speed of innovation and patient safety is a delicate one from a societal perspective, but with our admonition to *do no harm*, the decision should be clear within the medical community. Innovative orthopedic technologies should be carefully scrutinized prior to broad clinical implementation. When at all feasible, these technologies should be evaluated with rigorous surgical trial best practices.

Chapters 2, 3, 4, 5, 6, 7, 8, 9, 10 and 11 cover topics that should be considered during trial design. While they are certainly relevant to trial conduct Chaps. 12, 13, 14 and 15 are marginally less vital. If investigators have not finalized their decisions for the topics in Chaps. 2, 3, 4, 5, 6, 7, 8, 9, 10 and 11, the trial will be very difficult if not impossible to complete. Therefore, we have chosen to separate them in this way. Chapters 16, 17 and 18 cover trial completion and are primarily focused on data integrity, statistical analysis, and reporting. Chapters 19, 20 and 21 cover regulatory standards for different parts of the globe, while the final chapters explore alternatives to surgical trials. Despite being the gold standard, sometimes randomized controlled trials are not the best choice to answer a particular research question.

## 1.2 Design Considerations

Perhaps the greatest challenge facing a surgical trial, but also the key to assuring the minimization of biased results is the issue of randomization (see Chaps. 2 and 3). Every patient enrolled should have an unbiased opportunity to receive one of the treatments offered. The problem, of course, is that patients do not generally like to have their treatment decision left to chance, especially when one or more of those decisions involves a knife, drill, or saw.

Therefore, the interventions being offered should be carefully considered. Further, given the substantial risk of a placebo effect, blinding should be implemented whenever feasible. This is most reasonable when alternative surgical interventions are being offered. A patient will not know what happened in the operating room. However, blinding of the patient, observer, clinical team, and/or statistician is not always feasible. These topics are explored in Chap. 4.

Of course, an adequate number of patients need to be recruited in order to successfully test the trial hypotheses (usually a combination of safety and efficacy but increasingly including a cost-effectiveness component as well). Therefore, in cooperation with a trained statistician, the investigators should determine the sample size needed for recruitment (Chap. 5). Then the hard work begins—recruiting enough patients to successfully complete the trial.

Once patients have been successfully recruited, consented, and enrolled, they will need to have their treatment allocated. This is best done randomly, though alternative methods do exist that may aid with minimizing bias while improving recruitment success (Chap. 6). Treatment allocation is further explored in Chap. 7.

A further challenge is that once a patient is enrolled, there is typically a period of time between that moment and treatment. If, in that interim, a patient assigned to surgery refuses surgery, or a patient assigned to non-operative treatment opts for surgery, the randomization can be compromised. This is an alarmingly common occurrence in surgical trials comparing surgical intervention to conservative management. In the SPORT Trial evaluating lumbar fusion, a full 40% of patients assigned to surgery did not have surgery within 12 months of recruitment [5]. This clearly has implications for the interpretability of results since intention-to-treat analysis is the best practice. Beyond this crossover, there is the issue of early failure. How are those patients managed throughout the trial? Both of these topics are addressed in Chap. 8.

As patients move through the trial from treatment to interim follow-up evaluations to final evaluation, life can sometimes get in the way. Patients may graduate, change jobs, move, get divorced, lose interest, any of these which can hinder complete follow-up. Strategies for optimizing follow-up given these challenges are explored in Chap. 9.

Other decisions that will influence all of the above are A) which outcomes measures are being evaluated for safety and efficacy, and B) how long follow-up will continue. With regard to outcome measures (Chap. 10), medicine and surgery have rapidly moved to patient-centered outcomes evaluation with patient-reported outcome measures (PROMs) being the most commonly used measure in orthopedic surgical trials. These PROMs present special challenges for follow-up since patients are required to take an active role in evaluating their health rather than passively returning for a clinic visit for imaging, blood work, and/or physical examination.

Many top orthopedic journals today require a minimum of 2 years follow-up for studies evaluating implantable medical devices. This provides time for full recovery from surgery and up to a year or more of usual use of the implant in daily life, which should help provide some evidence of risk of early failure due to flawed engineering or technical difficulty with appropriate implantation. However, this also provides a challenge for investigators hoping to optimize recruitment and capture PROMs. Therefore, when designing a surgical trial it is important to consider how long the follow-up period should last (Chap. 11). The 2-year results of clinical observation with the Gore-Tex ACL suggested that there may have been a problem, but it was not entirely clear due to the small number of patients available for study [1]. Similarly, failure rates at 2 years for metal-on-metal implants were elevated compared to other implant designs but not alarmingly so and this trend was more quickly visible in large national registries rather than in smaller trials [2]. Safety outcomes are usually the most difficult to measure. Therefore, investigators should think carefully about potential alternative biomarkers that may signal signs of trouble. For example, in the case of metal-on-metal hip implants, serum metal ion levels increased faster than the implants failed [3].

## 1.3 Trial Conduct and Completion

While RCTs are the gold standard, they are also some of the most carefully regulated studies in the world since patient care is being randomized. Therefore, ethical approval is of utmost importance prior to study initiation (Chap. 11).

Perhaps the greatest threat to unsuccessful trial completion is a lack of adequate resources. Personnel, equipment, time, and costs should all be carefully considered to ensure that the trial can be successfully completed (Chap. 12).

Most ethics panels will require an independent adverse event monitoring board to determine whether the trial continues or is terminated early due to patient safety concerns or overwhelming evidence of the superiority of one treatment over the other. Chapter 13 provides best practice guidelines for adverse event reporting.

Winding down a trial is every bit as important as the prior steps. The data should be properly secured and audited. All proper documentation should also be provided to the appropriate parties (e.g., notices to ethics committees). Chapter 14 covers Trial Closeout.

Prior to conducting analysis of trial data, the data should be cleaned and if necessary appropriate imputation strategies should be implemented (Chap. 15). Finally, the a priori statistical analysis plan should virtually always be used to answer the research questions. These analysis plans should not be deviated from except under extraordinary circumstances. A guide to trial statistical analysis best practices is covered in Chap. 16.

Recent work by the EQUATOR network has created universal reporting standards for many different study design types. The CONSORT Statement (Chap. 17) provides the roadmap for trial reporting and is highly relevant to surgical trials as well as other medical interventions.

Regulatory guidance varies by region of the world with the US (Chap. 18) and EU having somewhat different criteria. Due to the international scope of ISAKOS, we also include an overview of the regulations that govern trials in Japan (Chap. 20), a country with a unique history of medical misadventures leading to regulatory change.

Finally, given that surgical trials are extremely challenging to undertake and successfully complete, we offer several study design alternatives that, while they do not necessarily adhere to the extremely rigorous standards of an RCT, may provide a practical alternative path to answering important surgical research questions. These are pragmatic trials (Chap. 21), prospective cohort studies (Chap. 22), and surgical registries (Chap. 23).

Our text concludes with a perspective from noted orthopedist, researcher, and journal editor, Professor Jón Karlsson on the future of surgical trials (Chap. 24). While the future is currently unknown, some challenges are on the horizon. As a professional society, we hope that we can meet them head-on to improve orthopedic patient care globally.

## 1.4 Final Thoughts

The need for surgical trials has never been greater as technological innovation is accelerating at a previously unimaginable pace. If we hope to provide the best care possible to our patients, we need to be sure that the evidence we use to make treatment decisions is of the highest quality possible. Until a better mousetrap is created, surgical trials remain our most rigorous option.

Onward and Upward.

## References

1. Paulos LE, Rosenberg TD, Grewe SR, Tearse DS, Beck CL. The GORE-TEX anterior cruciate ligament prosthesis. A long-term follow-up. Am J Sports Med. 1992;20(3):246–52. https://doi.org/10.1177/036354659202000302.
2. Kwon YM, Jacobs JJ, MacDonald SJ, Potter HG, Fehring TK, Lombardi AV. Evidence-based understanding of management perils for metal-on-metal hip arthroplasty patients. J Arthroplast. 2012;27(8 Suppl):20–5. https://doi.org/10.1016/j.arth.2012.03.029.
3. Drummond J, Tran P, Fary C. Metal-on-metal hip arthroplasty: a review of adverse reactions and patient management. J Funct Biomater. 2015;6(3):486–99. https://doi.org/10.3390/jfb6030486. PMID: 26132653; PMCID: PMC4598667.
4. https://www.fda.gov/medical-devices/premarket-submissions-selecting-and-preparing-correct-submission/premarket-notification-510k. Last visited 9 Jan 2024.
5. Weinstein JN, Tosteson TD, Lurie JD, et al. Surgical vs nonoperative treatment for lumbar disk herniation: the Spine Patient Outcomes Research Trial (SPORT): a randomized trial. JAMA. 2006;296(20):2441–50. https://doi.org/10.1001/jama.296.20.2441.

# Addressing the Challenges to Surgical Randomization

2

Dan Cohen, Casey Wang, Graeme Matthewson, Andrew Duong, and Olufemi R. Ayeni

## 2.1 Introduction

Randomized controlled trials (RCTs) are generally considered to be at the top of the echelon in terms of level of evidence and clinical applicability of clinical research results. These trials are best suited for research questions that are already well-developed in terms of demonstrating safety and possible efficacy of an intervention but still require high-quality evidence before recommending broad changes to clinical practice guidelines.

### 2.1.1 Importance of Randomization

The process of randomization is the key component that differentiates RCTs from strictly observational clinical studies. In the setting of therapeutic RCTs, randomization removes the treatment decision from the clinical care team and leaves it up to chance, which allows for a high degree of trust in the eventual results being due to the intervention being studied rather than biases that may not be balanced between groups if usual care pathways were respected. This is particularly important in surgical trials given the increased potential for bias as will be discussed throughout this chapter.

The most important features of randomization are that it truly allocates treatment randomly and that assignments are tamper proof so that neither intentional nor unintentional factors can influence treatment assignment. The goal of randomization is to ensure that factors such as age, sex, race, and other patient characteristics are distributed at random in order to prevent any bias from influencing associations between intervention and outcome. In addition, it allows for both unknown and unmeasured prognostic factors to have a similar likelihood of appearing in any potential treatment allocation group due to the random nature of group assignment. Forms of bias that are reduced or prevented due to randomization include confounding bias, selection bias, performance bias, attrition bias, detection bias, and reporting bias, among others (see Table 2.1 for definitions of these biases).

### 2.1.2 Forms of Bias

#### 2.1.2.1 Confounding Bias

In the case of confounding bias, this is defined as a situation in which a spurious association between exposure and outcome is observed as a

D. Cohen · C. Wang · G. Matthewson · A. Duong
Division of Orthopaedic Surgery,
Department of Surgery, McMaster University,
Hamilton, ON, Canada

O. R. Ayeni (✉)
Division of Orthopaedic Surgery,
Department of Surgery, McMaster University,
Hamilton, ON, Canada

Department of Health Research Methods,
Evidence, and Impact, McMaster University,
Hamilton, ON, Canada


S. Lyman et al. (eds.), *Introduction to Surgical Trials*,
https://doi.org/10.1007/978-3-031-77563-5_2

**Table 2.1** Forms of bias

| Form of bias | Definition |
|---|---|
| Confounding bias | Spurious association between exposure and outcome is observed as a result of a third factor that is associated with both exposure and outcome |
| Selection bias | Systematic difference between baseline characteristics of the groups that are compared |
| Performance bias | Differences that occur due to knowledge of intervention allocation in participants or investigator |
| Attrition bias | Systematic difference between study groups due to the number and the way that participants are lost from study groups |
| Detection bias | Systematic difference between study groups in how outcomes are determined due to knowledge of which outcome was received |
| Reporting bias | Systematic difference between study groups due to selective reporting of data by the research team |

result of a third factor that is associated with both exposure and outcome and is driving this association [1]. For example, let us explore the hypothetical case control study of patients undergoing ACL reconstruction with either quadriceps or hamstring tendon autograft to examine if post-operative graft re-rupture rates are higher with quadriceps compared to hamstring tendon autograft. It is well known that patients with generalized ligamentous laxity secondary to connective tissue disorders are more likely to sustain a graft re-rupture event. Let us assume that patients with ligamentous laxity are also more likely to receive a quadriceps tendon graft. The results of this study may show an increased re-rupture rate in patients undergoing reconstruction with quadriceps tendon autograft; however, this association may be spurious as patients in the quadriceps tendon group are also more likely to have ligamentous laxity which may be driving this observation. Hence, with randomization, we increase the probability that both known and unknown confounding factors are balanced between treatment arms and any group differences in these factors are due to chance alone.

### Selection Bias

Similar to confounding bias, selection bias also results in a systematic difference between baseline characteristics of the groups that are compared. For example, in the case of ACL reconstruction surgery, if surgeons are able to preferentially assign patients to a particular treatment arm (e.g., quadriceps vs hamstring tendon autograft), then they may preferentially assign patients to a particular intervention based on certain baseline characteristics such as age, sex, sport, or other variables which are confounders and may spuriously demonstrate an association between treatment and outcome.

Selection bias remains a challenge even in an RCT, because individual surgeon equipoise may differ from the trial's inclusion/exclusion criteria and a surgeon may choose not to enroll an eligible patient if they believe strongly that one intervention or the other is the best choice for that patient. Beyond educating participating surgeons on the biases induced by this individual equipoise conundrum, a further method to prevent this non-enrollment risk is to adequately conceal the allocation sequence, which is of critical importance even in the face of adequate randomization. If surgeons are able to identify which treatment arm patients will be allocated to, they may consciously or subconsciously elect to exclude them from the study [2].

### Concealment of Allocation

An example of inappropriate concealment of allocation potentially affecting the results of an otherwise well-designed RCT was a previously published general surgery trial comparing open versus laparoscopic appendectomy. Patients were appropriately randomized to their respective treatment arms using a random numbers table system and their allocated treatment group was placed in a sealed envelope that was opened just prior to the surgery [3]. In this trial, the attending surgeon's presence was required for laparoscopic, but not open procedures. Therefore, the study ran smoothly during the daytime, but during the night, in order to prevent calling in the senior surgeon, the junior residents developed a method wherein they held the translucent envelopes containing the patient's concealed allocation against the light and ensured to only open the envelope that assigned patients to the open treatment group and the next case to come during the daytime would receive the passed-along envelope allocated to the laparoscopic group [4]. However, this could potentially bias outcomes if attending surgeons, who performed more laparoscopies during the day, were more skilled than the junior surgeons, who performed the open surgery at night. Therefore, in order to ensure concealment of allocation, envelopes should be avoided. If they are used, one should ensure they are opaque and sealed, opened sequentially only after patient identifiers are written on the envelope, and kept in a locked and secure place [5]. In addition, it is recommended to use pressure sensitive or carbon paper inside the envelope to transfer information to the assigned allocation to create an audit trail and also to place cardboard or aluminum foil inside the envelope in order to prevent assignment detection via lighting techniques [6]. Another way to ensure proper concealment of allocation is through central randomization in which the individual recruiting the patient contacts a central methods center by phone or secure computer when group assignment is needed [7].

## 2.1.3 Randomization

### 2.1.3.1 Simple Randomization

In general, randomization involves generating a list of random numbers, usually by a computer program, that are completely independent of each other so that one cannot predict the next number in a sequence. Simple randomization involves pairing the randomly generated numbers to a randomly generated treatment group. This randomization method works very well in large trials, but in studies with smaller sample sizes, this can result in an imbalanced assignment of treatment groups due to a different number of patients in each group simply due to chance. For example, when randomizing 20 patients, the probability of a 12:8 or more imbalanced split between treatment groups nears 20%, whereas when randomizing 100 patients, the probability of a 60:40 split or greater is approximately 5% [8]. This is an especially important problem to consider in surgical trials where patient recruitment may be much more difficult. Open secret: People don't like the likelihood of being cut open left to chance.

### 2.1.3.2 Block Randomization

Another form of randomization is block randomization where randomization is performed within equal sized study blocks (e.g., 6 patients per block with 3 assigned to the experimental group and 3 to the standard treatment group). This method evenly assigns patients to each treatment group within each study block so that imbalance is eliminated so long as complete blocks are enrolled. Even if a partial block is enrolled when the trial concludes, only that single block has the potential for being imbalanced. The block sizes may vary depending on the number of treatment groups and the number of patients included in the study; however, it is generally advised to use larger block sizes when possible as this reduces predictability so that researchers cannot guess the next patient assignment [8, 9]. It is also possible to vary the block size randomly over the course of the study to help maintain concealment of allocation. For example, the first block is of 8 patients, the second of 4, and so on.

### 2.1.3.3 Cluster Randomization

Cluster randomization relies on the allocation of whole facilities or groups of participants to treatment groups as opposed to a single individual [10]. This form of randomization is sometimes more feasible particularly when looking to implement new guidelines or forms of care at the population level and also may be useful to prevent contamination where participants in the control arm receive the intervention from patients in the intervention arm [11]. From a statistical standpoint, these trials require much larger sample sizes as the assumption that outcomes between individuals are not correlated no longer holds true [11]. An example of this trial design was a study of 118 general surgery programs in the United States assessing whether different work-hour policies affect patient outcomes [12]. In this trial, the surgical programs were divided into three strata based on the rates of adverse outcomes and then each program with their included residents was randomly assigned to different treatment groups. In this example, it would not have been feasible to use any other trial design as it would not be possible to randomize patients at the individual level since it would not be possible to mix different work-hour policies within the same program. In addition, it provides protection against contamination since oftentimes multiple residents look after the same patients and if an adverse outcome is experienced, it would be difficult to associate it with a particular resident.

#### 2.1.3.4 Stratified Randomization

Stratified randomization is performed when investigators want to ensure that a certain important prognostic variable is equally allocated among treatment arms. This technique is extremely important for reducing selection bias and is done by subdividing patients into specific strata based on predefined inclusion and exclusion criteria and then generating a separate randomization list for each stratum [8]. An example of this randomization technique is in an orthopedic surgery trial examining early arthroscopic shoulder stabilization versus rehabilitation on the rates of re-dislocation in patients with acute first-time traumatic shoulder dislocation [13]. This trial included 40 total patients and used a block randomization technique with block sizes of 2 and 4. Given the close correlation between patient age and risk for shoulder dislocation, as well as the differences in outcomes based on surgical technique, patients were further stratified by age group and treating surgeon [13]. This is especially important in this case, as given the small sample size in this trial the risk for selection bias is much higher.

Another important consideration in the randomization process of surgical trials is ensuring to account for clustering which represents a variation in outcomes based on the treating surgeon or center [14]. For example, surgeons with more experience or fellowship training may have better outcomes than more junior surgeons, or different surgeons may have different surgical techniques or preferences resulting in better outcomes in some domains and worse outcomes in others. Certain surgical centers may have better outcomes than others due to differences in patient population or other unknown or unmeasurable factors which is especially important to consider in multi-center RCTs. In order to account for these differences, researchers can use stratified randomization techniques in order to evenly distribute patients into the respective treatment groups. A recently published systematic review that reviewed 246 surgical RCTs found that 50% of trials stratified their randomization technique to account for surgeon or center differences [14]. Moreover, of the 130 multi-center trials, 61% stratified by center, while just 6% of the 162 multisurgeon trials stratified by surgeon [14]. However, there is evidence in a large cohort study of cardiac patients that 95% of variation in outcomes is related to patient factors, while surgeon and center only contributed 2% and 3%, respectively [15]. However, this was a cardiac specific study which may not be generalizable to all surgical trials. We, therefore, would recommend that surgical trial designers attempt to stratify by center and/or surgeon, particularly when studying surgical procedures that require a high degree of technical skill or are known to have steep learning curves or strong volume–outcome relationships (Table 2.2).

Regardless, when performing any stratification technique, it is particularly important to assure adequate sample size (see Chap. 5) and tailor the statistical analysis (see Chap. 17) to account for the stratification factors. Not doing so may result in an underpowered study, which could result in an incorrect conclusion that treatment has no benefit [16]. In a large systematic review of 258 RCTs, 63% of trials performed stratified randomization based on either center or a specific variable, and of these trials only 26% reported adjusting their primary analysis for stratification by center [16].

#### 2.1.3.5 Minimization

Stratified randomization techniques are useful when trying to balance between important prognostic variables in larger trials; however, in

**Table 2.2** Randomization techniques

| Form of randomization | Strengths | Weaknesses |
|---|---|---|
| Simple randomization | Easy and least predictable | May result in unbalanced allocation in smaller trials |
| Block randomization | Excellent for smaller and pilot trials in order to ensure a balanced number of patients in each group | More easily predictable if one can guess the block sizes |
| Cluster randomization | Useful when looking to implement new guidelines or forms of care at the population level and helps prevent contamination | Potential for selection bias, complex design, loss of statistical power |
| Stratified randomization | Allows one to ensure equal allocation of a certain important prognostic variable among treatment groups | More difficult to analyze as requires statistical correction |
| Minimization | Allows one to perform stratified randomization in smaller trials | Prone to selection bias and significantly jeopardizes concealment of allocation |

smaller trials, this may not always be possible. Therefore, a possible alternative with smaller sample sizes is minimization where the treatment allocation to the next participant in a trial depends on the previously enrolled participant [17]. Essentially, with this technique, the first participant is allocated to a treatment group at random, and each subsequent allocation depends on how to achieve optimal balance between groups for important prognostic factors and whenever treatment groups are deemed to be in a balanced state, the next included participant is allocated via simple randomization [17]. The main drawback with this technique is the potential for selection bias, as researchers can easily predict which treatment group patients will be allocated to.

## 2.2 Conclusion

Overall, surgical trials do pose a multitude of challenges with respect to randomization, particularly related to RCTs limited to smaller sample sizes, the need to adjust for important prognostic factors, and difficulty with ensuring concealment of allocation. However, several effective methods and randomization techniques exist in order to address these challenges and minimize bias as much as possible.

## References

1. Braga LHP, Farrokhyar F, Bhandari M. Practical tips for surgical research. Can J Surg. 2012;55:132–8.
2. Mansournia MA, Higgins JPT, Sterne JAC, Hernán MA. Biases in randomized trials: a conversation between trialists and epidemiologists. Epidemiology. 2017;28:54–9.
3. Hansen JB, Smithers BM, Schache D, Wall DR, Miller BJ, Menzies BL. Laparoscopic versus open appendectomy: prospective randomized trial. World J Surg. 1996;20:17–20.
4. Bhandari M, Devereaux PJ. Issues in the design and conduct of randomized trials in surgery. 2004;2:7.
5. Farrokhyar F, Karanicolas PJ, Thoma A, Simunovic M, Bhandari M, Devereaux PJ, Anvari M, Adili A, Guyatt G. Randomized controlled trials of surgical interventions. Ann Surg. 2010;251:409–16.
6. Schulz KF, Grimes DA. Allocation concealment in randomised trials: defending against deciphering. Lancet. 2002;359:614–8.
7. Dettori J. The random allocation process: two things you need to know. Evid Based Spine Care J. 2010;1:7.
8. Randelli P, Arrigoni P, Lubowitz JH, Cabitza P, Denti M. Randomization procedures in orthopaedic trials. Arthroscopy. 2008;24:834–8.
9. Pocock SJ. Allocation of patients to treatment in clinical trials. Biometrics. 1979;35:183–97.
10. Puffer S, Torgerson DJ, Watson J. Cluster randomized controlled trials. J Eval Clin Pract. 2005;11:479–83.
11. Fayers PM, Jordhøy MS, Kaasa S. Cluster-randomized trials. Palliat Med. 2002;16:69–70.
12. Bilimoria KY, Chung JW, Hedges LV, et al. National cluster-randomized trial of duty-hour flexibility in surgical training. NEJM. 2016;374:713–27.

13. Kirkley A, Werstine R, Ratjek A, Griffin S. Prospective randomized clinical trial comparing the effectiveness of immediate arthroscopic stabilization versus immobilization and rehabilitation in first traumatic anterior dislocations of the shoulder: long-term evaluation. Arthroscopy. 2005;21:55–63.
14. Conroy EJ, Rosala-Hallas A, Blazeby JM, Burnside G, Cook JA, Gamble C. Randomized trials involving surgery did not routinely report considerations of learning and clustering effects. J Clin Epidemiol. 2019;107:27–35.
15. Papachristofi O, Klein AA, Mackay J, Nashef S, Fletcher N, Sharples LD, et al. Effect of individual patient risk, centre, surgeon and anaesthetist on length of stay in hospital after cardiac surgery: Association of Cardiothoracic Anaesthesia and Critical Care (ACTACC) consecutive cases series study of 10 UK specialist centres. BMJ Open. 2017;7:e016947.
16. Kahan BC, Morris TP. Reporting and analysis of trials using stratified randomisation in leading medical journals: review and reanalysis. BMJ. 2012;345:e5840.
17. Altman DG, Bland JM. Treatment allocation by minimisation. BMJ. 2005;330:843.

# 3 Randomization Strategies

Madison Thompson, Ziqing Yu, and Susan Odum

## 3.1 Introduction

Randomized controlled trials (RCTs) are the gold standard research design to determine the clinical efficacy or clinical effectiveness of new medical interventions [1, 2]. There are three key methodological features of RCTs that are thought to produce the most credible results: randomization, blinding, and a control or comparison intervention [3–5]. This chapter focuses on randomization, which is a process of randomly assigning, or allocating, study participants to the different intervention groups [3–5]. Random allocation means there is no predictable pattern to how study participants are assigned to intervention groups—assignment is solely due to chance [3–5].

When designing a RCT, the goal is to maximize the validity of the study findings. If internal validity is the primary goal, then investigators aim to minimize the effect that confounding variables may have on the outcome [4, 5]. By controlling these covariates and confounders, the more confidence we have that the differences in the outcome are due to the treatment under investigation. If external validity is the primary goal, then investigators aim to create groups that are representative of the patient population [4, 5]. Selecting the most effective and efficient randomization schema can improve the internal and external validity of a RCT.

## 3.2 Biases Introduced By Non-random Treatment Assignment

Successful randomization produces study groups that are statistically similar with respect to both known and unknown covariates by reducing or avoiding selection bias and accidental bias which prohibit determining a causal relationship between the treatment and the desired treatment effect [4–8]. Without random assignment, researchers are left to choose the intervention to which study participants are assigned. Bias may be introduced when researchers select the treatment for any given study participant. For example, if a surgeon-investigator prefers treatment A for patients with more severe injuries and patients with more severe injuries have more complications than patients with less severe injuries, then comparisons in complications between Treatment A and B will be confounded by injury severity

M. Thompson
Georgetown University School of Medicine, Washington, DC, USA
e-mail: mct91@georgetown.edu

Z. Yu · S. Odum (✉)
Department of Orthopaedic Surgery, Atrium Health Musculoskeletal Institute, Charlotte, NC, USA
e-mail: ziqing.yu@atriumhealth.org; susan.odum@atriumhealth.org


S. Lyman et al. (eds.), *Introduction to Surgical Trials*,
https://doi.org/10.1007/978-3-031-77563-5_3

and may decrease the magnitude of the true treatment effect. This is known as selection bias which threatens the external validity of the study findings [5–9]. At its core, selection bias occurs when study groups are not representative of the population as a whole [5–9].

Accidental bias encompasses all bias stemming from unknown or unmeasured covariates that ultimately impact study outcome [5–10]. Unsurprisingly, the introduction of such biases to RCTs threatens the internal validity of the study findings by introducing bias that masks the true treatment effect [5–10]. A review by Schulz and Grimes [11] found that effect size is exaggerated by as much as 40 percent when participants are not randomly assigned to treatment groups.

Historically, manual methods such as coin flips [5, 8, 12, 14–18], throwing dice [5, 8, 13–18], and even drawing cards [5, 8, 13–18] have been employed. Currently, these methods have been systematized by automated computer programs which are now routinely employed [5, 8, 12–18]. In this chapter, common randomization methods, including simple randomization, block randomization, stratified randomization, and adaptive randomization are reviewed. Each method is described along with its advantages and disadvantages. The selection of a randomization method is essentially based on clinical trial/study design that will produce interpretable and statistically valid results.

## 3.3 Randomization Strategies

### 3.3.1 Simple Randomization

Simple randomization is based on a single process with fixed probabilities to assign study participants to different groups. The most common method of simple randomization is flipping a fair coin, which has an equal chance of landing on either "heads" or "tails." In a study comparing two groups, flipping a coin gives each study participant a 50% chance, or 0.5 probability, of being assigned to either group. Therefore, the side of the coin determines the group assignment. If the coin lands with "heads" showing, the participant is assigned to group one, and, if "tails" is showing, the participant is assigned to group two [5, 8, 12–18]. While flipping a coin is simple and easy to implement, it can create imbalanced groups [5, 8, 12–21] (Fig. 3.1). This imbalance can be due to differences in frequencies of participants in each group, or allocation imbalance, and/or clinical imbalances of important patient characteristics, or covariates [5, 8, 12–21]. The law of large numbers theorem states that as the number of coin flips approaches infinity, the frequency of the two outcomes approaches the true probability, which is 0.5 with a fair coin flip [23]. Therefore, using simple randomization methods with small sample sizes is not recommended. Block randomization or stratified randomization are preferred methods for small sample sizes, because these methods assure creation of more balanced groups when sample sizes are limited [5, 8, 12–21].

### 3.3.2 Block Randomization

The block randomization method is used to avoid unequal numbers of participants assigned to each group, which may occur when employing simple randomization methods. In a block randomization schema, participants are assigned to the open (current unfilled) block, then randomly assigned to a treatment group within the assigned block [5, 8, 14–18] (Fig. 3.2). Best practice recommends that the study statistician creates the block randomization plan and does not inform the study investigators of the block size to maintain blinding [5, 8, 14]. The statistician should select a number of blocks which is a multiple of the number of study groups. Smaller block sizes improve the ability to control the allocation balance [5, 8, 14]. For example, when designing a randomization schedule for a RCT of 20 subjects, the statistician can create 5 blocks of 4 subjects. When randomly allocating 20 participants to one 5 blocks, and then one of the two groups, within each block, the allocation balance will never be off by more than 2 subjects (e.g., the first 2 subjects of an open block assigned to one treatment), which is helpful in case the trial is stopped early due to early stopping rules or another unexpected logistical challenge.

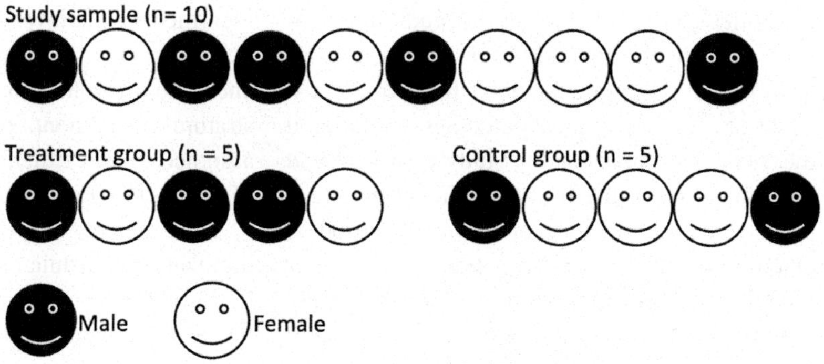


**Fig. 3.1** Simple randomization of ten individuals

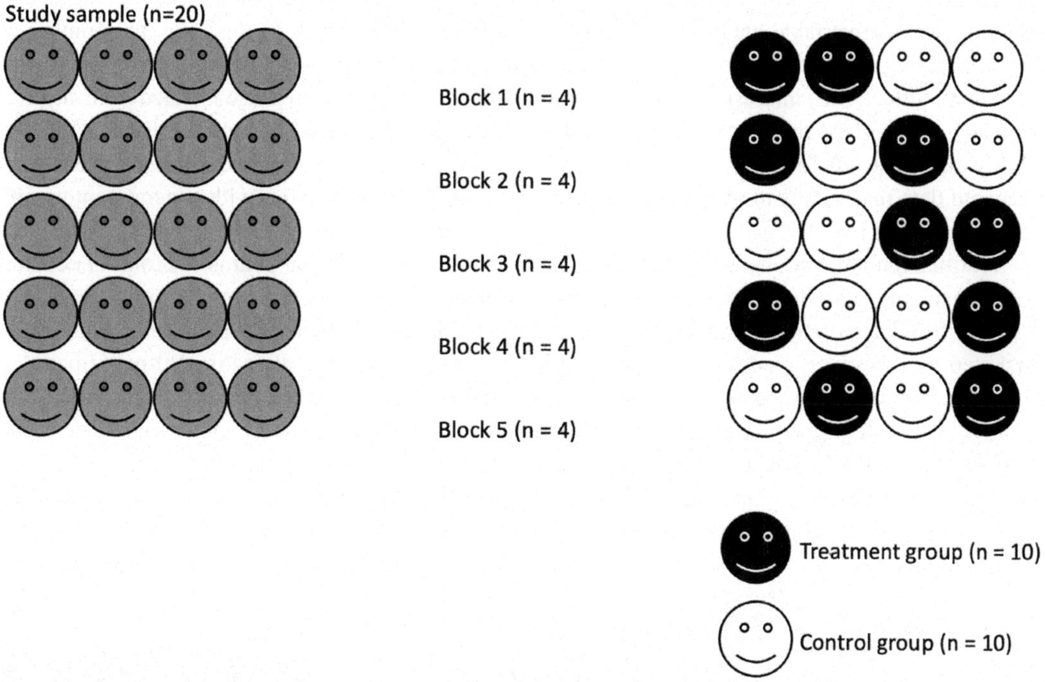


**Fig. 3.2** The process of block randomization for a clinical trial of 20 individuals

In an extension of block randomization, the size of the blocks can randomly vary in order to help maintain blinding of study personnel and assure that the blocks cannot be gamed [5, 8, 14, 16–18]. In the above example of 5 blocks of 4 subjects, the investigator responsible for treatment assignment may intuit that the blocks contain 4 patients and then resets. If a clinical investigator lacks true equipoise and really wants a specific patient to be assigned to their preferred treatment, they can potentially determine what the last assignment in a block will be if they know the block size. Varying the block size prevents this potential protocol breach. In the above example, the random block assignments could be: 6, 6, 2, 4, and 2. The larger blocks at the beginning make it more difficult to determine block size and are only used earlier in the study recruitment period when early stopping is less likely to occur [5, 8, 14, 16–18].

### 3.3.3 Stratified Randomization

While block randomization mitigates allocation imbalance, stratified randomization methods are preferred to balance important participant characteristics [5, 7–11]. Prior to the study intervention, individuals have different characteristics that may be prognostic factors, which would possibly vary with the clinical outcomes or confound the association between the study treatment and the clinical outcome. It is more likely that such prognostic factors will be more evenly distributed among groups with simple randomization or blocked randomization methods for large study samples [5, 7–11]. Furthermore, with large sample sizes, the bias created by the variability in the confounders and covariates can be mitigated with stratified or multivariable analyses to adjust for the effects of prognostic factors and isolate the treatment effect of interest. However, with smaller sample sizes the heterogeneity, or variability, in these characteristics may introduce bias into data that results in misleading or incorrect conclusions [5–11].

Stratified randomization methods are designed to mitigate the bias due to confounding [5–7, 14–19]. Similar to a block randomization, the first step of a stratified randomization method is to assign participants to a stratum, which is a group that is categorized by a covariate or confounder [5, 8, 14–19]. This may be a patient factor, such as health status, or a logistical consideration such as the study site where the treatment is to take place. These strata should be identified by the investigators based on prognostic factors either known or hypothesized to influence the outcomes of interest. Subsequent to stratum assignment, participants are randomly assigned to a treatment group within the stratum [5, 8, 14–19] (Fig. 3.3).

For example, when designing a stratified randomization schedule for a RCT of 20 individuals, the investigator can create three strata based on the characteristics of the anterior crucial ligament (ACL) injury; for example, isolated ACL, ACL with meniscal tear, or ACL with meniscal tear and cartilage defect. In this case, the number of patients assigned to a stratum can vary by stratum. For example, because isolated ACL injuries occur less frequently than ACL injuries with concomitant meniscal tears and cartilage defects, it is likely that ACL injuries with concomitant meniscal tears and cartilage defects will dominate the recruited cohort. The goal is twofold: (1) overall balanced treatment assignment and (2) balanced treatment assignment within each stratum.

When randomly allocating 20 participants to one of the three strata (e.g., isolated ACL, ACL with meniscal tear, ACL with meniscal tear and cartilage defect), and then one of the two groups, within each block, we can be assured that the treatment allocation will be balanced within each stratum. Separating patients into balanced

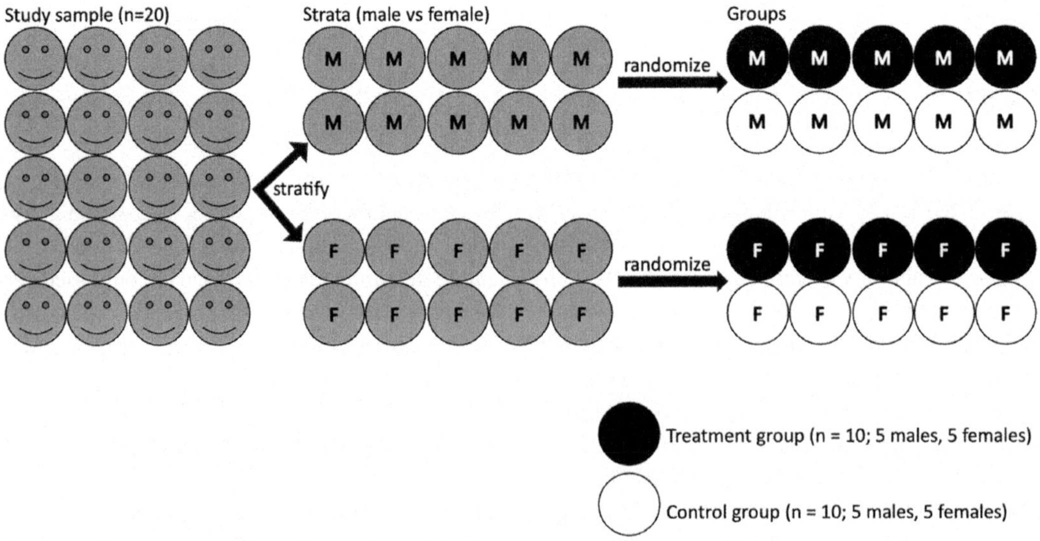


**Fig. 3.3** The process of stratified randomization for a clinical trial of 20 individuals

groups, or strata, based on prognostic factors and then randomizing patients to treatment t groups within strata, improves the internal validity of the RCT [9].

### 3.3.4 Stratified Block Randomization

As you can probably guess, stratified block randomization combines stratified randomization with block randomization. Research subjects are first assigned to a stratum based on a prognostic factor believed to influence outcomes independent of treatment. Once that assignment is made, the subjects are entered into the currently open block within that stratum and then randomized to a treatment group [5, 8, 14–19]. This solution both assures balance of the prognostic factor between treatment groups and the balance of treatment groups in the overall study sample [5, 8, 14–19].

### 3.3.5 Adaptive Randomization

In theory, more advanced adaptive randomization methods, such as biased coin design and response-adaptive randomization, overcome allocation imbalance by dynamically adjusting the allocation probabilities as each patient is enrolled [5, 8, 10, 20–22]. Furthermore, these methods allow the research team to monitor group balance in real time. Introduced in 1971 by Bradley Efron, the goal of biased coin design is to create equally sized groups by increasing the allocation probability to favor the group with fewer participants at the time that randomization is executed [10]. Let us consider a scenario, whereby, the first enrolled study patient is randomized using a "fair" coin flip with a 0.5 probability of assignment to either the treatment or the control group. If the first study patient is randomly allocated to the control group, then the second enrolled study patient will be randomized with a "biased" coin that decreases the allocation probability to the control group and increases the allocation probability to the treatment group [5, 8, 10, 20, 21]. By employing a biased coin flip that dynamically adjusts the allocation probabilities at the time each study patient is randomly allocated will ensure equal group sizes [20, 21].

Response-adaptive randomization is another common method of adaptive randomization. Instead of adjusting allocation probabilities based on prior group assignment, response-adaptive randomization methods dynamically adjust allocation probabilities based on the prior participants' response to trial intervention [20, 21]. This actually reflects how medicine is practiced: once new information is obtained, that knowledge is applied to current patients [20, 21].

### 3.3.6 Randomization to Three or More Groups

Thus far, the chapter has focused on RCTs comparing two groups; however, these randomization methods also apply to RCTs comparing more than two groups. The probabilities of allocation will vary as the number of groups vary. If study participants have equal chances of assignment, they would have a 0.5 probability of assignment to one of the two groups, a 0.333 probability of assignment to one of the three groups, a 0.25 probability of assignment to one of the four groups, and so on. The probabilities of group assignment have to sum to 1, but they don't have to be equivalent for all groups [5, 14–18]. While varying the allocation probabilities can introduce selection bias, there may be feasible and ethical reasons to do so. Therefore, it is critical that this decision is based on science and ethics [5, 8]. Let us consider a surgeon designing a RCT to compare three ACL surgical reconstruction techniques. One technique is the surgeon's standard of care with evidence of 90% effectiveness. The other two surgical repair techniques use suture anchor methods that are new for the surgeon. The research team may choose to design the randomization schema such that 50% of the study patients will be randomly allocated to the standard of care surgical technique, and 25% allocated to each of the new surgical techniques.

## 3.4 Ethical and Feasibility Considerations

Designing a surgical trial with internally and externally valid findings depends on a successful randomization method. Selecting the most appropriate randomization method and designing the best randomization schema is necessary for success. However, there are also ethical and logistical considerations.

One of the primary ethical considerations that is closely tied to randomization is equipoise. Each study has its own study equipoise, which is determined by the inclusion/exclusion criteria and the treatment assignments [24, 25]. Clinical investigators who commit to enrolling patients in a study should adhere to the study equipoise. Maintaining this equipoise is vital to the generalizability of the study findings. If each clinical investigator adheres to their own internal, or personal clinical equipoise, then they may consciously or unconsciously enroll only those subjects who meet their own personal equipoise rather than the broader study equipoise [24, 25]. In situations where surgeons are unwilling to comply with the study equipoise, they should decline to participate.

Prior to beginning a RCT, it is good practice to conduct a feasibility study, or a pilot study, to ensure that it is ethically and logistically possible to successfully conduct the proposed trial [26, 27]. During this pilot study, the research team will determine whether the key methodological design components and study activities are logistically feasible and will synergistically function properly to successfully complete the full trial [26, 27]. The research team should assess whether clinicians have equipoise and study participants are willing to accept the random assignment of the proposed treatments. Additionally, the research team can test the software used to generate the randomization schedule and allocate study participants to groups. It is also critical that all members of the care team are aware that the patient is in a RCT and how all required study procedures are conducted [26, 27]. This provides the research team an opportunity to ensure that all aspects of the randomization process and methods can be properly conducted and to make changes to improve study processes prior to initiating the full, definitive trial.

## 3.5 Conclusion

Randomization is a key methodological feature of the gold standard research design, the randomized controlled trial. Randomization reduces or eliminates sources of bias that jeopardize the validity of study findings. Successful randomization produces study groups that are statistically similar with respect to both known and unknown characteristics, or covariates, of the study participants.

Without randomization, researchers are left to choose the intervention to which study participants are assigned. Investigators who don't have personal clinical equipoise may be prone to choose one treatment over another for different patients. This can result in selection bias which threatens the external validity or generalizability of study findings. Without random allocation, both known and unknown covariates that are associated with the study outcome may be imbalanced within the study groups. This accidental bias threatens the internal validity of the study findings by introducing bias that masks the true treatment effect. When designing a RCT, selecting the most appropriate randomization is critical. While simple randomization methods, such as a fair coin toss, are easy to design and implement, these methods can produce groups with unequal sample sizes and unbalanced distributions of covariates. Blocked randomization and stratified randomization methods were developed to mitigate the imbalance that occurs with simple randomization methods. While these methods may be more complicated, many software solutions exist to simplify them. Additionally, there are more advanced, adaptive randomization methods to mitigate imbalances that rely on information about the previously enrolled study participants to dynamically adjust the allocation probabilities for each enrolled individual.

## References


1. Hadorn DC, Baker D, Hodges JS, Hicks N. Rating the quality of evidence for clinical practice guidelines. J Clin Epidemiol. 1996;49(7):749–54.
2. Altman DG, Schulz KF, Moher D, et al. The revised CONSORT statement for reporting randomized trials: explanation and elaboration. Ann Intern Med. 2001;134(8):663–94.
3. Friedman LM, Furberg CD, DeMets DL. Fundamentals of clinical trials. 4th ed. New York: Springer; 2010. https://doi.org/10.1007/978-1-4419-1586-3.
4. Matthews JNS. Introduction to randomized controlled clinical trials. 2nd ed. Boca Raton: Chapman and Hall/CRC; 2006. https://doi.org/10.1201/9781420011302.
5. Rosenberger WF, Lachin JM. Randomization in clinical trials: theory and practice. Hoboken: Wiley; 2015.
6. Altman DG, Bland JM. Statistics notes. Treatment allocation in controlled trials: why randomise? BMJ. 1999;318(7192):1209. https://doi.org/10.1136/bmj.318.7192.1209. PMID: 10221955; PMCID: PMC1115595.
7. Sverdlov O, Rosenberger W. Randomization in clinical trials: can we eliminate bias? J Clin Invest. 2013;3:37–47. https://doi.org/10.4155/CLI.12.130.
8. Berger VW, Bour LJ, Carter K, Chipman JJ, Everett CC, Heussen N, Hewitt C, Hilgers RD, Luo YA, Renteria J, Ryeznik Y, Sverdlov O, Uschner D, Randomization Innovative Design Scientific Working Group. A roadmap to using randomization in clinical trials. BMC Med Res Methodol. 2021;21(1):168. https://doi.org/10.1186/s12874-021-01303-z. PMID: 34399696; PMCID: PMC8366748. https://www.ncbi.nlm.nih.gov/pmc/articles/PMC8366748/.
9. Kahan BC, Rehal S, Cro S. Risk of selection bias in randomised trials. Trials. 2015;16:405. https://doi.org/10.1186/s13063-015-0920-x.
10. Efron B. Forcing a sequential experiment to be balanced. Biometrika. 1971;58(3):403–17. https://doi.org/10.2307/2334377. JSTOR. Accessed 15 Dec 2023.
11. Schulz KF, Grimes DA. Generation of allocation sequences in randomised trials: chance, not choice. Lancet. 2002;359:515–9.
12. Amberson JB, McMahon BT, Pinner M. A clinical trial of sanocrysin in pulmonary tuberculosis. Am Rev Tuberc. 1931;1931(24):401–35.
13. Dettori J. The random allocation process: two things you need to know. Evid Based Spine Care J. 2010;1(3):7–9. https://doi.org/10.1055/s--0030-1267062. PMID: 22956922; PMCID: PMC3427961.
14. Kang M, Ragan BG, Park J-H. Issues in outcomes research: an overview of randomization techniques for clinical trials. J Athl Train. 2008;43(2):215–21.
15. White SJ, Freedman LS. Allocation of patients to treatment groups in a controlled clinical study. Br J Cancer. 1978;37(5):849–57.
16. Kalish LA, Begg CB. Treatment allocation methods in clinical trials: a review. Stat Med. 1985;4(2):129–44. https://doi.org/10.1002/sim.4780040204. PMID: 3895341.
17. Randelli P, Arrigoni P, Lubowitz JH, Cabitza P, Denti M. Randomization procedures in orthopaedic trials. Arthroscopy. 2008;24(7):834–8. https://doi.org/10.1016/j.arthro.2008.01.011. Epub 2008 Mar 21. PMID: 18589273.
18. Altman DG, Bland JM. How to randomise. BMJ. 1999;319(7211):703–4. https://doi.org/10.1136/bmj.319.7211.703. PMID: 10480833; PMCID: PMC1116549.
19. Kernan WN, et al. Stratified randomization for clinical trials. J Clin Epidemiol. 1999;52(1):19–26.
20. Ning J, Huang X. Response-adaptive randomization for clinical trials with adjustment for covariate imbalance. Stat Med. 2010;29(17):1761–8. https://doi.org/10.1002/sim.3978. PMID: 20658546; PMCID: PMC2911996.
21. Hu F, Rosenberger WF. The theory of response–adaptive randomization in clinical trials. New York: Wiley; 2006.
22. Freedman B. Equipoise and the ethics of clinical research. N Engl J Med. 1987;317(3):141–5. https://doi.org/10.1056/NEJM198707163170304. PMID: 3600702.
23. Revesz R. In: Birnbaum ZW, Lukacs E, editors. The laws of large numbers, Probability and mathematical statistics: series of monographs and textbooks, vol. 4. New York: Academic Press; 1968. ISBN: 1483269027, 9781483269023.
24. Ubel PA, Silbergleit R. Behavioral equipoise: a way to resolve ethical stalemates in clinical research. Am J Bioeth. 2011;11(2):1–8. https://doi.org/10.1080/15265161.2010.540061. PMID: 21337264.
25. Lyman S, Nakamura N, Cole BJ, Erggelet C, Gomoll AH, Farr J 2nd. Cartilage-repair innovation at a standstill: methodologic and regulatory pathways to breaking free. J Bone Joint Surg Am. 2016;98(15):e63. https://doi.org/10.2106/JBJS.15.00573.
26. Arain M, Campbell MJ, Cooper CL, Lancaster GA. And what is a pilot or feasibility study? A review of current practice and editorial policy. BMC Med Res Methodol. 2010;10:67. https://doi.org/10.1186/1471-2288-10-67.
27. Abbott JH. The distinction between Randomized Clinical Trials (RCTs) and preliminary feasibility and pilot studies: what they are and are not. J Orthop Sports Phys Ther. 2014;44(8):555–8. https://doi.org/10.2519/jospt.2014.0110.

# 4 Surgical Trial Design: Interventions and Blinding

Madison Thompson and Stephen Lyman

*Quis, quid, ubi, quibus auxiliis, cur, quomodo, quando*

*—Cicero*

## 4.1 Introduction

In grade school, many were taught the 5W's (and 1 H): who, what, when, where, why, how. Cicero in fact formalized these questions, in hexameter no less, before the start of the first millennium. These questions, albeit seemingly simple, can often be overlooked when planning, executing, and publishing surgical RCTs. Just as important as it is to enumerate the details of interventions in surgical trials, it is also critical to blind trial participants from such information to prevent bias.

## 4.2 Interventions

Interventions in surgical studies can range from subtle modifications in surgical approach to pioneering innovations that redefine medical practice. With such a wide range of potential areas to investigate, it is no surprise that the studies to investigate these techniques are often multifaceted and complex. Not only do the surgeries themselves have the potential to vary greatly but management of the pre- and postoperative periods also leaves substantial room for variability. In order for surgeons to confidently accept, and more importantly adopt, findings of surgical RCTs, interventions need to be not only consistent across the study but also replicable.

### 4.2.1 Types of Interventions

Surgical trials are often conducted to compare different techniques, tools, and even management practices. Furthermore, such interventions can occur both inside and outside of the operating theater. Table 4.1 identifies common examples of the various types of interventions studied in surgical RCTs as well as provides examples of how these interventions can be executed at various stages of the surgical process.

M. Thompson (✉)
Georgetown University School of Medicine, Washington, DC, USA
e-mail: mct91@georgetown.edu

S. Lyman
Hospital for Special Surgery, New York, NY, USA

Medical Education, Kyushu University School of Medicine, Fukuoka, Japan
e-mail: LymanS@hss.edu


S. Lyman et al. (eds.), *Introduction to Surgical Trials*,
https://doi.org/10.1007/978-3-031-77563-5_4

**Table 4.1** Examples of interventions in surgical RCTS

| | Preoperative | Intraoperative | Postoperative |
|---|---|---|---|
| Procedural | Effect of prehabilitation programs on outcomes in knee arthroplasty | Comparison of surgical approaches in shoulder arthroplasty | Early active mobilization following hip arthroplasty |
| Device | Use of virtual reality training to improve surgical performance | Comparison of prosthetic devices in ankle arthroplasty | Intermittent compressive devices for deep venous thrombosis prophylaxis |

### 4.2.2 Learning Curve

In studies investigating different surgical procedures, it is important to factor in the effect of the surgeon's learning curve with any new procedure. The process of performing surgery is an intricate endeavor, demanding a high degree of expertise and skill. However, this expertise can significantly differ not only among different surgeons but also within the same surgeon over time. Such variations in skill levels, experience, and even the stage of training of the surgical team members can wield a substantial impact on the validity of the trial's findings.

Similarly, it is also important to recognize that in studies investigating entirely new practices, the process of mastering a novel skill in a clinical setting often involves a period of trial and error. Consequently, attributing the observed results solely to the introduced intervention can become challenging, as the effects of the learning process become intertwined with the intervention's actual impact. Mehta et al. demonstrated the staggering difference in risk of repeat surgery based on surgeon career volume [1] (Fig. 4.1a). Similarly, Marchand et al. found that operative time significantly decreased based on time since introduction to novel technology [2] (Fig. 4.1b).

Various approaches to help minimize the effect of the learning curve, including mandating a predefined number of cases be performed preceding the trial or skill assessment via direct observation, video, or even specimen quality ranking, have been proposed [3].

### 4.2.3 Co-interventions

Concomitant interventions, or co-interventions, must also be accounted for. Standard practice in clinical trials is for only one aspect, i.e., material of prosthetic, to vary. However, co-interventions such as perioperative analgesia and postoperative physical therapy can greatly affect patient outcomes, though these practices (if not the main intervention of the study) are not always standardized. Bias and confounding can occur when such variables that may affect outcomes are not balanced in trial arms. Therefore, it is imperative to standardize ancillary interventions such as pain management, anesthesia, and physical therapy.

### 4.2.4 Pragmatic Versus Explanatory Trials

When designing surgical RCTs, it is important to consider the scope of each trial. The pragmatic-explanatory continuum indicator summary (PRECIS) tool was developed to help distinguish between the different classifications of trials based on their objectives [4]. In pragmatic trials, the aim is to establish the effectiveness of an intervention in the "real world." Best practices certainly exist, but there is still much left to the discretion of the patient care team. Such co-interventions can be considered inevitable, and thus allowable, in "real world" settings of pragmatic trials and thus need not be as heavily regulated. In contrast, explanatory trials aiming to establish novel interventions under ideal settings should have far more rigid protocols to control for these external factors.

### 4.2.5 Reporting

A fundamental facet of replicability is adequate reporting. Whether a trial is pragmatic or explanatory, for instance, can greatly guide the interpretation and generalizability of its findings. Beyond categorizing the trial, actually detailing the interventions performed is paramount. A meta-

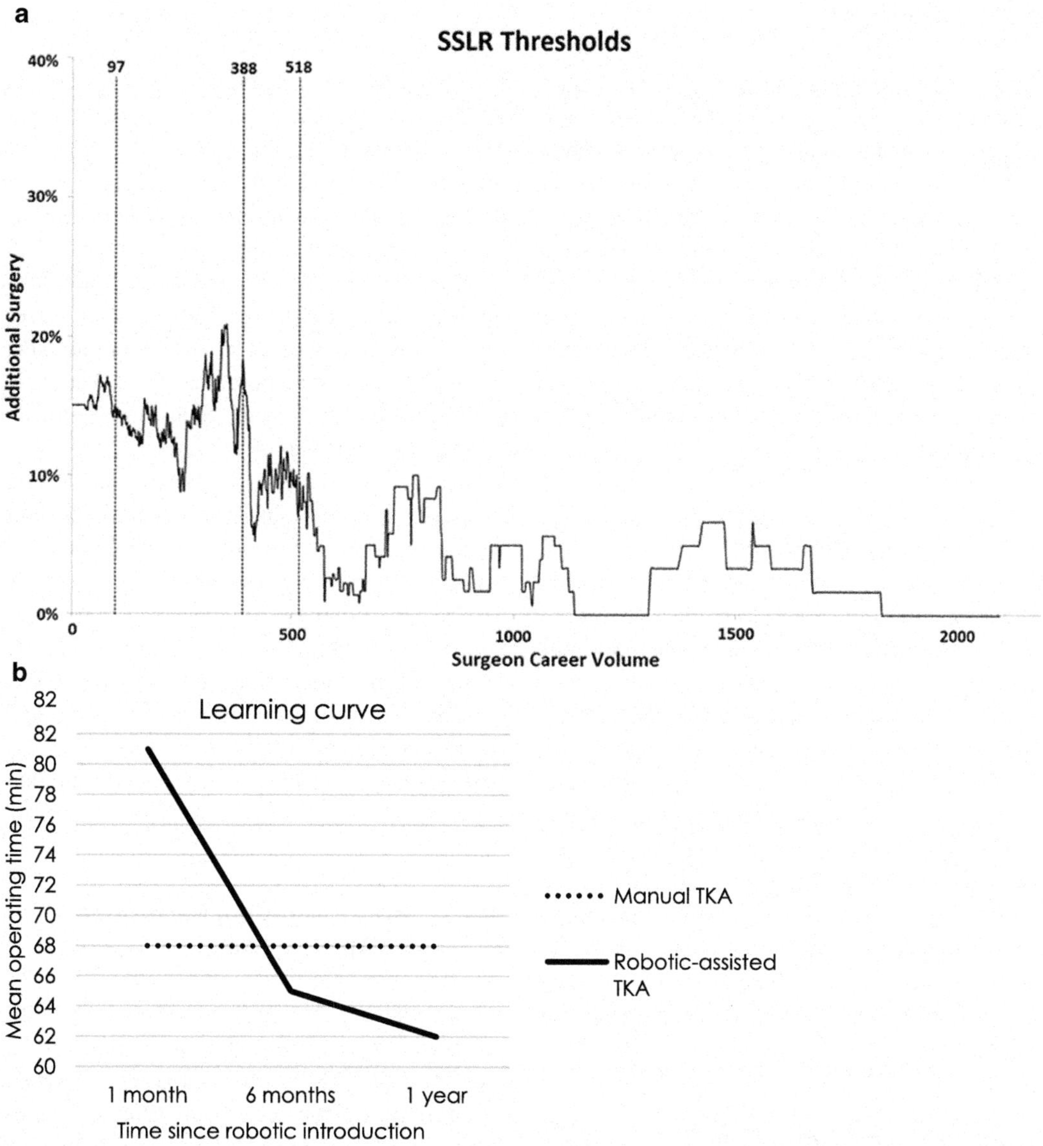


**Fig. 4.1** Learning curves in surgery. (**a**) Frequency of additional surgery based on surgeon career volume. (Courtesy of Mehta et al. [1]). (**b**) Mean operating time versus time since introduction to robot technology. (Adapted from Marchand et al. [2])

analysis of surgical RCTs found that nearly one-fifth of trials did not describe surgical interventions beyond naming them, i.e., open vs laparoscopic appendectomy [5]. Of the trials that did describe their interventions, not even half mentioned any sort of standardization of such practices, i.e., dissection or closure technique, let alone reported on any co-interventions such as anesthesia delivery or postoperative care. This, of course, leaves much open to various interpretations by surgeons and readers in general.

To combat this, Hoffmann and colleagues created the Template for Intervention Description and Replication (TIDieR) checklist [6]. The checklist expands upon the recommendations in the CONSORT [7] and SPIRIT [8] statements to create more specific guidelines regarding reporting of surgical interventions.

## 4.3 Blinding

Once the study interventions are decided upon (and an appropriate reporting plan devised), it is of paramount importance to also prevent information about these interventions from biasing those involved in the RCT. Blinding, as the name suggests, is the act of concealing, or masking, such information. While at first glance this statement appears rather simple, it leaves much left to unpack. What exactly gets blinded? How? And from whom? Perhaps there is some irony in that we, too, are often blinded to the complexity this term entails.

### 4.3.1 What Is Blinding?

Blinding is widely agreed to be the "process by which information that has the potential to influence study results is withheld from one or more parties involved in a research study" [9]. It is distinct from allocation concealment, which is the "process by which investigators and participants enrolled in a clinical study are kept unaware of upcoming group assignments until the moment of assignment" [9]. The critical difference is that allocation concealment occurs before randomization into the treatment group, thus minimizing selection bias, and blinding occurs after, with the goal of mitigating performance and detection bias (Fig. 4.2).

### 4.3.2 Who Gets Blinded?

In a surgical clinical trial, the list of key players includes patients, surgeons, data collectors, outcome assessors, and statisticians. Ideally, every one of these roles would be blinded, though of course this is not always feasible. Probst et al. found that in a meta-analysis of 378 surgical RCTs, outcome assessors (i.e., physical therapists evaluating mobility) were the most frequently blinded (26%), followed by patients (25%) [10]. Perhaps unsurprisingly, blinding surgeons was rather difficult, if even feasible at all, resulting in only 2% of surgeons being blinded in clinical trials. Of note, the odds ratio for reporting significant outcomes in trials with unblinded versus blinded surgeons was 13.7. Put more plainly, the odds of a study publishing significant results to support their hypothesis was 13.7 times higher if the surgeon knew what treatment group the patients were assigned to. This alarming demonstration of bias is the crux of why blinding is so important in surgical trials.

Granted, blinding surgeons and even other study contributors is not always feasible. Logistical and ethical constraints certainly pose a valid barrier at times; however, a disappointing number of studies still elected not to blind contributors even when it was still considered plausible [9].

### 4.3.3 How Is Blinding Performed in Surgical Trials?

Blinding in surgical trials is admittedly more difficult than in pharmaceutical trials, where pills, liquids, or injections can be formulated to appear identical even if the active ingredient is different. Boutron et al. [11] delineated the various, and often creative, techniques that surgical trials over the past decades have utilized to allow for at least some degree of blinding. Over half of the studies employed the use of sham procedures (Fig. 4.3).

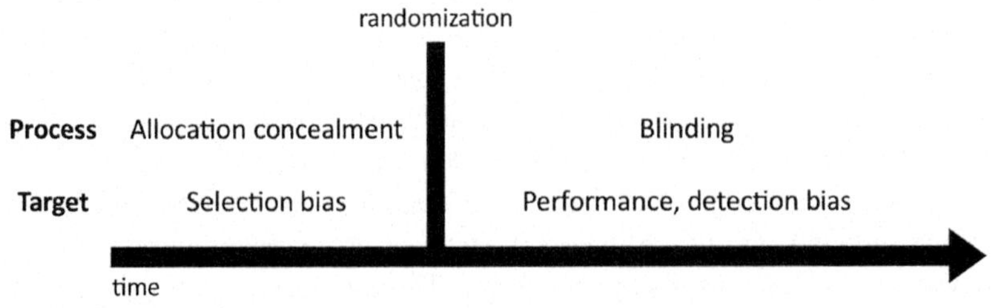


**Fig. 4.2** Allocation concealment versus blinding

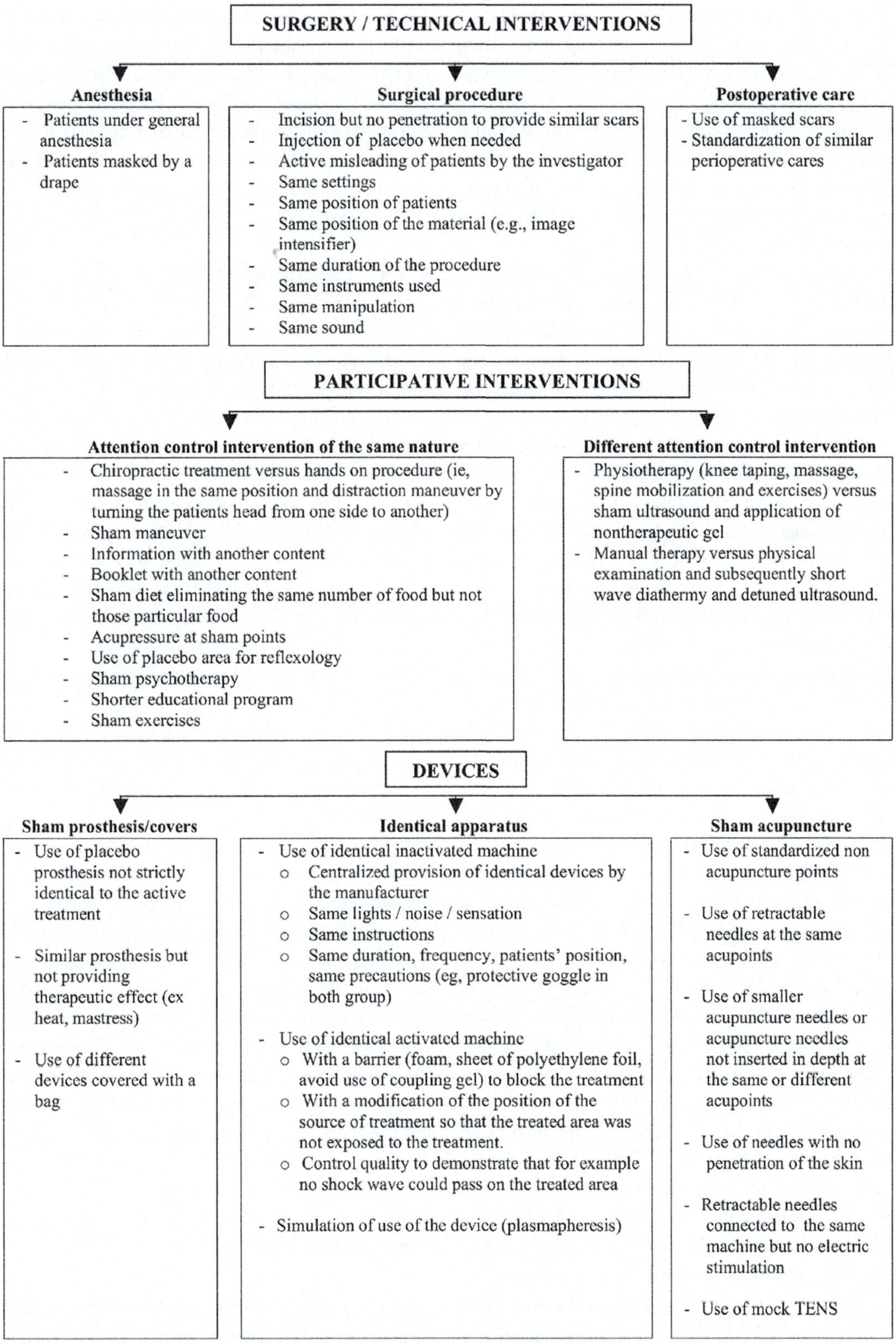


**Fig. 4.3** Sham procedure techniques. (Courtesy of Boutron et al. [11]. Reproduced under the terms of the Creative Commons Attribution License, which permits unrestricted use, distribution, and reproduction in any medium, provided the original author and source are credited)

These sham procedures often include stimulating the surgical intervention, including replicating lights and sounds of the OR, and even going so far as making superficial incisions to imitate arthroscopic surgical entry sites. While most studies employed techniques to blind participants to their assigned treatment groups, a small portion of projects opted to blind participants from the study hypothesis altogether [11].

Some trials have even managed to blind the surgeons. In a trial on lower back pain, surgeons inserted an intradiscal catheter into every subject. From there, an independent nurse connected the catheter to a generator that either transmitted electrothermal energy (treatment group) or simply did nothing (control group). By ensuring the generator displayed the same light sequence and produced the same noises regardless of electrothermal energy transmission, the surgeons were effectively unaware of which treatment their patients received [9]. If blinding the surgeons is not feasible, however, removing the surgeons from the remainder of postoperative care serves as an alternative method to reducing potential bias [9, 11].

Blinding of data collectors and outcome assessors is frequently achieved via the use of outside parties not privy to the study hypothesis, or at the very least group assignment. For instance, utilizing independent evaluators such as a physical therapist who measures changes in range of motion status post-knee arthroplasty without knowing of which prosthesis was used can help prevent detection bias [10]. Alternatively, a physical barrier such as an opaque sleeve or fabric over the possible surgical site can also serve to mask the nature of the intervention, if any occurred at all. Particularly in the case of outcome assessors, many trials opt to employ centralized adjudication committees [11]. These groups of experts are formed with the purpose of conducting independent reviews of the diverse subjective or intricate endpoints within clinical research. These endpoints often encompass tasks like assessing medical images, evaluating patient-reported outcomes, and analyzing adverse events.

While it is relatively straightforward to blind independent statisticians to a study's hypothesis or group assignment, it is important to acknowledge that there is often an overlap in roles within a study. For instance, the individual responsible for collecting patient data (such as Timed Up and Go scores) might also be in charge of analyzing and statistically modeling the findings. Therefore, maintaining blinding throughout the various stages of the study is of utmost importance.

### 4.3.4 Potential for Bias

Numerous meta-analyses have concluded that a lack of blinding in surgical RCTs leads to significant overestimation of treatment effect [10–13]. In studies utilizing patient-reported outcomes, non-blinded patients exaggerated the effect size by over 100% [12]. Data on the effect of unblinded outcome observers also points in this direction [9]; however, analysis is limited by the lack of transparent reporting in publications. If studies do not explicitly state which parties were blinded, as was the case in almost half of the trials reviewed by Probst et al. [10], they cannot be property evaluated.

All too often, studies employ buzzwords like double-blinded or triple-blinded when describing study design but fail to delineate which specific parties were actually blinded. If we consider the 5 parties previously described (patients, surgeons, data collectors, outcome assessors, and data analysts), this allows for 10 combinations in which 2 parties are blinded—all technically double-blinded studies, no? Surprisingly, in a survey of 200 trial authors, investigators found as many as 15 different operational meanings of the term "double-blind," yet nearly every author reported feeling confident that their definition was the most widely used [14]. The updated CONSORT statement in 2010 recommended doing away with the use of the double/triple blind terminology altogether, encouraging "explicit reporting of blinding status" [7].

## 4.4 Conclusion

Surgical RCTs demand careful consideration of interventions and blinding strategies. This collective effort bolsters the credibility of surgical research, ensuring its reliability and significance in advancing medical understanding and patient care. The sway of the learning curve underscores the impact of individual expertise on outcomes, while co-interventions like analgesia and physical therapy necessitate standardization to curb bias. Just as Cicero's timeless questions remain relevant, so too do the principles of transparent and replicable interventions in the realm of surgical RCTs.

## References


1. Mehta N, Chamberlin P, Marx RG, Hidaka C, Ge Y, Nawabi DH, Lyman S. Defining the learning curve for hip arthroscopy: a threshold analysis of the volume-outcomes relationship. Am J Sports Med. 2018;46(6):1284–93. https://doi.org/10.1177/0363546517749219.
2. Marchand KB, Ehiorobo J, Mathew KK, Marchand RC, Mont MA. Learning curve of robotic-assisted total knee arthroplasty for a high-volume surgeon. J Knee Surg. 2022;35(4):409–15. https://doi.org/10.1055/s-0040-1715126.
3. Karanicolas PJ, Farrokhyar F, Bhandari M. Practical tips for surgical research: blinding: who, what, when, why, how? Can J Surg. 2010;53(5):345–8.
4. Loudon K, Treweek S, Sullivan F, Donnan P, Thorpe KE, Zwarenstein M. The PRECIS-2 tool: designing trials that are fit for purpose. BMJ. 2015; https://doi.org/10.1136/bmj.h2147.
5. Blencowe NS, Mills N, Cook JA, Donovan JL, Rogers CA, Whiting P, Blazeby JM. Standardizing and monitoring the delivery of surgical interventions in randomized clinical trials. Br J Surg. 2016;103(10):1377–84. https://doi.org/10.1002/bjs.10254.
6. Hoffmann TC, Glasziou PP, Boutron I, Milne R, Perera R, Moher D, Altman DG, Barbour V, Macdonald H, Johnston M, Lamb SE, Dixon-Woods M, McCulloch P, Wyatt JC, Chan AW, Michie S. Better reporting of interventions: template for intervention description and replication (TIDieR) checklist and guide. BMJ. 2014; https://doi.org/10.1136/bmj.g1687.
7. Moher D, Hopewell S, Schulz KF, Montori V, Gøtzsche PC, Devereaux PJ, Elbourne D, Egger M, Altman DG. CONSORT 2010 explanation and elaboration: updated guidelines for reporting parallel group randomised trials. BMJ. 2010;340:c869. https://doi.org/10.1136/bmj.c869.
8. Chan AW, Tetzlaff JM, Altman DG, Laupacis A, Gøtzsche PC, Krleža-Jerić K, Hróbjartsson A, Mann H, Dickersin K, Berlin JA, Doré CJ, Parulekar WR, Summerskill WS, Groves T, Schulz KF, Sox HC, Rockhold FW, Rennie D, Moher D. SPIRIT 2013 statement: defining standard protocol items for clinical trials. Ann Intern Med. 2013;158(3):200–7. https://doi.org/10.7326/0003-4819-158-3-201302050-00583.
9. Monaghan TF, Agudelo CW, Rahman SN, Wein AJ, Lazar JM, Everaert K, Dmochowski RR. Blinding in clinical trials: seeing the big picture. Medicina (Kaunas). 2021;57(7):647. https://doi.org/10.3390/medicina57070647.
10. Probst P, Zaschke S, Heger P, Harnoss JC, Hüttner FJ, Mihaljevic AL, Knebel P, Diener MK. Evidence-based recommendations for blinding in surgical trials. Langenbeck's Arch Surg. 2019;404(3):273–84. https://doi.org/10.1007/s00423-019-01761-6.
11. Boutron I, Guittet L, Estellat C, Moher D, Hróbjartsson A, Ravaud P. Reporting methods of blinding in randomized trials assessing nonpharmacological treatments. PLoS Med. 2007;4(2):e61. https://doi.org/10.1371/journal.pmed.0040061.
12. Hróbjartsson A, Thomsen AS, Emanuelsson F, Tendal B, Rasmussen JV, Hilden J, Boutron I, Ravaud P, Brorson S. Observer bias in randomized clinical trials with time-to-event outcomes: systematic review of trials with both blinded and non-blinded outcome assessors. Int J Epidemiol. 2014;43(3):937–48. https://doi.org/10.1093/ije/dyt270.
13. Lilford R, Braunholtz D, Harris J, Gill T. Trials in surgery. Br J Surg. 2004;91(1):6–16. https://doi.org/10.1002/bjs.4418.
14. Haahr MT, Hróbjartsson A. Who is blinded in randomized clinical trials? A study of 200 trials and a survey of authors. Clin Trials. 2006;3(4):360–5. https://doi.org/10.1177/1740774506069153.

# Sample Size and Power Considerations for Surgical Trials

# 5

Michael Parides and Stephen Lyman

## 5.1 Introduction

It is essential that investigators planning an RCT collaborate with an experienced biostatistician to aid with study design, conduct, and statistical analysis. A key component of the design phase of any RCT is the determination of the necessary sample size required to successfully achieve the study aims. This, of course, is true for any study, but it is especially true for RCTs due to the substantial time and resources needed for their execution. As we will describe, sample size requirements differ with different trial objectives. An experienced biostatistician will be able to translate clinical hypotheses into statistical hypotheses, determine the appropriate statistical methods to evaluate those hypotheses, and compute the necessary sample size.

M. Parides (✉)
Hospital for Special Surgery, New York, NY, USA
e-mail: paridesm@hss.edu

S. Lyman
Hospital for Special Surgery, New York, NY, USA

Medical Education, Kyushu University School of Medicine, Fukuoka, Japan
e-mail: LymanS@hss.edu

## 5.2 Research Objectives and Study Types

Randomized clinical trials (RCTs) are heterogeneous with the specific objectives of the study impacting how sample sizes are calculated. The classical paradigm for RCTs is geared toward drug development, progressing along well-defined phases (i.e., Phase I, II, III, IV). However, these may not be readily applicable to RCTs of surgical procedures or devices where objectives such as defining a dose–response curve toxicity are not relevant. Orthopedic procedures or devices are more often investigated through confirmatory (Phase II) or exploratory trials (Phase III), with the goal of establishing superiority or non-inferiority.

Confirmatory trials are intended to provide a definitive answer—for example, safety and/or efficacy. Standard design parameters are typically used: alpha = 0.05; power = 90%; with clearly defined endpoints, effect sizes, and target populations.

Exploratory studies often have many objectives beyond establishing safety and/or efficacy. For example, the goal may be to establish the appropriate endpoint to be used in a future confirmatory trial, to obtain preliminary data on safety and effectiveness, on the variability of potential endpoints, or to assess optimal eligibility criteria. Multiplicity of inferential statistical testing is common in exploratory trials and less strict


S. Lyman et al. (eds.), *Introduction to Surgical Trials*,
https://doi.org/10.1007/978-3-031-77563-5_5

control of Type I error is often justifiable (i.e., the alpha-level may exceed 0.05).

Establishing superiority of an experimental intervention compared to a control is a standard aim of RCTs. However, demonstrating non-inferiority (equivalence) is a common goal in surgical trials as procedures and devices often need only to be equivalent, not superior, to accepted standards of care to obtain regulatory approval (see Chap. 19).

Contrary to the common misperception, demonstrating non-inferiority and showing that procedures or devices are truly equivalent requires a larger sample size than a superiority study. While effect size is used to determine the sample size for superiority trials, the non-inferiority margin is used to determine the sample size in non-inferiority trials. This non-interiority margin is an estimate of the threshold below which an intervention would be considered "worse" than an alternative treatment.

Of note, defining the non-inferiority margin is particularly important when testing procedures or devices, as setting it in advance will potentially permit the analysis to be switched from superiority to non-inferiority, even after the study has been initiated, without inflating the Type I error probability. A recommended resource for further reading on non-inferiority studies follows, at the end of this chapter.

## 5.3 Statistical Power

Power analysis refers to the estimation of the required sample size to achieve sufficient statistical power, that is, to detect an effect of when it truly exists. The power of a study depends on several factors, including the Type I error rate (the significance level (alpha)), the variability of data, the effect size, and the allocation ratios. As described below, researchers must carefully consider the trade-offs and find an optimal balance that allows them to achieve the desired statistical power while still maintaining a feasible and manageable sample size.

Power is a probability. It is the probability that a null hypothesis is rejected when it is in fact false. In statistical hypothesis testing, the failure to reject a false null hypothesis is referred to as a Type II error. If at the end of a trial, the null hypothesis is not rejected, the correctness of that decision is never known. Investigators only know what the power of the study was, or the probability that a Type II error would occur, and then only if the assumptions made to compute power were valid and the trial was rigorously conducted. Therefore, it is essential that sample size assumptions are empirically based and thoughtful, and that the power is large enough to confidently conclude that a negative result can be ascribed to a lack of treatment benefit.

Therefore, investigators should strive to design confirmatory clinical trials with power of 90% if possible. Many trials, especially surgical trials, are designed with 80% power, a value generally accepted as the minimal adequate power. This difference is larger than it may appear. Even though a trial with 90% power has a relative power increase of 12.5% compared to a trial with 80% power, it reduces the probability of a Type II error by 50% (from 20% to 10%).

A trial's Type I error rate is the probability of incorrectly rejecting the null hypothesis (i.e., it is the probability of a false positive finding). It defines the threshold to judge whether results, summarized as a p-value or observed significance level, are consistent with the null hypothesis. Type I errors are generally considered to be more egregious than Type II errors (false negative findings), especially in confirmatory trials, and so are chosen to be small; almost always 0.05. In exploratory trials, especially those designed as "Go-No Go" experiments to decide whether to proceed to a confirmatory trial, or not, larger probabilities of false positive findings, as high as 20%, may be acceptable.

## 5.4 Effect Size

The effect size is the magnitude of the difference between experimental treatment and control treatments deemed to be clinically important. It provides a standardized measure of the clinical impact of the intervention under investigation. In confirmatory studies of efficacy, the effect size should be the minimal clinically important difference (MCID) that would lead to a change in practice; it should not be the expected effect, or necessarily selected to replicate differences observed in prior studies, especially if those studies were non-randomized. Preliminary data are useful in determining whether the presumed benefit of the experimental treatment is likely to exceed the minimal clinically important difference. For a definition of MCID and related concepts of patient acceptable symptom state (PASS) and minimal detectable change (MDC), please see Chap. 10.

Effect size and sample size have an inverse relationship. A larger effect size is detectable with a smaller sample size for any pre-specified level of power, while smaller effect sizes require larger sample sizes to achieve the same level of power. Confirmatory clinical trials with negative results are difficult to interpret unless they are adequately powered to detect effect sizes representing the minimal clinically important difference.

While all randomized trials are often challenging to design and conduct, the difficulties presented by surgical trials make them prone to be smaller, and possibly underpowered trials, based on the use of overly optimistic effect sizes.

## 5.5 Variability of Endpoints

The variation in outcome measures, or endpoints, reflects the inherent differences that exist among individuals within the study population. This variation can stem from genetic diversity, environmental factors, lifestyle differences, or the heterogeneous nature of the medical condition being studied.

The magnitude of variation directly influences the precision required to detect treatment effects with adequate statistical power. If the variation is large, a larger sample size is necessary to increase precision, i.e., the level of accuracy or reliability in estimating the study's outcomes or treatment effects. Conversely, if the variation is small, a smaller sample size will be sufficient to detect meaningful differences between treatment groups.

Sample size calculations are approximations that depend on accurate assumptions about variability (standard deviations). Misspecification of variability may lead to misspecification of the necessary sample size. Assumptions concerning variability are often derived from previous studies, whether from investigators' own preliminary data or from the literature. In exploratory studies, they may simply reflect educated guesses. Closely following a trial's protocol helps to ensure that additional variability is not introduced into the measurement of outcomes.

## 5.6 Allocation Ratios

The allocation ratio in an RCT refers to the proportion of participants assigned to different treatment groups within a study. In a simple two-arm trial, the allocation ratio might be 1:1, with an equal number of participants in the treatment and control groups. This is the most efficient design and is consistent with the notion of clinical equipoise: the accepted belief of the medical community that there is insufficient evidence in favor of one treatment or another in a randomized trial. Equipoise provides the ethical basis for using randomization to determine how patients will be treated in the trial.

The efficiency of an RCT refers to the total sample size needed to detect an effect with prespecified power and Type I error. In trials with two arms (treatment groups), equal allocation yields the smallest total sample size compared to other allocation schemes. For example, a 2:1 allocation scheme, where patients would be twice as likely to be randomized into one arm than the other, results in a relative 12% increase in the total sample size compared to what it would be with 1:1 allocation. For 3:1 allocation, the increase is 33%.

There are scenarios where unequal allocation ratios may be advantageous, especially in exploratory trials, even though it leads to an increased total sample. In some cases, unequal allocation may be necessary to obtain an adequate amount of safety information about a new therapy given practical limits on a trial's total sample size.

Randomizing a greater proportion of patients to the new therapy could allow investigators to better determine its potential risk–benefit profile. Additionally, in cases where there may be strong patient preferences for a new therapy, such as in cases where the standard therapy has limited effectiveness and a new therapy appears promising, or if randomization is between a medical versus a surgical intervention, unequal allocation ratios may facilitate recruitment.

In some clinical trials, the allocation ratio may change over the course of the trial such that there is a greater probability for new participants to be randomized into the better performing arm given observed results up to that point. This dynamic allocation approach, where randomization probabilities change according to the accruing outcome data, is referred to as response adaptive randomization. The approach is controversial, with adherents arguing that it is a more ethical manner to assign treatments since patients are more likely to receive the treatment that is apparently better, and critics concerned about the potential bias that might be introduced if there are time trends in either the patient population being enrolled or in the delivery of therapy. For example, surgical therapies may improve with experience, due to improvements (learning) from increased experience of the surgeon with new procedures or devices or from improved post-operative patient management.

## 5.7 Non-adherence and Loss to Follow-up

Sample size estimates need to consider the real-world possibility that non-adherence and/or loss to follow-up leads to smaller effective sample sizes, undermining the intended power of the study, as well as the integrity of the randomization. Non-adherence refers to participants deviating from the assigned treatment protocol (see Chap. 8). These deviations may lead to incomplete or missing data, attenuate estimates of treatment differences, and affect the balance of the randomization. Loss to follow-up occurs when participants discontinue their involvement in the study or cannot be assessed for outcomes during the study period (see Chap. 9). Patient behavior, adverse events, or logistical challenges are factors which may contribute to non-adherence or loss to follow-up.

Adding a reasonable number of patients to the estimated sample size beyond what the power analysis would deem necessary is a common practice used to ensure adequate power when incomplete data are expected. However, simply adding patients does not address the potential for bias, which can be introduced when patients leave a study for specific and potentially systematic reasons. For example, consider the situation where patients with worse outcomes tend to drop out more frequently because they were less capable of or interested in returning for follow-up. If worse outcomes are more likely with the control group, an analysis of only patients with complete data could lead to a biased estimate of benefit for a new treatment and a reduction in power.

Intention-to-treat (ITT) analysis should be used to mitigate the potential bias introduced by non-adherence and loss to follow-up (see Chap. 17). In ITT analysis, participants are analyzed according to their originally assigned treatment groups, regardless of whether they adhered to the treatment or completed the study. ITT also requires that all randomized patients be included in the analysis. This requires imputation of missing data, such as the use of multiple imputation models (see Chap. 16). This approach maintains the integrity of the randomization process and reflects the real-world conditions of clinical practice. An experienced biostatistician can help develop a plan to mitigate the effects of missing data, assess its potential impact on a study's power, and consider its effect on sample size.

## 5.8 Interim Analysis

In many confirmatory trials, the design allows for conducting analyses before all the anticipated outcomes have been observed. These additional analyses, referred to as interim analyses, allow for the possibility to terminate a trial early should the accumulating results provide sufficient information to answer the trial's primary question. Interim analyses must account for the certain Type I error inflation associated with the repeated analysis of data. A variety of approaches have been proposed to maintain the Type I error rate at the desired level when interim analyses are planned. The most common class of approaches are referred to as group sequential approaches and generally incorporate an alpha spending function to distribute the total Type I error across the interim looks. More generally, adaptive clinical trials allow for pre-determined changes to the design of clinical trials based on the results of an interim analysis, including increasing the sample size to maintain power, dropping a treatment arm in trials of more than two arms, and changing the allocation ratio. Frequently, adaptively designed trials utilize Bayesian designs. Bayesian approaches incorporate uncertainty about parameters of interest (e.g., mean differences) and update those probabilities based on the observed data. It is critical that if interim analyses or adaptations are planned, that the trial's sample size estimate accounts for them.

## 5.9 Variable Types

Numerous formulas exist for determining sample size and a variety of software packages exist that implementing these formulas to determine sample size. The specific formula used depends primarily on the type of outcome. Outcomes variables are generally broken into two main types: continuous and discrete. Discrete variables can further be classified as binary (only two possible responses, e.g., yes/no, dead/alive, septic/aseptic), nominal (no inherent order, e.g., indication for revision surgery), or ordinal (ordered/hierarchical, e.g., Kellgren-Lawrence osteoarthritis grade). For each of these various types of variables, different statistical methods are used for analysis and different sample size calculations have been developed.

A further consideration for continuous variables is whether they are normally distributed. Do they follow a classic bell-shaped curve or are they skewed in some way? Fortunately, the central limit theorem ensures that even for relatively small sample sizes, resulting test statistics will be approximately normally distributed, whatever the distribution of the underlying data. However, for smaller surgical trials this becomes an additional consideration for both the statistical plan and sample size calculation.

The normality question is particularly important when patient reported outcome measures (PROMs) are used as outcomes in surgical trials. Due to the success of many common orthopedic procedures, post-operative PROMs scores may be highly skewed, calling into question the use of statistical methods with normality assumptions. Your biostatistician collaborator will know how to deal with these issues.

## 5.10 Other Statistical Considerations

Occasionally, the focus of a clinical trial may be on comparing paired observations, especially in exploratory single arm trials meant to establish proof of concept. For example, interest may be on testing whether functional outcomes such as PROMs scores or range of motion are improved post-treatment compared to pre-treatment. Measurements obtained on the same individual (paired data) will almost certainly not be independent. This dependence must be accounted for in determining sample size, as well as in the analysis. An extension of paired data is the situation where more than two repeated measures are obtained on trial participants. Such data are generally analyzed using relatively sophisticated models for longitudinal data and sample size estimates focused on the ability to detect changes in the trajectory of outcomes over time in a single group, or on the differences in the trajectory over time between groups.

In some trials, the outcome of interest is the time to occurrence of an event of interest, such as the duration of implant survival or the time to revision surgery. Sample size calculations, and analysis, are complicated by the fact that the outcome of interest is not observed in all patients (i.e., for some patients, the outcome is censored). Sample size estimation for time to event data first determines the number of events required to detect an effect size of interest with the desired power and Type I error rate. The total number of patients then follows from estimated probability that a patient experiences the event of interest.

## 5.11 Conclusion

RCTs are considered the "gold standard" for assessing the efficacy and benefit of treatments because when properly designed, rigorously conducted, and appropriately analyzed, RCTs yield unbiased estimates of both the benefit and risk of experimental treatments. One of the most critical elements of the design of RCTs is sample size: the number of patients required to ensure a high probability of achieving the trial's objectives. Sample size estimation requires the specification of several items, including the primary endpoint, null hypothesis, effect size, and the error probabilities for false negative and false positive conclusions—the Type I and Type II error rates.

Thoughtful sample size calculations allow investigators to design a study, which balances the need for ethical involvement of human subjects with the desired statistical rigor of the anticipated findings, in the face of real-world limitations. While some of the parameters may seem formulaic, specific considerations, which affect sample size estimation will have critical impacts on the integrity and validity of the study design and results. A *boiler plate* approach will not suffice to ensure that a study design is ethical and rigorous for the intervention and patients being studied.

There are numerous texts and review articles that address sample size calculations in detail. Here we sought to provide a very general and heuristic presentation of key concepts as it is beyond the scope of our intent to lay out all the various approaches to calculating sample size. We urge clinical investigators to contact a biostatistician to collaboratively design clinical trials to ensure scientific rigor.

### Practical Recommendations

### Estimates and Simulations

An online sample size calculator can be a useful tool to estimate the required number of patients during the phase of study design. Although they cannot substitute for a knowledgeable statistician collaborator, an online calculator can help the research team understand how the number of patients might change, based on various outcomes or other design parameters, which are being considered. The authors recommend the Vanderbilt University Medical Center Power and Sample Size Calculation tool:

https://biostat.app.vumc.org/wiki/Main/PowerSampleSize

### A Step-by-Step Guide to Using Another Online Calculator (https://www.sealedenvelope.com)

Kim J, Seo BS. How to calculate sample size and why. Clin Orthop Surg. ;5(3):235–42. https://doi.org/10.4055/cios.2013.5.3.235. Epub 2013 Aug 20. PMID: 24009911; PMCID: PMC3758995.

To optimize study design further, surgeon-researchers could also consider asking their statistician collaborator to fun full simulations, using software such as the "simr" package in R. Simulations can be used not only to investigate the impact of basic statistical parameters such as sample sizes, effect sizes, or data variability and distribution but also real-world considerations such as recruitment or drop-out rates.

### Further Reading

The authors recommend the following resources, including step-by-step guides, focused discussions of specific topics and textbooks, which provide more in-depth coverage of the principles of power analysis and sample size calculations than is covered in this chapter.

Concept Paper and Detailed Statistical Guideline for Clinical Trials from the International Council for Harmonisation of Technical Requirements for Pharmaceuticals for Human Use (ICH).

https://database.ich.org/sites/default/files/E9-R1_EWG_Concept_Paper.pdf

https://database.ich.org/sites/default/files/E9_Guideline.pdf

The International Council for Harmonisation of Technical Requirements for Pharmaceuticals for Human Use (ICH) was formed in 1990 with a mission to achieve greater harmonisation worldwide to ensure that safe, effective, and high quality medicines are developed and registered in the most resource-efficient manner. Harmonisation is achieved through the development of ICH Guidelines *via* a process of scientific consensus with regulatory and industry experts working side-by-side.

## Step-by-Step Guides for Determining Power and Sample Size During Study Design

Staffa SJ, Zurakowski D. Statistical power and sample size calculations: a primer for pediatric surgeons. J Pediatr Surg 2020;55(7):1173–1179. https://doi.org/10.1016/j.jpedsurg.2019.05.007. Epub 2019 May 16. PMID: 31155391.

Guller U, Oertli D. Sample size matters: a guide for surgeons. World J Surg 2005 May;29(5):601–5. https://doi.org/10.1007/s00268-005-7921-y. PMID: 15834629.

## An Example Illustrating How to Assess Power and Sample Size in Published Research

Cadeddu M, Farrokhyar F, Thoma A, Haines T, Garnett A, Goldsmith CH; Evidence-Based Surgery Working Group. Users' guide to the surgical literature: how to assess power and sample size. Laparoscopic vs open appendectomy. Can J Surg 2008;51(6):476–82. PMID: 19057738; PMCID: PMC2592579.

## For Further Reading on Non-inferiority Studies

https://trialsjournal.biomedcentral.com/articles/10.1186/1745-6215-12-106

## Review of the Mathematical Calculations of Sample Size

Wittes J. Sample size calculations for randomized controlled trials. Epidemiol Rev 2002;24(1):39–53. https://doi.org/10.1093/epirev/24.1.39. PMID: 12119854.

## Recommended Textbooks

Fundamentals of Clinical Trials
Lawrence M. Friedman, Curt D. Furberg, David L. DeMets
https://doi.org/10.1007/978-1-4419-1586-3
Springer-Verlag New York 2010
ISBN978-1-4419-1586-3
Published: 09 September 2010

Clinical Trials: A Methodologic Perspective
Steven Piantadosi
First published:8 July 2005
Print ISBN:9780471727811 | Online ISBN:9780471740131 | https://doi.org/10.1002/0471740136
2005 John Wiley & Sons, Inc.

Determining Sample Size and Power in Research Studies
JP Verma, Priyam Verma
Springer Singapore
First Published: 21 July 2020
Print ISBN: 978-981-15-5206-9 | Online ISBN: 978-981-15-5204-5
https://doi.org/10.1007/978-981-15-5204-5

## This Site Provides an Excellent Bibliography for Additional Reading

https://www.oxfordbibliographies.com/display/document/obo-9780199828340/obo-9780199828340-0296.xml

# Optimizing Recruitment in Randomized Controlled Trials

# 6

Amit Meena and Alan Getgood

## 6.1 Introduction

The evidence provided by randomized controlled trials (RCTs) is very reliable for evaluating the effects of a health care intervention. However, the successful conduct of an RCT can be hindered by difficulties in subject recruitment and retention. Inadequate recruitment leads to reduced statistical power and lack of precision in detecting significant effects of the intervention under investigation, which may result in an incorrect conclusion that can have far-reaching impact on the utilization of the technology or future use of the treatment under investigation. This can be seen as an ethical and moral dilemma, with patients undergoing a trial procedure, the results of which may never be appropriately analyzed due to the lack of successful recruitment [1]. Furthermore, the inability to complete a trial can be seen as a waste of valuable resources, including healthcare and research funding. Slow recruitment also causes delays, which can affect the impact of the study as the standard of care can change over time. It also increases costs, which in turn can even result in failure of the successful completion of trials.

RCT findings may have important regulatory and clinical decision-making effects, the success of which is dependent on employing efficient and effective methods for recruiting participants. Several strategies have been devised to facilitate adequate and timely recruitment of participants to RCTs. This chapter will highlight some of the techniques that have been described to improve subject recruitment to research studies, as well as detail many of the techniques that we employ to ensure successful subject recruitment and study completion within our own research practice.

The key recruitment strategies are broken down into three main areas of focus:

- Study methodology
- Subject education
- Incentivization

The aim of this chapter is to describe these strategies and where appropriate provide evidence as to their effectiveness.

## 6.2 Study Methodology

The design of a study is fundamental to its successful completion. The full scope of study design will be explored in other chapters within

A. Meena
Fowler Kennedy Sport Medicine Clinic, Western University, London, ON, Canada
e-mail: ameena@uwo.ca

A. Getgood (✉)
Aspetar Sports Medicine Hospital, Doha, Qatar
e-mail: alan.getgood@uwo.ca


S. Lyman et al. (eds.), *Introduction to Surgical Trials*,
https://doi.org/10.1007/978-3-031-77563-5_6

this book. In this section, we will focus on study design elements that are important in order to optimize subject recruitment and retention.

***Is the Research Question Interesting and Relevant for Target Subjects*** One of the first tasks that one faces when designing a study is to develop the research question. A well-built research question will often follow the PICO format, that is (1) the Patient problem or Population; (2) the Intervention; (3) the Comparison (if there is one); and (4) the Outcome(s). Our experience is that the more relevant the research question is to the target population, then the greater the likelihood is that they will be more interested in taking part in the study. As such, when designing the research question we should think about whether the study will be exciting for subjects to be involved in and is it a clinical problem that they can relate to? If you are not sure, a pilot feasibility study can be performed to determine the rate and likelihood of successful recruitment. If two or more treatment options are being compared, then one must determine if these options are both standard of care or if one is a new technology/treatment. Will subjects be blinded to treatment allocation? What about outcome measures? Simple questionnaires are more easy to perform than undergoing lengthy investigations such as magnetic resonance imaging, or invasive measures such as synovial fluid aspiration or blood draw. Equally, large numbers of questionnaires with multiple questions can be laborious to complete. All of these questions need to be considered to determine the level of interest for the target population and whether the study will be a significant burden on them, which could influence recruitment as well as retention.

***Study Design*** It is known that a clinical study having active arms of treatment has higher rates of recruitment when compared with a placebo-controlled study [2]. Furthermore, patients show increased rates of participation when they are aware of their treatment mode even if it is predetermined randomly. As such, open trials have been shown to have greater patient buy-in than blinded studies [3]. This shines light on the anxiety issues of unknown treatments which can often lead to reduced clinical trial participation. A study by Caldwell et al. demonstrated that unblinded trial designs have higher consent rates as compared to the blinded trial designs as there is no element of the fear of the unknown [4]. However, the relative loss to follow-up in both arms of an unblinded trial possibly jeopardizes the resulting study validity, as patients drop out more easily if they are not satisfied with the treatment group they were allocated. This further speaks to the importance of retention as well as recruitment.

Being part of a randomized trial may be the only way to get access to a new technology, for example, in a phase two or three regulatory study. If this is the case, one way to help boost trial participation is by providing preferential randomization to the trial technology, such as in a 2:1 ratio. Potential candidates may be more likely to opt in as they believe that they are getting a higher chance of receiving the type of experimental treatment, which may be desirable. However, studies show that the consent rates are not influenced by the likelihood of receiving the experimental treatment or not getting the placebo, indicating that patients' decisions for participation in clinical studies are not affected by the type of treatment they are going to receive [5].

A more controversial strategy is the use of randomization prior to consent, the so-called Zelen study design [6]. This can be utilized more easily when the two comparative treatments are both judged to be standard of care. Experimental treatments can also be tested but should only be included if knowing that being part of a randomized trial would influence the outcome of the study leading to bias. The patient is randomized at screening and then forwarded on to the specific physician for that treatment where they receive informed consent for that procedure or treatment modality. This type of study design is most applicable for questions regarding real-world treatment or intervention effects under conditions of incomplete adherence [7]. While controversial, Zelen designed this study type to increase participant engagement and recruitment in real-world studies, trying to counteract the issues of patient and physician preference for treatment arms. That said, they are poorly suited to address explanatory or efficacy questions and more often preferred for addressing pragmatic or policy questions.

***Do Participating Investigators Have Equipoise in Regard to Treatment Groups?*** It is vital that all participating investigators have equipoise as to the nature of the treatment groups. In the example of a surgical trial, where surgery A is being compared to surgery B, if a surgeon has a clear preference of one arm over another, it would be unethical to recruit patients to the study. Ensuring equipoise is vital to ensure that all potential subjects are approached/screened and that certain individuals are not excluded that will result in selection bias.

***Consent Process*** There are multiple ways in which potential subjects may be approached and inclusion in an RCT proposed. One systematic review demonstrated that the best way to increase recruitment to a study was telephone contact following the delivery of mailed letter or email [3]. This is of course very dependent on the type of trial, and in particular, the type of interventions being studied. The majority of trials that our clinic is involved revolve around surgical treatments. As such, patients are seen by participating surgeons in clinic. All patients presenting with the problem under investigation are pre-screened for eligibility. They are in turn flagged for potential recruitment. Once they are seen by the participating surgeon and the inclusion/exclusion criteria are met, thereby indicating that they are eligible for recruitment, the participating surgeon approaches them with the study concept. The use of an investigator pitch can be very helpful. It is vital that this pitch is not coercive, but the pros and cons of being part of a study can be highlighted. The patient is then introduced to the research assistant where more details are provided, including a full letter of information that details all pertinent information regarding trial participation. This material should be presented in a way that the patient can easily understand (i.e., layman's terms). Consent is then completed by the research assistant.

***Do the Study Sites Have Appropriate Research Infrastructure?*** Successful trial design and subject recruitment is very dependent on having appropriate research infrastructure. Different levels of infrastructure are required as to whether the site is leading a trial or acting as a participating recruitment center. Appropriate staffing levels, funding, and external resources for collecting outcomes are essential. The study site selection should be made based on predetermined criteria. The sites should meet these criteria which can be confirmed by means of site initiation visits. Adequate oversight from the trial sponsors/lead investigators/monitor should be in place to ensure smooth functioning of these sites. Sites must be able to pre-screen subjects to check for eligibility so as to capture as many possible eligible subjects as possible.

Aspects of site infrastructure are also critical for subject retention. We studied factors that were associated with subject loss to follow-up from a large multicenter RCT [8]. We found that study site, and therefore site infrastructure, was a key predictor of loss to follow-up. This suggested that sites with less research support performed worse in maintaining subject retention in trials.

## 6.3 Education Tools

Participant education is a mandatory part of the consent process for research studies. However, its value goes beyond just informed consent. Increasing the awareness of the health problem under study for potential participants has been demonstrated to increase consent rates by engaging subjects in the learning process [9]. Education strategies that focus on the health issue under study, such as through the provision of questionnaires, videos, educational sessions, and interactive programs have been successfully implemented [10–12]. In contrast, strategies that focus on understanding the clinical trial process have not been shown to improve consent rates.

***Delivery of Trial Information*** The mode of delivery of information to potential participants can play a role in improving recruitment to RCTs. Various methods can be used to deliver trial information. Providing a video alongside written information leads to an improved willingness to participate in a study compared with written information alone. Interactive computer presentations can also improve recruitment. The presence of a research assistant who is available to answer questions along with an interactive audio-visual presentation has slightly better chances of participant recruitment, compared with just the research assistant [13]. Recruitment can also be enhanced by delivering verbal education sessions in the participants native language before presenting the consent as compared with print materials alone [14].

***Mode of Contact*** Using telephone reminders to follow up on written invitations has been demonstrated to improve subject recruitment [15]. SMS messages containing quotes from existing recruits when texted to potential participants have also been seen to improve recruitment of new participants when compared with the standard written invitation. Interestingly, the role of the recruiter has also shown no evidence of affecting recruitment rates [14]. It would appear that the substance of information provided is the chief factor that increases the rate of recruitment, rather than when, how, or who provides the information. From our own experience, having buy-in from the surgeon investigator is extremely important to get the patient to believe in the study subject and need for research. The information delivery and consent process is then performed by the research assistant, with the surgeon investigator always available if further questions need to be addressed.

***Increasing Patient Awareness*** In a world of social medial, it has never been easier to disseminate information to the public and therefore potential trial subjects. Awareness regarding a disease or a new condition under study can be spread by using various social media platforms with the help of targeted advertising, information videos, and by reaching out to online user groups that are shared by people suffering from the same orthopedic conditions. Mainstream media can also be utilized to advertise recruitment, such as placing information advertisements in newspapers or having investigators interviewed on local television or radio shows. However, many of these formats can come with a financial cost and the trial team must be aware for the potential low return on investment as there are several studies that show that publicizing a trial has not resulted in a significant increase in recruitment rates, which remained nearly constant [16].

## 6.4 Incentivization

The concept of incentivizing subjects to participate in a trial is not uncommon but can be applied in a variety of forms, of which it is vitally important that any incentive offered is in no way coercive [17]. Non-financial incentivization includes feedback on the trial progress and outcome of the trial. Participants may receive information that they may not otherwise get when being outside of a trial, such as their own specific data on their rehabilitation post-surgery using the research tools that we are employing in the study. However, this is of course dependent on the study design and the level of blinding. We also find that patients can be extremely motivated by the fact that they are helping advance science by being part of a research study. As such, it is important that they are aware that their participation may not directly help them but could go on to indirectly help other people in the future.

Financial incentives can be in the form of provision of payments for out of pocket expenses that have been incurred while being part of a study, such as parking or food. Different rules around what can be offered to participants often exist in many countries and jurisdictions and should be explored within your own research ethics board. For example, research participants may be offered compensation for out of pocket expenses but may not be able to be compensated for their time. While monetary perks to participants have been shown to increase recruitment rates, the amount of money does not seem to be that important [18].

## 6.5 Author Strategies for Successful Recruitment and Retention of the Subjects in an RCT

The following strategies were utilized to boost recruitment during the design and implementation of the ISAKOS sponsored Stability study, an RCT comparing anterior cruciate ligament reconstruction (ACLR) with or without lateral extra-articular tenodesis (LET) in young patients at high risk of re-injury [19]. The sample size target for this study was 600 patients; therefore, multiple strategies were employed to enroll participants in a timely manner.

**Maximizing Subject Recruitment**

1. The research question targeted a young healthy population who wished to return to sport. One of the major issues faced by this patient population was the risk of re-injury. As such, the intervention (LET) and the primary outcome focused on reducing rotatory laxity and the risk of re-injury which was of interest to the target population.
2. Multiple sites were engaged in the study that had appropriate research infrastructure already in place. They were all familiar with research practice and had appropriate levels of staffing to undertake a successful study.
3. Regular remote and in person investigator meetings were held to ensure buy-in and education for investigators.
4. Recruitment materials, such as recruitment scripts, flyers, and laminated reference cards that summarize eligibility criteria were developed and distributed to the sites.
5. As part of the clinical monitoring plan, we closely monitored recruitment every month at each of the sites. Sites that achieved or exceeded the recruitment goals were permitted to recruit more subjects beyond their enrollment target, while for those sites that lagged in recruitment, we worked closely with them to increase enrollment. Strategies to improve recruitment varied based on the barriers encountered by the site on a case-to-case basis. If gross recruitment for the study lagged behind targeted enrollment, we could have considered adding sites, re-allocating financial support for additional sites from those sites that are not meeting recruitment projections or have been terminated from the study.
6. Pre-screening was completed the day before clinic to make sure we flagged potentially eligible subjects. Research assistants were then present in clinic and touched base with the recruiting surgeons to ensure all eligible subjects were approached for trial inclusion.

**Maximizing Subject Retention**

Participants that are lost to follow-up are a major concern in any study [8]. We factored in a 15% loss to follow-up in the Stability Study sample size collection. However, by employing the following techniques we achieved a 5% loss to follow-up rate.

1. The provision of a research assistant to collect complete demographic information from the participant at the time of enrollment and to update the contact information at each subsequent follow-up visit. We utilize a specific site tracker to record study details and participant information. This includes information such as upcoming appointment time (which we remind them by phone or email), what has been completed, or what needs to be completed as well as any additional information that may pertain to the participant or their involvement in the study. This tracker is updated daily/weekly.
2. The patient is made aware of the time commitments required for participation at the time of taking the informed consent by the surgeon and research assistant. Any study activities (such as questionnaires) that can be completed ahead of time at home are sent to the participant prior to the appointment to limit the time commitment in clinic. Relevant questions are answered so that the participant fully understands their responsibilities before signing the consent form.
3. The project coordinator and quality control lead at the data management company can pro-

actively monitor participant retention using the web-based data management system. Missing data reports can be shared with the site research assistant and principal investigator on a monthly basis for adjudication and resolution.

4. The data management software can be used effectively as they offer a participant tracker report that the research assistant at each site can generate. This feature assists the site with planning and tracking participant visits. In addition to these texts and emails, we will also send personalized emails from our email accounts. These personalized emails sometimes help response rates as people are more likely to ignore a computer rather than someone they have met in person.
5. The data management software can send an automatic email or text message to participants (who have opted into this feature) regarding upcoming and overdue appointments. Multiple attempts to contact non-responders can be utilized.
6. Each participant is provided with a secure personalized login. The data management software records the date, time, and user information in the audit log so that the electronic information can serve as a primary data source. The audit log also tracks initial data values, updated data values, and reasons for changes made to updated data values. Providing this option allows the research team to collect patient-reported data when participants cannot physically attend a follow-up (e.g., vacation).
7. In the event of it being difficult to get patients back to clinic, or if they were not responding to calls from the research team, members of the surgical team would personally call the patient and ask them to return for follow-up. If they were unable to return to clinic, then information regarding adverse events could be collected and patient-reported outcomes collected remotely.

## 6.6 Conclusion

A number of strategies can be utilized to boost subject recruitment in randomized controlled trials. These mainly revolve around study design, potential subject education, and making participation in the study an appealing proposition. Subject retention is equally as important, as hitting the recruitment target is only good if those subjects reach the study endpoint, achieving statistical power to answer the research question.

## References


1. Halpern SD, Karlawish JH, Berlin JA. The continuing unethical conduct of underpowered clinical trials. JAMA. 2002;288(3):358–62.
2. Caldwell PH, Butow PN, Craig JC. Parents' attitudes to children's participation in randomized controlled trials. J Pediatr. 2003;142(5):554–9.
3. Treweek S, Pitkethly M, Cook J, Fraser C, Mitchell E, Sullivan F, et al. Strategies to improve recruitment to randomised trials. Cochrane Database Syst Rev. 2018;2(2):MR000013.
4. Caldwell PH, Hamilton S, Tan A, Craig JC. Strategies for increasing recruitment to randomised controlled trials: systematic review. PLoS Med. 2010;7(11):e1000368.
5. Myles PS, Fletcher HE, Cairo S, Madder H, McRae R, Cooper J, et al. Randomized trial of informed consent and recruitment for clinical trials in the immediate preoperative period. Anesthesiology. 1999;91(4):969–78.
6. Zelen M. A new design for randomized clinical trials. N Engl J Med. 1979;300(22):1242–5.
7. Simon GE, Shortreed SM, DeBar LL. Zelen design clinical trials: why, when, and how. Trials. 2021;22(1):541.
8. Firth AB, Bryant DM, Johnson AM, AMJ G, STABILITY 1 Study Group. Predicting patient loss to follow-up in the STABILITY 1 study: a multicenter, international, randomized controlled trial of young, active patients undergoing ACL reconstruction. J Bone Joint Surg. 2022;104(7):594.
9. Losina E, Wright J, Katz JN. Clinical trials in orthopaedics research. Part III. Overcoming operational challenges in the design and conduct of randomized clinical trials in orthopaedic surgery. J Bone Joint Surg Am. 2012;94(6):e35.
10. Kendrick D, Watson M, Dewey M, Woods AJ. Does sending a home safety questionnaire increase recruitment to an injury prevention trial? A randomised controlled trial. J Epidemiol Community Health. 2001;55(11):845–6.
11. Du W, Mood D, Gadgeel S, Simon MS. An educational video to increase clinical trials enrollment among breast cancer patients. Breast Cancer Res Treat. 2009;117(2):339–47.
12. Ellis PM, Butow PN, Tattersall MH. Informing breast cancer patients about clinical trials: a randomized clinical trial of an educational booklet. Ann Oncol. 2002;13(9):1414–23.

13. Hutchison C, Cowan C, McMahon T, Paul J. A randomised controlled study of an audiovisual patient information intervention on informed consent and recruitment to cancer clinical trials. Br J Cancer. 2007;97(6):705–11.
14. Free C, Hoile E, Robertson S, Knight R. Three controlled trials of interventions to increase recruitment to a randomized controlled trial of mobile phone based smoking cessation support. Clin Trials. 2010;7(3):265–73.
15. Treweek S, Mitchell E, Pitkethly M, Cook J, Kjeldstrom M, Taskila T, et al. Strategies to improve recruitment to randomised controlled trials. Cochrane Database Syst Rev. 2010;4(1):MR000013.
16. Pighills A, Torgerson DJ, Sheldon T. Publicity does not increase recruitment to falls prevention trials: the results of two quasi-randomized trials. J Clin Epidemiol. 2009;62(12):1332–5.
17. Martinson BC, Lazovich D, Lando HA, Perry CL, McGovern PG, Boyle RG. Effectiveness of monetary incentives for recruiting adolescents to an intervention trial to reduce smoking. Prev Med. 2000;31(6):706–13.
18. Halpern SD, Karlawish JH, Casarett D, Berlin JA, Asch DA. Empirical assessment of whether moderate payments are undue or unjust inducements for participation in clinical trials. Arch Intern Med. 2004;164(7):801–3.
19. Getgood AMJ, Bryant DM, Litchfield R, Heard M, McCormack RG, Rezansoff A, et al. Lateral extra-articular tenodesis reduces failure of hamstring tendon autograft anterior cruciate ligament reconstruction: 2-year outcomes from the STABILITY Study Randomized Clinical Trial. Am J Sports Med. 2020;48(2):285–97.

# 7 Treatment Allocation

Bálint Zsidai, Alexandra Horvath, Jón Karlsson, and Eric Hamrin Senorski

## 7.1 Introduction

In orthopedics, randomized controlled trials (RCT) constitute the highest level of evidence (Level 1) and the proportion of articles published based on RCTs in the field of orthopedic sports medicine have steadily risen to approximately 10% during the last 20 years [1]. Conducting an RCT comparing the efficacy of different interventions requires thorough understanding of several key concepts pertinent to the treatment allocation process. Evaluating the effects of interventions requires the carefully planned elimination of potential residual biases, which may lead to invalid conclusions about the efficacy of the therapy being evaluated. Surgical trials are inherently difficult to randomize, and blinding of all individuals involved in the investigation is often impossible. Additionally, potential subjects may be less likely to be open to random allocation of treatment choice, especially when an existing operative or non-operative intervention may already be well established. This chapter provides an overview of the concepts required to conduct patient allocation to treatment groups of a surgical RCT.

## 7.2 Randomization

Randomization is the process ensuring the allocation of trial participants into experimental and control groups in a manner dictated by random chance, ruling out the effect of selection bias or

B. Zsidai
Department of Orthopaedics, Institute of Clinical Sciences, Sahlgrenska Academy, University of Gothenburg, Gothenburg, Sweden

Sahlgrenska Sports Medicine Center, Gothenburg, Sweden

A. Horvath
Sahlgrenska Sports Medicine Center, Gothenburg, Sweden

Department of Internal Medicine and Clinical Nutrition, Institute of Medicine, Sahlgrenska Academy, University of Gothenburg, Gothenburg, Sweden

J. Karlsson
Department of Orthopaedics, Sahlgrenska University Hospital, Sahlgrenska Academy, Gothenburg University, Gothenburg, Sweden

E. H. Senorski (✉)
Sahlgrenska Sports Medicine Center, Gothenburg, Sweden

Department of Health and Rehabilitation, Institute of Neuroscience and Physiology, Sahlgrenska Academy, University of Gothenburg, Gothenburg, Sweden
e-mail: eric.hamrin.senorski@gu.se


S. Lyman et al. (eds.), *Introduction to Surgical Trials*,
https://doi.org/10.1007/978-3-031-77563-5_7

confounding factors, such as patient age, sex, smoking status, body mass index, and various other possible effect modifiers. Without this process, patient allocation into different treatment groups may be disproportionate, introducing prejudices that potentially impact the ultimate conclusions of a surgical trial [2]. Without randomization, patients enrolled into two different treatment groups may differ in terms of age, preinjury activity level, motivation to return to sport, and various other unknown factors, which may affect the treatment outcomes measured in the study. While some confounding variables may be accounted for during statistical analysis, systematic elimination of bias through randomization mitigates the introduction of biases that may otherwise remain undetected. In order to achieve random allocation of patients, numbers may be generated manually by flipping a coin, using the day of the week or pulling a number from a hat. However, these methods may easily be influenced and rendered non-random and should be avoided. Today, computer-generated number sequences and tables are the gold standard of the randomization process [3].

It is important to mention that using patient data from medical charts, such as date of birth and identification numbers, is considered" quasi-randomization," which does not truly randomize a patient population and is therefore not recommended [3]. Several methods are available for the randomization of trial participants in a manner that eliminates residual biases arising from confounding variables, thereby creating random groups with near-identical distribution of patient-related factors [4]. The chosen method is usually determined based on the requirements of the given clinical trial scenario. However, in general, randomization enables researchers to conduct statistically robust studies with an optimal number of recruited patients.

Randomization techniques using a fixed allocation of treatments generate experimental and control groups by assigning a probability ratio (e.g., 1:1 or 2:1) to the placement of a participant in one group or the other. Although predefined ratios other than 1:1 are often argued to introduce bias, the economic advantage of allocating a smaller proportion of patients to the experimental treatment, which is often paid for by the trial itself, is sometimes cited as a rationale for groups of unequal sizes [5]. Fixed allocation randomization can further be divided into the following subtypes:

- *Simple randomization* is the least complex and predictable method and can be executed using computer-generated random numbers or randomization tables. While this is the most commonly employed randomization technique in large RCTs, this method is less reliable in ensuring bias prevention and balanced group-characteristics in trials with smaller sample sizes.
- *Block randomization* is favorable in trials where an equal number of participants are required between groups and the total number of eligible patients is expected to be limited. Allocation sequences are generated in a way which eliminates group imbalances, usually through the creation of equal sized blocks of sizes that are multiples of the number of available treatment groups in the study. For instance, in a trial with two intervention groups (A and B) that randomizes participants in groups of four, six possible sequence combinations are generated (AABB, ABBA, ABAB, BAAB, BABA, and BBAA). Selection of a random number will then determine the combination (block) according to which the next four patients will be assigned. This process is repeated for the next four patients until all subjects have been assigned to a group based on the a priori sample size goal. This assures that if a trial is stopped early, a relatively balanced number of patients will have been allocated to each treatment arm.
- *Stratified randomization* strives to overcome the issue of selection bias caused by random imbalances between intervention groups. This is accomplished by dividing the sample population according to predetermined prognostic variables (covariates) prior to randomization. Following stratification, participants are assigned to groups using block randomization. Although it generally provides an elegant

strategy for controlling the impact of covariates on the outcomes of a study, this method may be problematic when a large number of covariates need to be taken into consideration. Proper group balance and improved statistical power and precision with a small number of trial participants may warrant the use of stratified randomization in small-scale trials. Conversely, simple randomization is usually sufficient in eliminating imbalances in studies with large patient samples.

In contrast to fixed allocation methods, adaptive allocation permits changes in the probability of randomization into one treatment group or another over time in order to achieve balanced covariates between patient groups or to assign new patients to the intervention group with a favorable response based on previous allocations:

- *Covariate adaptive randomization* can be advantageous in small trials, where simple randomization could result in statistically significant between-group differences in some covariates [6, 7]. Moreover, it ensures real-time adjustment of group imbalances during the recruitment process. Covariates are identified prior to the trial start, and the assignment of patients to treatment groups occurs in a sequence that maintains a between-group balance in terms of these variables.
- *Response adaptive randomization* is an adaptive randomization technique based on patient response to an intervention. Successively recruited patients are assigned to the treatment group that provides superior results based on previous patient responses during the surgical trial. A positive treatment response means the next patient will be allocated to the same group, while a negative response will assign the subsequent patient to another intervention group [7].

A pitfall of fixed allocation in small-sized trials is the unequal distribution of variables and confounders between treatment groups, leading to the misinterpretation of study results. Randomization by adaptive allocation provides a solution to avoid this by keeping track of the distribution of covariates. New participants are assigned to groups based on keeping these covariates balanced across the intervention groups.

## 7.3 Control Groups

The choice of the control treatment against which the efficacy or efficiency of a surgical intervention is measured is crucial during the trial design process. The gold standard in an RCT is a placebo control. However, in the context of surgical trials, implementation of a placebo essentially means performing sham surgery, which is a topic of ethical debate, especially when a standard treatment of known effectiveness already exists. The ethical concerns associated with sham surgery include but are not limited to (1) violation of the trust between doctor and patient, (2) potential exposure to the unnecessary risks of performing the sham operation, (3) implications of informed consent, and (4) withholding the current standard of care from patients that could otherwise benefit.

Additionally, while recent reports have highlighted the growing relevance and frequency of sham surgery in orthopedic trials, poor recruitment and high drop-out rates diminish the quality of these studies [8, 9]. Nonetheless, sham surgery, when implemented, may be able to provide valuable information in terms of the utility of surgical interventions and may eventually prevent unnecessary exposure of patients to the risks associated with a procedure of unknown effectiveness. Examples of such RCTs are the Finnish Degenerative Meniscal Lesion Study (FIDELITY) comparing arthroscopic meniscectomy with sham surgery [10], and another surgical RCT comparing osteoarthritis treatment using arthroscopic lavage or debridement with sham surgery [11].

Other types of treatment groups are more typically used in surgical trials, specifically no treatment or an active treatment control group [12]. The choice of a control group largely depends on the state of clinical evidence in terms of the effectiveness of the currently available treatments. In the simplest case, there is true equipoise (i.e., an expert consensus that neither treatment arm is more beneficial than the other) about the effectiveness of two treatment modalities, allowing randomization into each group with the goal of identifying the intervention resulting in superior outcomes. The intervention groups of the STABILITY trial [13] serve as a clear illustrative example of this type of design. A novel surgical intervention, in this case lateral extra-articular tenodesis (LET) in combination with single-bundle, hamstring tendon anterior cruciate ligament reconstruction (ACL-R), was compared with an active control treatment of single-bundle, hamstring tendon ACL-R, with the aim of determining whether the addition of LET is superior in reducing ACL-R graft failure [14]. As ACL-R is considered the standard of care in young active patients, this is a well-chosen control group to measure outcomes when equipoise exists about the effectiveness of another intervention.

## 7.4 Allocation Concealment

Allocation concealment refers to the process of implementing the allocation sequence assigned to recruited patients in a way that excludes the possibility of introducing further bias [7]. This process entails withholding the treatment allocation of enrolled subjects from those conducting the trial. Today, distance randomization is the most widely accepted approach to allocation concealment. This requires the enrolling individual to access a third-party telephone or web-based service, which then completes the random allocation process in a centralized and secure manner, shielded from the influence of the investigators. Previously, opaque envelopes have been used to conceal participant group assignment from team members of a study. While there is contrasting evidence in terms of the effectiveness of this practice in maintaining investigator blinding [15, 16], concealed envelopes may be subject to manipulation and their use is therefore not recommended with modern electronic solutions available [12].

## 7.5 Non-randomized Allocation

In situations when large-scale implementation of randomization is not feasible due to geographic or logistical limitations, non-randomized allocation may be used to evaluate the outcomes of a new intervention compared with a control group. The main drawback of non-randomized allocation in surgical trials is that patient groups are generally subject to multiple confounding variables, which become difficult to adjust for using this strategy [7]. Moreover, the non-random patient selection process may also be biased due to tampering by study personnel or imbalanced allocation of "healthier" patients into one intervention group, which is why non-randomized allocation is not generally favored in surgical trial design [7]. However, non-randomized allocation may be necessary on certain levels of the study design and may introduce some bias:

- *Surgeon-level randomization*: A single- or multicenter randomized controlled trial may often subject to the participation of few or even a single surgeon from a given surgical center. In such cases, participants are per definition not equally randomized in terms of the operating surgeon compared to centers with trial participation by a large number of surgeons.
- *Site-level randomization*: Typically, patients who participate in multicenter RCTs are assigned to a site closest to their home to facilitate commute and compliance to follow-up visits. Consequently, truly random allocation in terms of study site is difficult to achieve and may compromise the ability of patients to participate in the RCT.

**Fact Box 7.1**

**Randomization:** Randomization is the process ensuring the allocation of trial participants into experimental and control groups in a manner controlled by random chance.

**Fixed Allocation Randomization:** Experimental and control groups are generated using a fixed probability ratio.

**Adaptive Allocation Randomization:** The probability of randomization into a group changes based on certain factors, such as the distribution of covariates or patient response to a treatment.

**Equipoise:** The consensus that neither treatment alternative in a study is superior compared with the others based on clinical expertise.

**Allocation Concealment:** It eliminates bias by withholding information about the treatment groups trial participants have been assigned to from those implementing the allocation sequence.

**Blinding:** It involves withholding information about the groups trial participants have been allocated to from (1) patients of the study population, (2) care-providers and outcome investigators, and (3) data collectors and analysts.

## 7.6 Blinding

Blinding in surgical RCTs refers to the process of hiding which treatment group study participants have been assigned to from one or several of the following stakeholders: (1) enrolled patients, (2) care-providers, (3) outcome data collection personnel, and (4) statistical analysts. Thus, a study may be single-, double-, triple-, or even quadruple-blinded based on the number of the previously stated parties kept unaware of participant group assignment. However, the updated Consolidated Standard of Reporting Trials (CONSORT) statement suggests the specific clarification of which parties are blinded in a study rather than using these general terms [17]. This is especially warranted when individuals assume multiple roles during the conduction of a trial (e.g., a participating surgeon also involved in outcome assessment). While trials should strive to blind as many of the involved parties as possible, surgical trials pose inherent challenges in achieving this, since surgeons cannot be blinded to the operation they are performing. In contrast, blinding of the remaining study participants is more practical and therefore encouraged. Surgical scars may be concealed from outcome assessors using sleeves or clothing, while deidentification of patient data using digital tools avoids any introduction of bias by data collection and/or analysis staff [12]. Regardless, recently performed reviews involving orthopedic trauma, general, and abdominal surgery have demonstrated that the frequency of blinding study contributors in surgical trials, where possible, has significant room for improvement [18, 19]. The crucial importance of blinding in randomized trials stems from the need to prevent biases introduced by participating patients, investigators, or other study personnel. Although both practices aim to eliminate probable biases, blinding must not be confused with allocation concealment. While the former is implemented following patient randomization in order to prevent detection and performance bias, the latter eliminates selection bias prior to patient randomization [7]. Of note, a quick method of unblinding must always be available in case severe complications of a treatment arise [20].

In many cases, blinding can be a straightforward procedure, but some orthopedic trials involving the comparison of operative and nonoperative treatments may face several difficulties and pitfalls in avoiding reporting and assessor bias. In the Meniscal Tear in Osteoarthritis Research (METEOR) trial [21], the efficacy of arthroscopic partial meniscectomy was compared to a standardized non-operative physical therapy protocol in patients with symptomatic meniscal tears and concurrent osteoarthritic pathology. The authors of this trial discuss that while assessor and participant blinding could have been established using sham surgery, the investigators opted not to use a placebo group, thereby avoiding the reluctance of patients to be randomized to sham surgery as well as the ethical issues surrounding sham procedures [21]. Instead, the investigators chose to mitigate observer bias by the use of a validated self-report questionnaire and the blinding of data analysts.

## 7.7 Conclusion

Taken altogether, subjects of a surgical RCT can be allocated to various treatment groups using fixed allocation (simple, block, or stratified randomization) and adaptive allocation (covariate or response) randomization techniques. Control groups used in surgical trials include placebo (sham surgery), no treatment, and active treatment groups. Allocation concealment prevents the introduction of selection bias by withholding the knowledge of which group a subject has been assigned to from the enrolling staff. Blinding is important to perform with respect to (1) enrolled patients, (2) care-providers, (3) outcome data collection personnel, and (4) statistical analysts in order to limit the impact of caregiver expectations as well as assessor and responder bias on outcome measures of a trial. The ethical issues surrounding blinding must always be carefully considered.

## References


1. Grant HM, Tjoumakaris FP, Maltenfort MG, Freedman KB. Levels of evidence in the clinical sports medicine literature: are we getting better over time? Am J Sports Med. 2014;42(7):1738–42. https://doi.org/10.1177/0363546514530863.
2. Schulz KF, Grimes DA. Generation of allocation sequences in randomised trials: chance, not choice. Lancet. 2002;359(9305):515–9. https://doi.org/10.1016/S0140-6736(02)07683-3.
3. Dettori J. The random allocation process: two things you need to know. Evid Based Spine Care J. 2010;1(3):7–9. https://doi.org/10.1055/s-0030-1267062.
4. Sterne JAC, Savovic J, Page MJ, Elbers RG, Blencowe NS, Boutron I, et al. RoB 2: a revised tool for assessing risk of bias in randomised trials. BMJ. 2019;366:l4898. https://doi.org/10.1136/bmj.l4898.
5. Peckham E, Brabyn S, Cook L, Devlin T, Dumville J, Torgerson DJ. The use of unequal randomisation in clinical trials—an update. Contemp Clin Trials. 2015;45(Pt A):113–22. https://doi.org/10.1016/j.cct.2015.05.017.
6. Suresh K. An overview of randomization techniques: an unbiased assessment of outcome in clinical research. J Hum Reprod Sci. 2011;4(1):8–11. https://doi.org/10.4103/0974-1208.82352.
7. Pawlik TMS, J. A. Clinical trials. In: Success in academic surgery. 2nd ed. Cham: Springer; 2020.
8. Louw A, Diener I, Fernandez-de-Las-Penas C, Puentedura EJ. Sham surgery in orthopedics: a systematic review of the literature. Pain Med. 2017;18(4):736–50. https://doi.org/10.1093/pm/pnw164.
9. Wall L, Hinwood M, Lang D, Smith A, Bunzli S, Clarke P, et al. Attitudes of patients and surgeons towards sham surgery trials: a protocol for a scoping review of attributes to inform a discrete choice experiment. BMJ Open. 2020;10(3):e035870. https://doi.org/10.1136/bmjopen-2019-035870.
10. Sihvonen R, Paavola M, Malmivaara A, Itala A, Joukainen A, Nurmi H, et al. Arthroscopic partial meniscectomy versus sham surgery for a degenerative meniscal tear. N Engl J Med. 2013;369(26):2515–24. https://doi.org/10.1056/NEJMoa1305189.
11. Moseley JB, O'Malley K, Petersen NJ, Menke TJ, Brody BA, Kuykendall DH, et al. A controlled trial of arthroscopic surgery for osteoarthritis of the knee. N Engl J Med. 2002;347(2):81–8. https://doi.org/10.1056/NEJMoa013259.
12. Musahl VK, Karlsson J, Hirschmann MT, Ayeni OR, Marx RG, Koh JL, Nakamura N. Basic methods handbook for clinical orthopaedic research. 1st ed. Berlin/Heidelberg: Springer; 2019.
13. Getgood A, Bryant D, Firth A, Stability G. The Stability study: a protocol for a multicenter randomized clinical trial comparing anterior cruciate ligament reconstruction with and without lateral extra-articular tenodesis in individuals who are at high risk of graft failure. BMC Musculoskelet Disord. 2019;20(1):216. https://doi.org/10.1186/s12891-019-2589-x.
14. Getgood AMJ, Bryant DM, Litchfield R, Heard M, McCormack RG, Rezansoff A, et al. Lateral extra-articular tenodesis reduces failure of hamstring tendon autograft anterior cruciate ligament reconstruction: 2-year outcomes from the STABILITY study randomized clinical trial. Am J Sports Med. 2020;48(2):285–97. https://doi.org/10.1177/0363546519896333.
15. Hewitt C, Hahn S, Torgerson DJ, Watson J, Bland JM. Adequacy and reporting of allocation concealment: review of recent trials published in four general medical journals. BMJ. 2005;330(7499):1057–8. https://doi.org/10.1136/bmj.38413.576713.AE.
16. Kennedy ADM, Torgerson DJ, Campbell MK, Grant AM. Subversion of allocation concealment in a randomised controlled trial: a historical case study. Trials. 2017;18(1):204. https://doi.org/10.1186/s13063-017-1946-z.
17. Moher D, Hopewell S, Schulz KF, Montori V, Gotzsche PC, Devereaux PJ, et al. CONSORT 2010 explanation and elaboration: updated guidelines for reporting parallel group randomised trials.

Int J Surg. 2012;10(1):28–55. https://doi.org/10.1016/j.ijsu.2011.10.001.

18. Karanicolas PJ, Bhandari M, Taromi B, Akl EA, Bassler D, Alonso-Coello P, et al. Blinding of outcomes in trials of orthopaedic trauma: an opportunity to enhance the validity of clinical trials. J Bone Joint Surg Am. 2008;90(5):1026–33. https://doi.org/10.2106/JBJS.G.00963.
19. Probst P, Zaschke S, Heger P, Harnoss JC, Huttner FJ, Mihaljevic AL, et al. Evidence-based recommendations for blinding in surgical trials. Langenbeck's Arch Surg. 2019;404(3):273–84. https://doi.org/10.1007/s00423-019-01761-6.
20. Kendall JM. Designing a research project: randomised controlled trials and their principles. Emerg Med J. 2003;20(2):164–8. https://doi.org/10.1136/emj.20.2.164.
21. Katz JN, Chaisson CE, Cole B, Guermazi A, Hunter DJ, Jones M, et al. The MeTeOR trial (Meniscal Tear in Osteoarthritis Research): rationale and design features. Contemp Clin Trials. 2012;33(6):1189–96. https://doi.org/10.1016/j.cct.2012.08.010.

# Crossover and Early Failure in Surgical Trials

8

Jason L. Koh

## 8.1 Introduction

Various types of clinical trial designs exist, but randomized controlled trials (RCTs) are considered the most rigorous and have the best ability to identify if there is a true difference between interventions. These RCTs have been the "gold standard" of assessment of treatment, since randomly assigned groups of patients are presumed to be comparable, mitigating the risk of pre-existing differences on outcomes, and theoretically the only differences in outcomes are related to the interventions provided [1–3]. Since patients are assigned to treatment arms randomly, both identified and unidentified factors that may impact results will be distributed evenly among the different groups, reducing the risk of biased outcomes and improving the validity of the trial.

Randomized clinical trials in surgery have been difficult to implement in practice for several reasons [4]. One of the key reasons is that the technical nature of surgery and the role of individual surgeon expertise can make it difficult to assess whether it is the assigned treatment or the performance of the procedure that results in differences in outcomes. This complexity is one of the reasons crossover can occur from a novel procedure to a more traditional one. However, there are other circumstances where there is a lack of treatment adherence. Beyond surgical or technical challenges, this lack of adherence may be the result of differences in patient preference, inability to receive assigned treatment in a timely manner, or early failure of the originally assigned treatment. Unplanned crossover of subjects from one treatment arm to another may create significant confounding effects in statistical analysis and can adversely impact the validity of the trial to adequately compare treatments. Various methods of analysis have been proposed to address the impact of crossover in trials, each with its own advantages and disadvantages.

### 8.1.1 Crossover

Crossover occurs when patients are assigned to one treatment arm but receive another. This is quite common in surgical trials [1–3]. *Deliberate* crossover can be a result of planned design—for example, in *crossover trials*, randomly assigned subjects receive two or more treatments in different order. These trials are typically performed for chronic diseases where the interventions are short term and not expected to have permanent effects (e.g., there is no "carry over" effect) [5]. Therefore,

J. L. Koh (✉)
Mark R. Neaman Family Chair of Orthopaedic Surgery, Orthopaedic & Spine Institute, Endeavor Health, Evanston, IL, USA

University of Chicago Pritzker School of Medicine, Chicago, IL, USA

Northwestern University McCormick School of Engineering, Evanston, IL, USA


S. Lyman et al. (eds.), *Introduction to Surgical Trials*,
https://doi.org/10.1007/978-3-031-77563-5_8

this type of crossover trial design is usually not feasible for surgical treatments, since most surgical procedures have permanent structural consequences. Crossover can also occur as a planned intervention; for example, as a planned salvage operation if there is early failure. This is occurring in the clinical trial of the Aesculap Novocart 3D autologous chondrocyte transplantation procedure, where if a patient is randomized to microfracture and if this treatment fails, they may be eligible to receive the chondrocyte transplantation [6]. Alternatively, crossover can be unplanned, which may confound analysis of results.

Unplanned crossover is quite common [3] and may occur for multiple reasons. One of the primary reasons is non-adherence to the study protocol as a result of patient preference. Unlike pharmaceutical trials where treatments are relatively easily blinded to the subjects by use of masking medications to appear identical, surgical trials are often characterized by vastly different patient experiences in the treatment arms (e.g., physical therapy compared to surgery, or open vs. arthroscopic techniques). Given these differences, patients often may have strong personal preferences for one treatment or another and lack equanimity between the arms of the trial. When patient preferences are not aligned with the assigned group, there is a higher likelihood of noncompliance, dropout, or crossover [7–9]. These effects can be very large. In the Spine Patient Outcomes Research Trial (SPORT) trial of lumbar stenosis, 33% of consented patients assigned to surgery did not have this procedure in the initial 2-year study period. Alternatively, 43% of patients assigned to nonoperative management underwent surgery. The investigators identified that patient treatment preferences in the crossover populations were stronger for the treatment that was actually received [10, 11]. Particularly when outcomes are subjective or patient reported, this preference may create a bias toward a more favorable result to the treatment due to confirmation bias. Additionally, ethical questions about patient autonomy can arise, since patients may be entering a trial with the goal of receiving a particular treatment.

Similarly, investigator preference can play a role in crossover. Investigators in surgical trials may have a strong interest or experience with a particular treatment, and this conscious or unconscious lack of equipoise (see Chap. 6) may result in protocol deviations [12, 13]. Surgical trials may be more prone to this type of crossover since treatments are often not blinded or are impossible to blind to the investigator, unlike many pharmaceutical trials where the intervention can be blinded effectively to all trial stakeholders. This investigator bias may have multiple potential effects. Investigator preference can affect decisions regarding patient eligibility or inadvertently bias allocation of patients to one treatment or another when one is felt to be superior or is more familiar. For example, surgeons may prefer surgical management, whereas non-surgeons may prefer nonoperative management. Surgeons may prefer one technique over another and may break protocol. Another risk is that there may be premature adjudication of a treatment (usually nonoperative) and subsequent crossover to the other (surgical) arm. These factors not only risk affecting the validity of the trial but also raise ethical concerns about the ethical treatment of subjects.

Another potential cause of crossover is the complex technical nature of many surgical treatments [13–15]. Surgery or other complex procedures typically involve multiple precise steps that require acquisition of skills and experience that take time and effort to achieve [16]. There is ample evidence that surgical outcomes are related to surgeon experience and case volume. Particularly with a new or investigational procedure (such as minimally invasive surgery), investigators may have varying expertise in the technical aspects of performing the operation. This may result in being unable to successfully perform an assigned procedure and subsequent crossover to the other intervention. This has been studied in multiple cardiac surgical studies where greater crossover away from newer techniques was found among less experienced surgeons [1]. Similarly, it has been noted that in surgical treatments of laparoscopic versus open surgery, early conversion to open surgery occurred with surgeons less experienced in laparoscopic techniques [3, 17]. Additionally, even if crossover does not occur, the relative individual variability in experience of investigators with each technique may play a role in the results. The net result is that outcomes may be attributed to a procedure itself but are actually related to the technical ability of the participating surgeons. Even with well-established techniques, surgical experience can be variable due to training, experience, and individual ability, which can have an effect on successful completion of the assigned treatment. For example, in the treatment of proximal humerus fracture, hemiarthroplasty or open reduction and internal fixation are two commonly performed techniques that have both been demonstrated to have good results, but surgeons typically have more proficiency or experience in one technique or the other due to personal experience [18]. This differential technical expertise can sometimes be addressed by study design, where patients are randomized to surgeons or participating centers (where a specific protocol compliant technique is dominant) rather than to specific treatments.

Patient factors interacting with the technical aspect of procedures can also have an effect on early crossover. Such conditions such as more severe disease or patient body habitus [19] may impact the technical ability to perform an assigned surgical procedure on a given patient. Garas reported that in gastrointestinal oncology surgery studies, patients that had crossover from minimally invasive to open surgery had more severe disease and higher comorbidities [3]. This was possibly related in part to the increased technical difficulty of trying to perform a procedure in a patient with more significant involvement. Instruments may not be designed for certain types of pathology, or, for example, in the case of arthroscopic instrumentation, may not be able to reach the hip joint in the morbidly obese. Implants may be only available in specific sizes and may not be appropriate for the body habitus of the patient.

Another factor that may contribute to unplanned crossover is the inability to receive the assigned treatment. This may be patient related due to unrelated medical illness such as cardiac or pulmonary disease. A patient may be deemed too high risk to undergo surgical management and therefore receives only nonoperative management. Alternatively, patients may delay elective surgical management for a period of time due to personal or social circumstances or even ambivalence about proceeding with a surgical intervention [20]. Another situation is when access to care is limited or variable. For example, operating rooms or specific surgical equipment may not be immediately available, which may affect outcomes, particularly in the setting of acute trauma surgery. This may make the groups less comparable as well as resulting in unplanned crossover to a nonsurgical or alternative treatment arm.

### 8.1.2 Early Failure as a Cause of Unplanned Crossover

A common cause of unplanned crossover is early failure of the assigned treatment. Surgical trials may have an arm with a less- or non-invasive treatment compared to a surgical procedure or compare two different surgical treatments. It is not uncommon for patients who have received one treatment to crossover to the other if expected results are not achieved by a pre-specified time-point or if the initial management is judged to be a failure. Failure can be a lack of sufficient improvement, further progression of disease, or worsening of symptoms. The UK FASHIoN trial of hip arthroscopy resulted in 16% of patients assigned to surgery not receiving a procedure and 8% of those assigned nonsurgical treatment receiving arthroscopy [21]. An even more striking degree of crossover was seen in the Danish study of anterior cruciate ligament (ACL) tears comparing early ACL reconstruction to nonoperative management with optional delayed reconstruction. Approximately 39% of the nonoperative group had ACL reconstruction within 2 years [22], and 51% had reconstruction within 5 years [23], largely due to patient and investigator determination that nonoperative management was unsatisfactory.

Non-adherence in surgical trials may also occur due to complexity or novelty of the procedure combined with individual surgeon experience resulting in early failure. As noted previously, this failure may occur during the course of performing the assigned procedure resulting in conversion to the other arm. Alternatively, lack of experience with performing the procedure may result in relatively worse outcomes, early failure, and subsequent revision with the alternate treatment as a rescue crossover. In an intent-to-treat analysis, the rescue procedure outcome would be credited to the assigned group.

### 8.1.3 Impact of Crossover

Crossover in surgical trials creates challenges to the interpretation of treatment effects, since randomized trials assume that the treatment groups are comparable and that differences in outcomes can be confidently related to differences in the assigned interventions rather than other factors. Crossover has a risk of introducing bias and can complicate interpretation of results.

### 8.1.4 Types of Bias Introduced by Crossover

Crossover can introduce bias into a trial by confounding the treatment effects. Patients who switch treatments may differ in terms of baseline characteristics, disease severity, or other factors that could affect outcomes [3, 20, 24]. This can lead to a dilution of the treatment effect or a masking of the true effect. Additionally, crossover can lead to carryover effects, where the treatment effect of the first intervention can affect the outcomes of the second intervention. Alternatively, crossover can lead to an underestimation of adverse effects if patients in the control group crossover to the intervention group and experience complications. This can further complicate the interpretation of the trial results. Several types of bias can occur:

(A) Selection Bias: Participants may self-select or investigators may select based on preference, medical conditions, response to treatment, experience, side effects, or other reasons into different treatment arms post-randomization, resulting in unequal distribution of confounding variables [25, 26].

(B) Performance Bias: Changes in behavior or additional treatments or complications in the crossover group can affect outcomes separately from the studied intervention.

(C) Attrition Bias: Differential dropout rates due to crossover can skew results, especially if the reasons for dropout are related to treatment efficacy or side effects.

### 8.1.5 Interpretation of Results

Crossover can make the interpretation of the trial results more challenging. Traditionally, randomized clinical trials have used the intention-to-treat (ITT) analysis, which includes all randomized patients *regardless* of whether they received the assigned treatment [20]. If there is significant crossover, many subjects will not receive the assigned interventions, which makes it difficult to attribute differences in outcomes to the particular intervention. Additionally, crossover disrupts the comparability of the groups. Movement of participants between groups can lead to an under- or overestimation of treatment effects. As a result, outcomes may be attributed to the wrong intervention. This can make it difficult to determine accurate conclusions about the efficacy and safety of the procedures. As Weinstein and Levin note "It has been said that the intention-to-treat principle actually tests a *policy* (emphasis added) of treatment rather than the treatment itself" [20] or as Hernan puts it "the *effect of assigned treatment* versus the *effect of treatment*" [27]. This is particularly relevant when there is substantial crossover, which in some surgical trials approaches 50%.

It is important to recognize that the ITT analysis as popularized by Peto in 1976 was in the context of oncology therapy trials where there was crossover by only "a few" patients, and "that detection of anything less extreme than 2:3 (mortality) is very difficult [28]." Statistically, it has been demonstrated that "In placebo-controlled RCTs, ITT analysis underestimate the treatment effect … In RCTs with an active comparator, ITT estimates can overestimate a treatment's effect in the presence of differential adherence" [27]. It has further been posited that "large scale crossover analyzed under the intention-to-treat principle further degrades statistical power," sometimes to the point that no differences can be identified [20].

Alternative approaches include per-protocol and as-treated analysis. The per-protocol (PP) analysis only includes patients who received the assigned treatment and excludes those who cross over [29]. This exclusion is a type of *censoring* of the data [30]. In some situations, the PP analysis includes patients until the time of crossover. PP analysis focuses on the intervention's effects under ideal conditions and minimizes confounding factors related to adherence and compliance. However, PP analysis may introduce selection bias, as patients who cross over may differ from those who do not in terms of baseline characteristics or disease severity. This sacrifices the benefits of randomization and may compromise generalizability. Typically, control patients cross over because of treatment failure (orthopedic trials) or because they become sicker (cardiac/oncology trials). This creates a bias in favor of control by withdrawing failures or potentially overestimating treatment effect if there are two intervention arms.

The as-treated (AT) analysis analyzes participants based on the treatment actually received, regardless of the initial randomization [31]. This turns the RCT into an observational study. This has several strengths. Similar to the PP analysis, it focuses on the intervention's effects. It captures the experiences of all participants, enhancing external validity of the results and potentially maintaining generalizability. It may reflect real-world scenarios, where patients may switch treatments. However, it can introduce confounding since the treatment groups may no longer be comparable due to crossover or non-adherence. The initial randomization is lost, and therefore, it is difficult to ascribe differences in outcomes exclusively to the treatment.

These approaches require additional statistical methods used in nonrandomized studies to account for potential differences between the two groups and mitigate the effect of confounding variables on the outcomes of the interventions. These can include Cox regression or other multivariate data analysis [29]. Over the last two decades, additional sophisticated statistical methods have been developed to address these situations where there is significant crossover. These include the inverse probability of censoring weighting (IP or IPCW) model which weights each patient, the rank-preserving structural failure time model (RPSFT) [30, 32], g-estimation, and instrumental variable (IV) weighting [27]. These tools can be used to reduce bias and allow treatment effects to be more clearly identified. These have been considered as valid by government health technology assessment bodies such as the National Institute for Health and Care Excellence (NICE) in the United Kingdom [32]. D'Amico identified that ITT analyses dilute treatment effect size for efficacy and safety, whereas the censored analysis created less predictable magnitude and direction of bias [33]. Hernan suggests that in situations where there is significant crossover, use of these multiple methods of analysis (ITT, PP, AT) with appropriate adjustment with IP weighting or g-estimation can provide additional information about the true effects of treatment [27].

### 8.1.6 Design Considerations

To minimize the impact of crossover on trial outcomes, several design considerations can be implemented. These can involve patient selection, investigator and site selection and training, and appropriate planning for statistical methods to address potential crossover.

#### 8.1.6.1 Statistical Trial Design

A statistician should be involved in clinical trial design. Preemptive planning for potential crossover events and statistical analysis of the data should be part of the trial design. At this time, essentially all RCTs will use ITT analysis, but strong consideration should be given to modern PP or AT approaches with appropriate IP or g-estimation. This should be described in the study protocol a priori to limit the likelihood of a trial being rejected at the publication state due to fatal protocol violations.

#### 8.1.6.2 Patient Selection

In many cases, crossover occurs as a result of patient-related factors. Stringent inclusion and exclusion criteria should be developed and adhered to, regarding potential complexity of procedure with regard to patient factors, general health, comorbidities, and willingness to adhere to assigned treatments. This helps establish that patients are suitable for the assigned intervention and decreases the likelihood that unplanned conversion to another treatment occurs. Patient willingness to adhere to assigned treatment is critically important for multiple reasons, including risk of crossover and respect for patient autonomy. Therefore, a robust and comprehensive informed consent process is critical to determine that (1) the patient is willing to adhere and (2) understands the importance of receiving the allocated treatment. Appropriate scripting of consent may be helpful. Recruitment for surgical trials is difficult and it is tempting for investigators to consent patients who might not be fully committed to the randomization protocol. Appropriate education and communication about the equanimity of the trial is important to help patients remain committed to compliant trial participation. If there is significant concern about compliance, the potential subject should not be enrolled.

#### 8.1.6.3 Investigator and Site Selection and Training

Investigators must demonstrate equipoise in the conduct of the trial and be aware of potential conscious or unconscious bias toward one arm or another. For surgical trials, it is important that the investigators have appropriate clinical ability to perform the procedural intervention. Lack of experience or expertise can result in unplanned crossovers if the planned procedure cannot be executed. Appropriate selection of investigators may involve careful screening to determine experience or expertise, training of investigators, group tutorials, or skills demonstration sessions. Investigators should be trained that equipoise is critical to avoid premature assessment of failure and to make a strong effort to maintain subject allocation. Each site should be evaluated for ability to carry out the designated intervention. Site clinical staff and investigator education can be standardized to help reinforce appropriate behavior.

#### 8.1.6.4 Conduct of the Trial

If possible, delays in providing the intervention should be avoided. A substantial gap between enrollment and performance of surgery may result in unexpected changes in patient condition or interest. Careful monitoring and communication with patients can help maintain understanding and adherence to the trial. Health evaluations, well-being checks, and investment in frequent patient communication increase the likelihood of remaining in the allocated group. Investigators should have regular meetings to assess trial conduct and monitor and prepare for possible crossover events. Crossovers should be clearly and accurately documented.

#### 8.1.6.5 Reporting of the Trial

As previously noted, ITT analysis is nearly universally performed for RCTs. Increasingly, PP and AT analysis is used to provide additional information regarding the outcomes of specified interventions. Crossovers should be clearly identified and care should be taken to avoid potentially misleading ITT analyses. Reporting of observational data [34] can be performed separately from RCT [10] even if they are from the same trial. Conclusions can be based upon the total analysis since each analytical method has its strengths and weaknesses.

## 8.2 Conclusions

Crossovers commonly occur in randomized surgical trials and may have significant effects on the interpretation of trial results. Crossovers can be the result of multiple factors from patient preference, investigator biases, or technical difficulty of the procedure itself. Appropriate study design and execution can help mitigate the number of crossover events. Additional statistical analyses such as per-protocol and as-treated that go beyond the commonly used intent-to-treat method may help provide more information about the effect of a surgical procedure in the setting of high crossover. These can supplemented with newer statistical tools such as IP or g-estimates, which require analysis by a trained statistician. A statistician should be involved in the design and as a co-investigator in any surgical trial.

## References

1. Gaudino M, Fremes SE, Ruel M, Di Franco A, Di Mauro M, Chikwe J, et al. Prevalence and impact of treatment crossover in cardiac surgery randomized trials: a meta-epidemiologic study. J Am Heart Assoc. 2019;8(21):e013711.
2. Losina E, Wright J, Katz JN. Clinical trials in orthopaedics research. Part III. Overcoming operational challenges in the design and conduct of randomized clinical trials in orthopaedic surgery. J Bone Joint Surg Am. 2012;94(6):e35.
3. Garas G, Markar SR, Malietzis G, Ashrafian H, Hanna GB, Zacharakis E, et al. Induced bias due to crossover within randomized controlled trials in surgical oncology: a meta-regression analysis of minimally invasive versus open surgery for the treatment of gastrointestinal cancer. Ann Surg Oncol. 2018;25(1):221–30.
4. Cook JA. The challenges faced in the design, conduct and analysis of surgical randomised controlled trials. Trials. 2009;10:9.
5. Carpenter JS, Storniolo AM, Johns S, Monahan PO, Azzouz F, Elam JL, et al. Randomized, double-blind, placebo-controlled crossover trials of venlafaxine for hot flashes after breast cancer. Oncologist. 2007;12(1):124–35.
6. NOVOCART 3D treatment following microfracture failure. Available from: https://www.clinicaltrials.gov/study/NCT03219307?intr=NOVOCART&rank=7.
7. Mittal R, Harris IA, Adie S, Naylor JM. Factors affecting patient participation in orthopaedic trials comparing surgery to non-surgical interventions. Contemp Clin Trials Commun. 2016;3:153–7.
8. Thorstensson CA, Lohmander LS, Frobell RB, Roos EM, Gooberman-Hill R. Choosing surgery: patients' preferences within a trial of treatments for anterior cruciate ligament injury. A qualitative study. BMC Musculoskelet Disord. 2009;10:100.
9. Arega A, Birkmeyer NJ, Lurie JD, Tosteson T, Gibson J, Taylor BA, et al. Racial variation in treatment preferences and willingness to randomize in the Spine Patient Outcomes Research Trial (SPORT). Spine (Phila Pa 1976). 2006;31(19):2263–9.
10. Weinstein JN, Tosteson TD, Lurie JD, Tosteson AN, Hanscom B, Skinner JS, et al. Surgical vs nonoperative treatment for lumbar disk herniation: the Spine Patient Outcomes Research Trial (SPORT): a randomized trial. JAMA. 2006;296(20):2441–50.
11. Weinstein JN, Lurie JD, Tosteson TD, Tosteson AN, Blood EA, Abdu WA, et al. Surgical versus nonoperative treatment for lumbar disc herniation: four-year results for the Spine Patient Outcomes Research Trial (SPORT). Spine (Phila Pa 1976). 2008;33(25):2789–800.
12. Kaur G, Hutchison I, Mehanna H, Williamson P, Shaw R, Tudur SC. Barriers to recruitment for surgical trials in head and neck oncology: a survey of trial investigators. BMJ Open. 2013;3(4):e002625.
13. Boutron I, Ravaud P, Nizard R. The design and assessment of prospective randomised, controlled trials in orthopaedic surgery. J Bone Joint Surg Br. 2007;89(7):858–63.
14. Simunovic N, Devereaux PJ, Bhandari M. Design considerations for randomised trials in orthopaedic fracture surgery. Injury. 2008;39(6):696–704.
15. Roman H, Marpeau L, Hulsey TC. Surgeons' experience and interaction effect in randomized controlled trials regarding new surgical procedures. Am J Obstet Gynecol. 2008;199(2):108 e1–6.
16. Alsagheir A, Koziarz A, Belley-Cote EP, Whitlock RP. Expertise-based design in surgical trials: a narrative review. Can J Surg. 2021;64(6):E594–602.
17. Garas G. ASO author reflections: induced bias due to crossover within randomized controlled trials in surgical oncology. Ann Surg Oncol. 2018;25(13):3889–90.
18. Rangan A, Handoll H, Brealey S, Jefferson L, Keding A, Martin BC, et al. Surgical vs nonsurgical treatment of adults with displaced fractures of the proximal humerus: the PROFHER randomized clinical trial. JAMA. 2015;313(10):1037–47.
19. Rihn JA, Radcliff K, Hilibrand AS, Anderson DT, Zhao W, Lurie J, et al. Does obesity affect outcomes of treatment for lumbar stenosis and degenerative spondylolisthesis? Analysis of the Spine Patient Outcomes Research Trial (SPORT). Spine (Phila Pa 1976). 2012;37(23):1933–46.
20. Weinstein GS, Levin B. Effect of crossover on the statistical power of randomized studies. Ann Thorac Surg. 1989;48(4):490–5.
21. Griffin DR, Dickenson EJ, Wall PDH, Achana F, Donovan JL, Griffin J, et al. Hip arthroscopy versus best conservative care for the treatment of femoroacetabular impingement syndrome (UK FASHIoN): a multicentre randomised controlled trial. Lancet. 2018;391(10136):2225–35.
22. Frobell RB, Roos EM, Roos HP, Ranstam J, Lohmander LS. A randomized trial of treatment for acute anterior cruciate ligament tears. N Engl J Med. 2010;363(4):331–42.
23. Frobell RB, Roos HP, Roos EM, Roemer FW, Ranstam J, Lohmander LS. Treatment for acute anterior cruciate ligament tear: five year outcome of randomised trial. BMJ. 2013;346:f232.

24. Gaudino M, Chikwe J, Bagiella E, Bhatt DL, Doenst T, Fremes SE, et al. Methodological standards for the design, implementation, and analysis of randomized trials in cardiac surgery: a scientific statement from the American Heart Association. Circulation. 2022;145(4):e129–e42.
25. Pincus T, Koch G, Lei H, Mangal B, Sokka T, Moskowitz R, et al. Patient Preference for Placebo, Acetaminophen (paracetamol) or Celecoxib Efficacy Studies (PACES): two randomised, double blind, placebo controlled, crossover clinical trials in patients with knee or hip osteoarthritis. Ann Rheum Dis. 2004;63(8):931–9.
26. Hui D, Zhukovsky DS, Bruera E. Which treatment is better? Ascertaining patient preferences with crossover randomized controlled trials. J Pain Symptom Manag. 2015;49(3):625–31.
27. Hernan MA, Hernandez-Diaz S. Beyond the intention-to-treat in comparative effectiveness research. Clin Trials. 2012;9(1):48–55.
28. Peto R, Pike MC, Armitage P, Breslow NE, Cox DR, Howard SV, et al. Design and analysis of randomized clinical trials requiring prolonged observation of each patient. I. Introduction and design. Br J Cancer. 1976;34(6):585–612.
29. Smith VA, Coffman CJ, Hudgens MG. Interpreting the results of intention-to-treat, per-protocol, and as-treated analyses of clinical trials. JAMA. 2021;326(5):433–4.
30. Adler AI, Latimer NR. Adjusting for nonadherence or stopping treatments in randomized clinical trials. JAMA. 2021;325(20):2110–1.
31. Moura L, Donahue MA, Yan Z, Smith LH, Hsu J, Newhouse JP, et al. Comparative effectiveness and safety of seizure prophylaxis among adults after acute ischemic stroke. Stroke. 2023;54(2):527–36.
32. Jonsson L, Sandin R, Ekman M, Ramsberg J, Charbonneau C, Huang X, et al. Analyzing overall survival in randomized controlled trials with crossover and implications for economic evaluation. Value Health. 2014;17(6):707–13.
33. D'Amico R, Bonafede E, Balduzzi S, Longo G, Guarneri V, Piacentini F, Moja L, Liberati A. Unplanned crossover in randomised controlled trials: consequences for efficacy and safety outcomes. Abstracts of the 19th Cochrane Colloquium; 19–22 Oct 2011. Madrid: Wiley; 2011.
34. Weinstein JN, Lurie JD, Tosteson TD, Skinner JS, Hanscom B, Tosteson AN, et al. Surgical vs nonoperative treatment for lumbar disk herniation: the Spine Patient Outcomes Research Trial (SPORT) observational cohort. JAMA. 2006;296(20):2451–9.

# Strategies to Optimize Follow-Up in Surgical Trials

9

Monica S. Vel, Ran Atzmon, Steven D. Jones, Kinsley Pierre, and Seth L. Sherman

## 9.1 Introduction

Surgical trials are often concerned with the long-term effects of an intervention [1–4]. Most surgical trials appear as randomized controlled trials (RCTs), prospective observational cohort studies (see Chap. 23), and/or open label trials [2, 5–12]. These studies involve pre- and post-intervention clinical visits and emphasize follow-up compliance rates to improve the generalizability of results to the broader population [3, 10–18]. However, when patients are lost to follow-up, there is a high risk of biased results [2, 5, 6, 9, 14, 16, 19–22]. Bias occurs when results are skewed toward one intervention for reasons unrelated to safety or effectiveness. This can result in spurious findings, which may have serious consequences for study accuracy, reproducibility, and generalizability [2, 5–7, 9, 14, 19–22].

Researchers have identified specific factors associated with incomplete follow-up, such as age, sex, travel time, language, health literacy, and many others [5, 17, 22–26].. This chapter aims to highlight and expand on the many ways one can maximize patient compliance by implementing strategies that focus on limiting the previously stated barriers, and therefore, minimizing the bias due to loss to follow-up [5, 6, 12, 14–16, 19, 20, 22, 24, 25, 27]. These strategies include constant and consistent communication between the research team and study participants, monetary incentives to compensate for the patient's time, and the utilization of enhanced communication methods (e.g., telehealth visits, online surveys, and translators) [5, 8, 12, 26, 28–31].

The authors thank Madison Thompson for her assistance in preparing the figures and table for this chapter.

M. S. Vel · R. Atzmon · S. D. Jones · K. Pierre
S. L. Sherman (✉)
Department of Orthopaedic Surgery,
Stanford University, Stanford, CA, USA
e-mail: shermans@stanford.edu

## 9.2 Risk Factors for Poor Patient Compliance

### 9.2.1 Background

Many researchers believe that less than 5% loss to follow-up is an adequate threshold to minimize bias and not affect the overall results of a study. Conversely, any loss to follow-up that exceeds 20% substantially increases bias and subsequently decreases the credibility of results [6, 14, 20, 22]. The current literature articulates that age, sex, travel time, language barriers, and many other factors can lead to reduced follow-up rates. When follow-up is lost, there is an imposed non-response and selection bias on the research. Non-response bias prevents a study group from being representative of the population due to drop-out and noncompliance rates [1, 8, 12, 19, 21, 28]. Similarly, selection bias compro-


S. Lyman et al. (eds.), *Introduction to Surgical Trials*,
https://doi.org/10.1007/978-3-031-77563-5_9

mises true randomization by not accurately reflecting the target population among its constituents. This also prevents a study's results from being generalizable to the broader population [2, 5–9, 16, 22]. These biases become more prevalent when there is a lack of communication, organization, and commitment from the research team and/or research subjects, which further influences loss to follow-up [2, 5–7, 14, 19, 21, 22, 25].

Subjects who are lost to follow-up are underrepresented in surgical trials because they tend to systematically differ from those who are not [4–6, 9, 10, 12–16, 20, 22, 24–26, 31]. Underrepresentation can harm the validity of a study and/or surgical intervention because it may result in losing crucial patient data, skewing the results in a specific direction. This can compromise generalizability and promote the previously highlighted biases [4, 6, 9, 11, 19, 20, 22]. The overall goal for researchers is to optimize follow-up visit compliance to enhance patient recovery and expand research utility. Identifying strategies to maximize compliance helps assure successful study completion and improves the clinical utility of the research findings [3, 5, 26, 32].

### 9.2.2 Age

Younger populations, defined as <30 years old, are less likely to follow-up after a surgical procedure. This may be because younger patients tend to recover more quickly and may feel that further follow-up is unnecessary. Younger populations also return to work and sport more rapidly than older populations which may also influence the rate of follow-up compliance [3, 5, 8, 28]. Conversely, older populations are more likely to adhere to follow-up protocols due to an increased awareness of overall health and recovery status. This in turn increases their effort to complete follow-up procedures [3, 8, 24].

### 9.2.3 Sex

Researchers have also found that sex plays a role in follow-up compliance. Male patients are at higher risk of follow-up loss than female patients. Indeed, younger male patients are at the highest risk for incomplete follow-up [8, 26, 28, 33]. Men are already noted to be at higher risk for noncompliance for other medical conditions. This is because they tend to have a lower perception of their conditions in comparison to women [34].Therefore, they are just as at risk for incomplete follow-up in surgical trials. Furthermore, women tend to visit their doctors more frequently than men; thus, they are more adherent with follow-up protocols [5, 34].

### 9.2.4 Forgetfulness

Other research articles have shown that loss to follow-up may also be due to the forgetfulness of the patient [35]. This is influenced by a lack of communication between the patient and the research team/providers. Patients may also assume that they do not need to return for further follow-up. Younger and older populations tend to both make this mistake. As previously mentioned, younger patients may neglect further follow-up due to quicker recovery time. In contrast, older patients may forget due to aging or other hindering health conditions [3, 8, 10, 35].

### 9.2.5 Distance

Distance and transportation to the hospital/clinic also play a significant role in follow-up compliance. Patients who live in rural settings or have moved to other regions away from their primary care location are less likely to complete their follow-up visits. Extensive commuting can be burdensome, so missing an appointment may outweigh the costs of the trip over the benefits of additional follow-up. As previously mentioned, some older individuals are more likely to maintain follow-up compliance, but various health conditions can make them incapable of commuting. This accounts for a minute percentage of incomplete follow-ups in this category [10, 26, 31].

### 9.2.6 Language

An additional barrier to follow-up compliance worth highlighting is language. Most questionnaires, also known as patient-reported outcome measures (PROMs), are written in English and therefore cater to English speakers or those who comprehend the English language. Some clinics, including ours, offer patient forms in alternative languages, such as Spanish and/or Mandarin, to accommodate language preferences [17, 22, 23]. However, this is still not enough to account for patients who do not speak any of those languages; hence, their data is lost [17, 23, 31].

### 9.2.7 Health Literacy

A final barrier that may lead to noncompliance in surgical trials is health literacy. This is defined as the ability to comprehend one's health information and execute decisions that allow one to have more control over their healthcare [36–41]. Lower health literacy is equivalent to a lesser understanding of a treatment. Health literacy is especially important in surgical trials because a participant must be able to fully understand pre- and postoperative procedures in order to comply with the protocol and make more advanced decisions about their care [40]. People who are more prone to having a reduced health literacy are those with disabilities, cognitive impairment, language barriers, and so on[43]. These detriments foster miscommunication between physicians and patients, thus leading to a decreased understanding of one's health. Due to this limited comprehension, participants are more likely to disengage with study protocols and procedures [36]. This leads to reduced follow-up rates because those who know less have little confidence when following up since they do not fully understand what is being explained to them [36–41].

## 9.3 Methods to Optimize Patient Compliance

### 9.3.1 Solutions for Age, Sex, and Forgetfulness Risk Factors

Many hospitals and clinics have implemented various strategies to combat the barriers to follow-up (see Table 9.1). As previously stated, younger patients, males, and the elderly are more prone to being lost to follow-up. The research team should provide repetitive communication through phone calls, emails, and text messages for these populations. This can encourage young and male patients to document their progress more consistently since they are more susceptible

**Table 9.1** Risk factors and solutions

| Risk factors | Solutions |
|---|---|
| Age | Send more follow-up reminders via email, text, and phone call. This seems to work for younger and older populations. However, younger populations are least likely to adhere to follow-up protocols |
| Sex | Monetary incentives may help men more than women |
| Forgetfulness | Send more follow-up reminders via email, text, and phone call. This seems to work for younger and older populations. However, older populations tend to be more forgetful |
| Distance | Telemedicine helps alleviate transportation constraints |
| Language barrier | Offering real-time translators online and PROMs in languages other than English helps minimize language barriers |
| Health literacy | Physicians must ensure that their patients have a full understanding of procedures by clarifying any questions, encouraging patients to ask further questions, and using laymen's terms instead of complex medical terminology |

to noncompliance due to quicker recovery rates. For the elderly, this constant communication can serve as a reminder to complete PROMs since they are more susceptible to forgetfulness, regardless of how vigilant they are about taking care of their health.

Researchers have also offered monetary incentives as a means of increasing follow-up rates in these populations, especially for males. This is because incentives promote reciprocity and may sway patients to complete their follow-up procedure if they otherwise may not. Incentives have been shown to be more successful for younger patients and men and less so for elderly patients and women. This is possibly due to younger and male patients having lower follow-up rates at baseline, making them more susceptible to simple incentive influence [3, 5, 8, 28].

Some researchers state that too much incentive can have undue influence on a patient's decision to participate in a trial which can lead to ethical concerns later on. Some patients complete study procedures due to pure altruism; however, others would not have completed any procedures if it was not for the monetary incentive involved [42, 43]. Others enroll because they do not have adequate healthcare or the funds for a particular procedure that a study will give them. Therefore, there is some selection bias on those who choose to participate and those who do not purely based on what a study has to offer. Additionally, patients may make their choice to participate solely based on the money being offered to them, which can cloud their judgment on the procedure itself. The whole point of the informed consent process is to give a person autonomy on their decision to participate. When large monetary incentives are involved, this autonomy may be compromised [42, 43].

### 9.3.2 Solutions for Distance and Language Barrier Risk Factors

Providers have utilized telemedicine as a solution to geographical and transportation constraints, as well as language barriers. This avenue of treatment has become more common since the start of the COVID-19 pandemic and continues to be widely used [29, 30]. Telehealth allows patients to meet their doctors on a secure online platform, usually offered by a treating institution and complete questionnaires online or via smart phone [3, 4, 12, 19, 26, 31, 44]. Additionally, PROMs are also provided via tablet, telephone, smartphone, or laptop. Furthermore, real-time translators can be used to effectively communicate with patients about their diagnosis and treatment options [3, 8, 29–31]. By providing these enhanced communication services, hospitals and clinics allow the patient to maintain an active role in their recovery without the burden of travel, which may also save on healthcare-related costs [3, 12, 26, 29–31, 44]. This helps foster a welcoming environment and increases the likelihood of follow-up compliance, although, of course, compliance remains imperfect.

### 9.3.3 Solutions for Low Health Literacy Risk Factors

In order to promote higher health literacy, providers must acknowledge the prevalence of lower health literacy [39, 40]. Physicians may assume their patient has an understanding of a specific procedure, without clarifying with them. This is why it's crucial for healthcare providers to encourage patients to ask questions about their treatments. Providers can then help clarify any misunderstandings along the way, further increasing patient knowledge and promoting health literacy. Additionally, researches state it is best to refrain from using complex medical terminology when speaking to patients of all calibers so that they do not get confused and/or discouraged when discussing treatment procedures with their physicians [39, 40].

## 9.4 Protocol Specified Follow-Up Visits

Hospitals and clinics adhere to standard protocols that specify time periods in which preoperative and postoperative visits should occur during a patient's recovery process [4, 8]. Patients are given PROMs to assess their functional abilities at that given timepoint. These PROMs are administered routinely and are designed to measure improvement over time and reflect aspects of patient health and satisfaction [1, 3, 8, 14, 17, 19, 34]. At a minimum, most PROM data is collected at the following timepoints: baseline (prior to intervention, i.e., surgery), at some interim timepoint during recovery, and once recovery is expected to be complete. Our sports medicine clinic at Stanford Medicine mirrors this schedule of administering PROMs. For example, patients undergoing anterior cruciate ligament (ACL) reconstruction receive questionnaires pre-operatively and at 2 weeks, 6 weeks, 3 months, 6 months, and 1 year post-intervention [10, 17]. Some studies even extend their follow-up periods up to 2, 5, or even 10 years, which most often occurs in surgical trials, as researchers are concerned with the long-term effects of an intervention [2, 4, 14, 17, 22–24].

If surgery is deemed necessary by the treating physician, a patient will be given baseline questionnaires to complete before the time of their operation. These pre-surgical questionnaires are administered electronically and serve as a threshold for future questionnaires administered to monitor the patient's post-surgical progress over time [2, 4, 8, 18, 23, 28]. Following surgical intervention, patients are monitored and given more questionnaires at subsequent visits. These post-surgical PROMs are also administered electronically and capture patient progress over time. Evidence shows that those who complete their PROMs once are more likely to do it again. This applies to general follow-up compliance among women and older populations, which is higher than that of younger and male populations.

## 9.5 Optimizing Follow-Up Visits

The hospitals and clinics with the highest follow-up rates keep constant communication with their patients, stay organized, and are committed to tracking patient progress. These steps help to ensure optimal recovery and make patients feel well cared for [1, 6, 21]. Furthermore, high follow-up compliance rates improve the utility of results and may validate previous findings or even uncover new ones [2, 5–7, 9, 12–14, 19–22].

Our Orthopaedic Sports Medicine Clinic at Stanford takes a similar patient-centered approach when delivering our care, which improves follow-up rates. All patients who come into the clinic are scheduled through the electronic health record. In addition, our online PROMs portal is integrated into our electronic health record. This PROMs portal is used for administering PROMs to all new patients as well as patients scheduled for follow-up. Once a patient is scheduled for a visit in the electronic health record scheduling system, they are also scheduled in the PROMs portal, which triggers questionnaires relevant to their visit. Once the questionnaires are activated, an email (see Fig. 9.1) will automatically be sent to them via the PROMs portal.

If a patient does not complete their questionnaires before the visit, the clinical research coordinator (CRC) will enter a kiosk code unique to the patient on the PROMs portal app using a Stanford-issued iPad, which will be given to the patient to complete their tasks when they arrive at the clinic (see Fig. 9.2). Once the patient completes their forms, the physician will review the results and proceed with the visit.

If the physician deems that surgery is necessary, the PROMs portal will automatically send pre-operative forms to the patient's email. The CRC will then ensure that the patient completes their forms before their operation. The CRC does this by sending a secure email via the electronic health record (see Fig. 9.3a, b) 2 weeks prior to surgery. The CRC will then check the PROMs portal the week of surgery to see if the patient has completed their required forms. If they have not, the CRC will forward the email to the treating physician. From there, the treating physician will contact the patient to emphasize the importance of this data in efficiently tracking their progress and monitoring their recovery.

In order to make sure that the patient has completed their forms, the CRC will check the patient-centered dashboard in the PROMs portal. All completed tasks will have a green check mark

**Fig. 9.1** Example email sent via PatientIQ database

Text version

**Tasks Outstanding**

Dear [patient name],

We look forward to seeing you at [org name] for your upcoming visit with your healthcare provider **Dr. [physician name]**. Prior to your visit, it is very important that you complete all the forms that have been assigned to ensure we have all the information to provide you with the highest quality of medical care. Please click on the "Start My Tasks" link below to begin.

If you are unable to complete your tasks prior to your appointment, please arrive at least 30 minutes early to your appointment to allow time to complete your forms.

Image version

**Tasks Outstanding**

Dear [patient name],

We look forward to seeing you at [org name] for your upcoming visit with your healthcare provider **Dr. [physician name]**. Prior to your visit, it is very important that you complete all the forms that have been assigned to ensure we have all the information to provide you with the highest quality of medical care. Please click on the "Start My Tasks" link below to begin.

If you are unable to complete your tasks prior to your appointment, please arrive at least 30 minutes early to your appointment to allow time to complete your forms.

next to them, thus indicating completion by the patient (see Fig. 9.4). Post-surgery, the Sports Medicine Clinic at Stanford has PROMs automatically emailed via the PROMs portal at 6 months, 12 months, 2 years, and 5 years, similar to other surgical trials [10, 17]. The CRC monitors postoperative compliance in the exact manner as pre-operative compliance.

If a patient is also a part of a research study in our department, they will be sent PROMs relevant to the research study with the earliest being sent 3 weeks post-intervention. Furthermore, our clinic sends out surgical and physician satisfaction forms to monitor patient-specific feedback.

Through constant communication with patients at the Stanford Sports Medicine Clinic, our follow-up rates have been relatively high. We have seen that follow-up remains highest before surgery and at the 2-year follow-up period. However, we start seeing declines in the middle at the 6-month mark and 1-year mark (see Fig. 9.5). This could be due to factors previ-

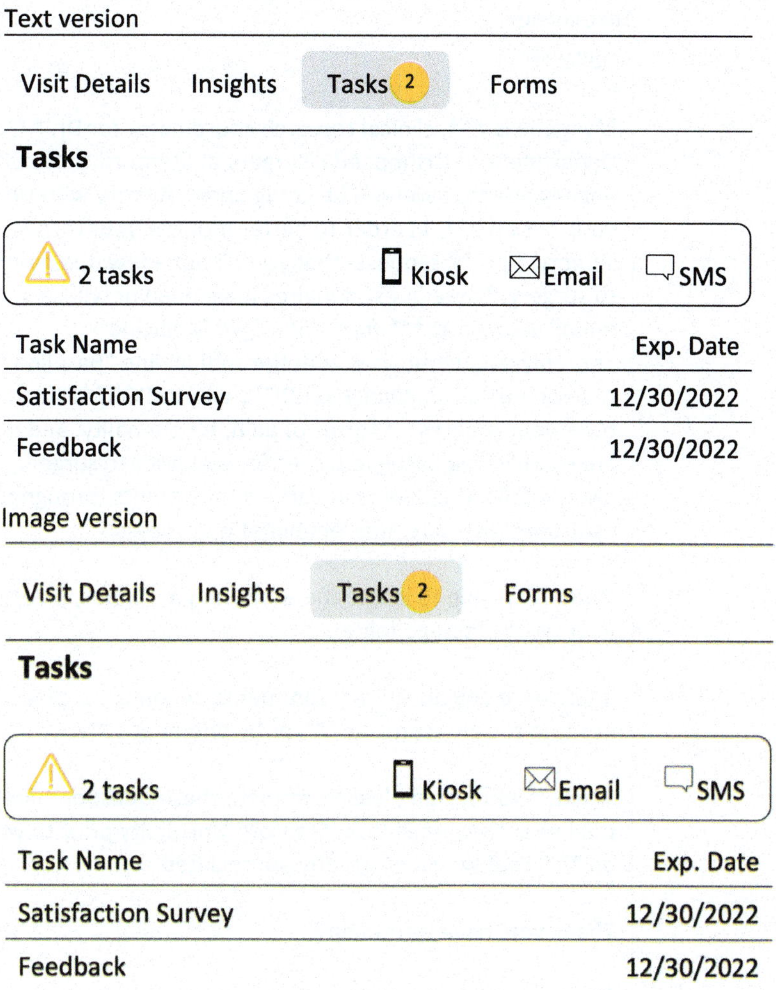


**Fig. 9.2** Patient dashboard of outstanding tasks

ously stated such as age, sex, travel time, or language barriers [3–5, 10, 13, 15, 17, 19, 22–26, 28, 31–33].

Without constant reminders, patients may forget to complete PROMs associated with follow-ups [2–4, 14, 17, 23, 26]. This emphasizes the importance of persistent communication and organization from the research team and treating providers. These factors influence follow-up compliance and may ultimately reduce bias in future research [2, 5–7, 14, 19, 21, 22, 25].

Text version

Hello ***

My name is ***, clinical research coordinator for Dr. *** in the Department of Orthopaedic Surgery at Stanford University. I understand that you will be going under surgery with Dr. *** for your *** on ***. In order to better monitor your recovery from surgery, Dr. *** requests that you fill out a few questionnaires prior to surgery. These questionnaires have been or will be sent to your e-mail address at *** from "Stanford Medicine <noreply@patientiq.io>" with the subject line "Baseline *** Assessment". Compliance is CRITICALLY IMPORTANT to help us track your progress in terms of pain, functionality, and mobility. We are establishing baseline scores for you prior to surgery, we will also be collecting scores at various time points throughout your post-operative care and rehabilitation process.

If you're unable to locate the e-mail in your inbox, please check your spam message folder.

If you have any questions, comments or concerns, please do not hesitate to contact me at *** or by phone at ***.

Again, if you would please complete these questionnaires by using the link in the e-mail from Stanford University prior to your surgery on ***, that would be greatly appreciated.

Thank you, have a good day.

***

Clinical Research Coordinator Associate
Department of Orthopaedic Surgery
Stanford University

**Fig. 9.3** Example email CRC sends via EPIC

Image version

Hello ***

My name is ***, clinical research coordinator for Dr. *** in the Department of Orthopaedic Surgery at Stanford University. I understand that you will be going under surgery with Dr. *** for your *** on ***. In order to better monitor your recovery from surgery, Dr. *** requests that you fill out a few questionnaires prior to surgery. These questionnaires have been or will be sent to your e-mail address at *** from "Stanford Medicine <noreply@patientiq.io>" with the subject line "Baseline *** Assessment". Compliance is CRITICALLY IMPORTANT to help us track your progress in terms of pain, functionality, and mobility. We are establishing baseline scores for you prior to surgery, we will also be collecting scores at various time points throughout your post-operative care and rehabilitation process.

If you're unable to locate the e-mail in your inbox, please check your spam message folder.

If you have any questions, comments or concerns, please do not hesitate to contact me at *** or by phone at ***.

Again, if you would please complete these questionnaires by using the link in the e-mail from Stanford University prior to your surgery on ***, that would be greatly appreciated.

Thank you, have a good day.

***
Clinical Research Coordinator Associate
Department of Orthopaedic Surgery
Stanford University

**Fig. 9.3** (continued)

**Fig. 9.4** Completed tasks on PatientIQ

Text version

Visit Details Insights Tasks **Forms**

**Forms**

| | Name | Date | Type | |
|---|---|---|---|---|
| | Dr. Sherman Patient | | Patient | ⤓ |
| √ | ASES | 09/28/2022 | Patient | ⤓ |
| √ | PROMIS Bank v2.0 | 09/28/2022 | Patient | ⤓ |
| √ | Shoulder SANE | 09/28/2022 | Patient | ⤓ |
| √ | Surgery Satisfaction | 09/28/2022 | Patient | ⤓ |
| √ | VAS Pain | 09/28/2022 | Patient | ⤓ |
| √ | Feedback | 09/20/2022 | Patient | ⤓ |
| √ | Satisfaction Survey | 09/20/2022 | Satisfaction | ⤓ |
| √ | Satisfaction Survey | 05/15/2022 | Satisfaction | ⤓ |
| | Sports Shoulder | 03/28/2022 | Clinical | ⤓ |

Image version


Visit Details Insights Tasks **Forms**

**Forms**

| | Name | Date | Type | |
|---|---|---|---|---|
| | Dr. Sherman Patient | | Patient | ⤓ |
| √ | ASES | 09/28/2022 | Patient | ⤓ |
| √ | PROMIS Bank v2.0 | 09/28/2022 | Patient | ⤓ |
| √ | Shoulder SANE | 09/28/2022 | Patient | ⤓ |
| √ | Surgery Satisfaction | 09/28/2022 | Patient | ⤓ |
| √ | VAS Pain | 09/28/2022 | Patient | ⤓ |
| √ | Feedback | 09/20/2022 | Patient | ⤓ |
| √ | Satisfaction Survey | 09/20/2022 | Satisfaction | ⤓ |
| √ | Satisfaction Survey | 05/15/2022 | Satisfaction | ⤓ |
| | Sports Shoulder | 03/28/2022 | Clinical | ⤓ |

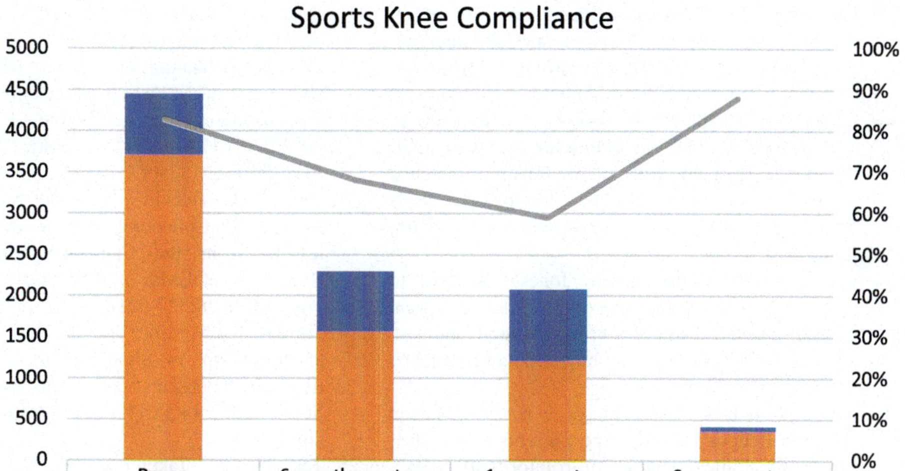


| | Preop | 6 months post-op | 1 year post-op | 2 years post-op |
|---|---|---|---|---|
| Tasks Expired | 736 | 731 | 858 | 49 |
| Tasks Complete | 3722 | 1581 | 1228 | 368 |
| Compliance Rate | 83% | 68% | 59% | 88% |

**Fig. 9.5** Sports knee compliance at Stanford Sports Medicine Clinic

## 9.6 Conclusion

Follow-up compliance is a primary issue in surgical trials [2, 3, 5–10, 14–16, 20, 25, 27, 32]. Hospitals and clinics have implemented telehealth, online PROMs, scheduled email reminders, and many other features to combat factors influencing loss to follow-up. However, we still see that there are many noncompliant patients [3, 4, 12, 19, 26, 29–31, 44]. These patients tend to systematically differ from those who are compliant, and, therefore, are underrepresented in published study results [4–6, 9, 10, 12–16, 20, 22, 24–28, 32]. This underrepresentation can prevent the results from being generalizable to the broader population, and in turn, increase the effects of bias while decreasing the validity of the study and/or intervention [4–7, 9, 14, 18–22]. A future goal is to be able to reach the highest percent of compliance possible, ideally 100%, in order to improve research utility and advance evidence-based care.

## References


1. Peters M, Crocker H, Jenkinson C, Doll H, Fitzpatrick R. The routine collection of patient-reported outcome measures (PROMs) for long-term conditions in primary care: a cohort survey. BMJ Open. 2014;4(2):e003968. https://doi.org/10.1136/bmjopen-2013-003968.
2. Bederman SS, Chundamala J, Wright JG. Randomized clinical trials in orthopaedic surgery: strategies to improve quantity and quality. JAAOS—J Am Acad Orthop Surg. 2010;18(8):454–63.
3. Marx RG, Wolfe IA, Turner BE, et al. MOON's strategy for obtaining over eighty percent follow-up at 10 years following ACL reconstruction. JBJS. 2022;104(3):e7. https://doi.org/10.2106/JBJS.21.00166.
4. Kaur M, Sprague S, Ignacy T, Thoma A, Bhandari M, Farrokhyar F. Practical tips for surgical research. Can J Surg. 2014;57(6):420–7. https://doi.org/10.1503/cjs.006314.
5. Madden K, Scott T, McKay P, et al. Predicting and preventing loss to follow-up of adult trauma patients in randomized controlled trials. J Bone Joint Surg Am. 2017;99(13):1086–92. https://doi.org/10.2106/JBJS.16.00900.
6. Sprague S, Leece P, Bhandari M, et al. Limiting loss to follow-up in a multicenter randomized trial in orthopedic surgery. Control Clin Trials. 2003;24(6):719–25. https://doi.org/10.1016/S0197-2456(03)00136-3.
7. Somerson JS, Bartush KC, Shroff JB, Bhandari M, Zelle BA. Loss to follow-up in orthopaedic clinical trials: a systematic review. Int Orthop. 2016;40(11):2213–9. https://doi.org/10.1007/s00264-016-3212-5.
8. Warwick H, Hutyra C, Politzer C, et al. Small social incentives did not improve the survey response rate of patients who underwent orthopaedic surgery: a randomized trial. Clin Orthop. 2019;477(7):1648–56. https://doi.org/10.1097/CORR.0000000000000732.

9. Farrokhyar F, Karanicolas PJ, Thoma A, et al. Randomized controlled trials of surgical interventions. Ann Surg. 2010;251(3):409–16. https://doi.org/10.1097/SLA.0b013e3181cf863d.
10. Leider M, Campbell R, Qadiri Q, Pastore L, Tjoumakaris F. Lost to follow-up: does it matter after arthroscopic rotator cuff repair (a matched cohort analysis of functional outcomes). JSES Int. 2021;6(2):275–8. https://doi.org/10.1016/j.jseint.2021.11.009.
11. Hoffmann MF, Sietsema DL, Jones CB. Lost to follow-up: reasons and outcomes following tibial plateau fractures. Eur J Orthop Surg Traumatol. 2016;26(8):937–42. https://doi.org/10.1007/s00590-016-1823-6.
12. Norquist BM, Goldberg BA, Matsen FAI. Challenges in evaluating patients lost to follow-up in clinical studies of rotator cuff tears*. JBJS. 2000;82(6):838.
13. Tariq MB, Vega JF, Westermann R, Jones M, Spindler KP. Arthroplasty studies with greater than 1000 participants: analysis of follow-up methods. Arthroplast Today. 2019;5(2):243–50. https://doi.org/10.1016/j.artd.2019.03.006.
14. Ueland TE, Carreira DS, Martin RL. Substantial loss to follow-up and missing data in National Arthroscopy Registries: a systematic review. Arthrosc J Arthrosc Relat Surg. 2021;37(2):761–770.e3. https://doi.org/10.1016/j.arthro.2020.08.007.
15. Choi JK, Geller JA, Patrick DA Jr, Wang W, Macaulay W. How are those “lost to follow-up” patients really doing? A compliance comparison in arthroplasty patients. World J Orthop. 2015;6(1):150–5. https://doi.org/10.5312/wjo.v6.i1.150.
16. Kristman V, Manno M, Côté P. Loss to follow-up in cohort studies: how much is too much? Eur J Epidemiol. 2004;19(8):751–60. https://doi.org/10.1023/B:EJEP.0000036568.02655.f8.
17. Schamber EM, Takemoto SK, Chenok KE, Bozic KJ. Barriers to completion of patient reported outcome measures. J Arthroplast. 2013;28(9):1449–53. https://doi.org/10.1016/j.arth.2013.06.025.
18. Ayers DC, Zheng H, Franklin PD. Integrating patient-reported outcomes into orthopaedic clinical practice: proof of concept from FORCE-TJR. Clin Orthop. 2013;471(11):3419–25. https://doi.org/10.1007/s11999-013-3143-z.
19. Ramkumar PN, Tariq MB, Spindler KP. Risk factors for loss to follow-up in 3,202 patients at two years after ACL reconstruction: implications for identifying health disparities in the MOON Prospective Cohort Study. Am J Sports Med. 2019;47(13):3173–80. https://doi.org/10.1177/0363546519876925.
20. Dettori JR. Loss to follow-up. Evid-Based Spine-Care J. 2011;2(1):7–10. https://doi.org/10.1055/s-0030-1267080.
21. Hutchings A, Neuburger J, Grosse Frie K, Black N, van der Meulen J. Factors associated with non-response in routine use of patient reported outcome measures after elective surgery in England. Health Qual Life Outcomes. 2012;10(1):34. https://doi.org/10.1186/1477-7525-10-34.
22. Zelle BA, Bhandari M, Sanchez AI, Probst C, Pape HC. Loss of follow-up in orthopaedic trauma: is 80% follow-up still acceptable? J Orthop Trauma. 2013;27(3):177–81. https://doi.org/10.1097/BOT.0b013e31825cf367.
23. Chenok K, Teleki S, SooHoo NF, Huddleston J, Bozic KJ. Collecting patient-reported outcomes: lessons from the California Joint Replacement Registry. eGEMs. 2015;3(1):1196. https://doi.org/10.13063/2327-9214.1196.
24. Torrens C, Martínez R, Santana F. Patients lost to follow-up in shoulder arthroplasty: descriptive characteristics and reasons. Clin Orthop Surg. 2022;14(1):112–8. https://doi.org/10.4055/cios21034.
25. Tejwani NC, Takemoto RC, Nayak G, Pahk B, Egol KA. Who is lost to follow-up?: a study of patients with distal radius fractures. Clin Orthop. 2010;468(2):599–604. https://doi.org/10.1007/s11999-009-0968-6.
26. Samade R, Colvell K, Goyal KS. An update on loss to follow-up after upper extremity surgery: survey of patient responses. Hand. 2021;16(1):104–9. https://doi.org/10.1177/1558944719840743.
27. Murray DW, Britton AR, Bulstrode CJK. Loss to follow-up matters. J Bone Joint Surg Br. 1997;79-B(2):254–7. https://doi.org/10.1302/0301-620X.79B2.0790254.
28. Brealey SD, Atwell C, Bryan S, et al. Improving response rates using a monetary incentive for patient completion of questionnaires: an observational study. BMC Med Res Methodol. 2007;7(1):12. https://doi.org/10.1186/1471-2288-7-12.
29. Nandra K, Koenig G, DelMastro A, Mishler EA, Hollander JE, Yeo CJ. Telehealth provides a comprehensive approach to the surgical patient. Am J Surg. 2019;218(3):476–9. https://doi.org/10.1016/j.amjsurg.2018.09.020.
30. Parisien RL, Shin M, Constant M, et al. Telehealth utilization in response to the novel coronavirus (COVID-19) pandemic in orthopaedic surgery. J Am Acad Orthop Surg. Published online April 7, 2020:10.5435/JAAOS-D-20-00339. 2020; https://doi.org/10.5435/JAAOS-D-20-00339.
31. Patterson JT, Albright PD, Jackson JH, et al. Travel barriers, unemployment, and external fixation predict loss to follow-up after surgical management of lower extremity fractures in Dar es Salaam, Tanzania. OTA Int. 2020;3(1):e061. https://doi.org/10.1097/OI9.0000000000000061.
32. Akl EA, Briel M, You JJ, et al. LOST to follow-up Information in Trials (LOST-IT): a protocol on the potential impact. Trials. 2009;10(1):40. https://doi.org/10.1186/1745-6215-10-40.
33. Williams DP, Price AJ, Beard DJ, et al. The effects of age on patient-reported outcome measures in total knee replacements. Bone Jt J. 2013;95-B(1):38–44. https://doi.org/10.1302/0301-620X.95B1.28061.

34. Rosenbaum JA, Blau YM, Fox HK, Liu XS, DiBartola AC, Goyal KS. Patient loss to follow-up after upper extremity surgery: a review of 2563 cases. Hand N Y N. 2019;14(6):836–40. https://doi.org/10.1177/1558944718787277.
35. Liu TC, Ohueri CW, Schryver EM, Bozic KJ, Koenig KM. Patient-identified barriers and facilitators to pre-visit patient-reported outcomes measures completion in patients with hip and knee pain. J Arthroplast. 2018;33(3):643–649.e1. https://doi.org/10.1016/j.arth.2017.10.022.
36. Leak C, Goggins K, Schildcrout JS, et al. Effect of health literacy on research follow-up. J Health Commun. 2015;20(0):83–91. https://doi.org/10.1080/10810730.2015.1058442.
37. Koch P, Schillmöller Z, Nienhaus A. How does health literacy modify indicators of health behaviour and of health? A longitudinal study with trainees in North Germany. Healthcare (Basel, Switzerland). 2021;10(1):2. https://doi.org/10.3390/healthcare10010002.
38. De Oliveira GS, McCarthy RJ, Wolf MS, Holl J. The impact of health literacy in the care of surgical patients: a qualitative systematic review. BMC Surg. 2015;15(1):86. https://doi.org/10.1186/s12893-015-0073-6.
39. Williams MV, Davis T, Parker RM, Weiss BD. The role of health literacy in patient-physician communication. Fam Med. 2002;47:118.
40. Roy M, Corkum JP, Urbach DR, et al. Health literacy among surgical patients: a systematic review and meta-analysis. World J Surg. 2019;43(1):96–106. https://doi.org/10.1007/s00268-018-4754-z.
41. Baur C. New directions in research on public health and health literacy. J Health Commun. 2010;15(sup2):42–50. https://doi.org/10.1080/10810730.2010.499989.
42. Singer E, Bossarte RM. Incentives for survey participation: when are they "coercive"? Am J Prev Med. 2006;31(5):411–8. https://doi.org/10.1016/j.amepre.2006.07.013.
43. Resnik DB. Bioethical issues in providing financial incentives to research participants. Theor Med Bioeth. 2015;5:35–41. https://doi.org/10.2147/MB.S70416.
44. Higgins J, Semple J, Murnaghan L, Sharpe S, Theodoropoulos J. Mobile web-based follow-up for postoperative ACL reconstruction: a single-center experience. Orthop J Sports Med. 2017;5(12):2325967117745278. https://doi.org/10.1177/2325967117745278.

# 10 Considerations in Choosing Outcome Measures

Isabel A. Wolfe and Robert G. Marx

## 10.1 Introduction

Over the years, a number of outcome measures have been used in orthopedic surgical trials to measure and compare treatment success. The objectives of research differ from the routine administration of patient-reported outcome measures (PROMs) in clinical practice, and therefore require special consideration [1]. Modern outcome evaluation has paid more attention to patients' perceptions of the treatment process, medical care, time of recovery, and return to prior level of activity [2–4]. This chapter will discuss considerations in choosing outcome measures, with a focus on patient-reported outcome measures, commonly used in surgical trials today.

## 10.2 Types of Outcome Measures

For many surgical procedures, possible outcome measures fall into the following main categories: imaging or radiographic analysis, implant survivorship analyses (if involving prostheses), surgeon-based outcome measures, performance-related assessments, and patient-reported outcome measures [5, 6]. Imaging or radiographic analysis, while relatively low cost and readily available, may not reflect the patient's perception of outcome. Radiographs can be useful to evaluate pre-operative pathology and to evaluate the implant over time [7]. However, there can be a lack of correlation between radiographic changes and patient symptoms, and inter- and intra-observer reliability can be poor in some cases [8]. Implant survivorship analysis, while a clear and objective measure of treatment success, does not account for poor patient outcomes if the implant is not revised.

Symptoms and physical examination findings collected by the surgeon are also used as outcome data. This data can be both objective (e.g., range of motion) and subjective (e.g., pain). Examples of surgeon-based outcome measures include the Harris Hip Score and the American Knee Society Score [9, 10]. These measures are often not validated, particularly in view of discrepancies in surgeon and patient ratings of health [8].

Considering these limitations and accompanying the overall shift toward patient-centered care, the use of patient-reported outcome measures (PROMs) has increased dramatically over the last 20 years [6]. PROMs are validated questionnaires that are completed by patients and can assess a wide range of outcomes. They are generally divided into different domains (e.g., pain, function, and satisfaction) and help identify patient-related issues that are relevant to functioning and activities in daily life [2, 3, 11].

I. A. Wolfe · R. G. Marx (✉)
Hospital for Special Surgery, New York, NY, USA
e-mail: info@drrmarx.com; marxr@hss.edu


S. Lyman et al. (eds.), *Introduction to Surgical Trials*,
https://doi.org/10.1007/978-3-031-77563-5_10

## 10.3 Which Outcome Measures Are Used?

A systematic review of primary outcome measures used in joint replacement RCTs between 2008 and 2013 showed that while significantly more trials in 2013 specified a primary outcome, the overall frequency of primary outcome reporting remains low and there is still wide heterogeneity in primary outcomes reported [12]. Of the knee studies included in this systematic review, 14/19 of the 2008 studies did not report a primary outcome measure, while 9/20 of the 2013 studies did not report a primary outcome measure. In 2008, studies that did report an outcome measure largely used surgeon-based and functional assessments, while in 2013, one study reported use of the Oxford Knee Score (PROM) as a primary outcome measure. A similar trend was seen in hip studies, with Harris Hip Scores and the WOMAC being used in several studies as primary outcome measures.

A 2017 analysis of outcome measures used in level 1 clinical ACL studies specifically also identified a wide variety of measures, including KT-1000, range of motion, graft retention, Lysholm, Tegner, and subjective IKDC scores [13]. The two most popular independent outcome measures were found to be report of the pivot-shift test (surgeon evaluation by physical exam), and inclusion of the Knee Injury and Osteoarthritis Outcome (KOOS) score (PROM).

## 10.4 PROMs

The first step in choosing the appropriate outcome measure is to consider the following questions: "What do I want to measure?", "What is the reason for assessment?", and "Who are the patients in this study?". It is necessary to determine what domains or constructs are to be measured (e.g., pain, physical function, quality of life), what patients are to be included, if outcome measures exist for this purpose, and if their use is feasible. Both general and specific PROMS should be considered. The PROMs should be easily understood by the patient and easily interpretable by the investigator [2].

In terms of quality, the PROMs used should be reliable, valid, and responsive [6, 14, 15]. There is extensive evidence that PROMS used in many areas of orthopedics are flawed or lack data on psychometric properties [6, 7, 16, 17]. An extension of CONSORT guidelines for patient-reported outcomes (PROs) has been developed to guide the reporting of PROs in RCTs. The CONSORT-PRO checklist contains five items to refer to when reporting the use of a PRO as a primary and secondary outcome measure [18]. The COSMIN checklist is also used as a set of criteria for assessing the measurement properties of PROMs [19].

Reliability refers to the precision of an outcome measure to make an assessment without measurement error. Validity involves the ability of an outcome measure to accurately measure what it is designed to measure. Finally, responsiveness is a measurement of an instrument's ability to detect changes over time. Careful evaluation of each of these properties is critical in determining the value of using a particular outcome measure for a given purpose [20].

Some PROMS are only validated for specific conditions or in certain languages and/or cultures. Other disadvantages/limitations include absence of a PROM collection infrastructure and a general lack of knowledge and confidence in using outcome measures [21]. Additionally, most PROMs are developed for the general population, and may not be as effective in certain specific populations. For example, athletes may reach a ceiling of function domain but are still not ready to return to sport [2]. In this case, additional outcome measures may be necessary. Finally, minimal clinically important difference (MCID) scores for outcome measures are frequently used evidence-based guides to gauge meaningful changes. A MCID score is defined as the minimal change in score on an outcome instrument that aligns with the patient's perception of beneficial change [22]. The MCID score is a point estimate that can either represent a change in the score or a particular value for the final score.

## 10.5 Summary

As surgical trials move toward comparative effectiveness evaluation, it is important to consider how effectiveness is determined. PROMs represent an opportunity to quantify a patients' posttreatment experience and to measure a variety of global, disease-specific, and joint-specific outcomes. In selecting PROMs for use, domains to be measured, patient populations of interest, validity, reliability, responsiveness, and feasibility must be carefully assessed.

## References


1. Gershon RC, Rothrock N, Hanrahan R, et al. The use of PROMIS and assessment center to deliver patient reported outcomes in clinical research. J Appl Meas. 2010;11:304–14.
2. Piedade SR, Filho MF, Ferreira DM, Slullitel DA, Patnaik S, Samitier G, Maffulli N. PROMs in sports medicine. In: Rocha Piedade S, Imhoff A, Clatworth M, Cohen M, Espregueira-Mendes J, editors. The sports medicine physician. Cham: Springer; 2019. p. 685–95.
3. Cappelleri JC, Zou KH, Bushmakin AG, et al. Patient-reported outcomes: measurement, implementation and interpretation. Boca Raton: Taylor & Francis; 2014. p. 331.
4. Black N. Patient reported outcome measures could help transform healthcare. BMJ. 2013;346:19–21.
5. deVet HCW, Terwee CB, Mokkink LB, et al. Measurement in medicine. Cambridge: University Printing House; 2011. p. 337.
6. Gagnier JJ. Patient reported outcomes in orthopaedics. J Orthop Res. 2017;35(10):2098–108.
7. Gagnier JJ, Huang W, Mullins M, et al. Measurement properties of patient-reported outcome measures used in patients undergoing Total hip arthroplasty: a systematic review. J Bone Joint Surg Rev. 2018;6(1):c2.
8. Wylde V, Blom AW. Assessment of outcomes after hip arthroplasty. Hip Int. 2009;19(1):1–7.
9. Harris WH. Traumatic arthritis of the hip after dislocation and acetabular fractures: treatment by mold arthroplasty. An end-result study using a new method of result evaluation. J Bone Joint Surg Am. 1969;51:737–55.
10. Noble PC, Scuderi GR, Brekke AC, et al. Development of a new Knee Society Scoring System. Clin Orthop Relat Res. 2012;470(1):20–32.
11. Wang D, Jones MH, Khair MM, et al. Patient reported outcome measures for the knee. J Knee Surg. 2010;23:137151.
12. Richards BL, Wall PDH, Sprowson AP, Singh JA, Buchbinder R. Outcome measures used in arthroplasty trials: systematic review of the 2008 and 2013 literature. J Rheumatol. 2017;44(8):1277–87.
13. Ahmad SS, Meyer JC, Krismer AM, Ahmad SS, Evangelopoulos DS, Hoppe S, Kohl S. Outcome measures in clinical ACL studies: an analysis of highly cited level I trials. Knee Surg Sports Traumatol Arthrosc. 2017;25(5):1517–27.
14. Terwee CB, Bot SDM, de Boer MR, et al. Quality criteria were proposed for measurement properties of health status questionnaires. J Clin Epidemiol. 2007;60:34–42.
15. Aaronson N, Alonso J, Burnam A, et al. Assessing health status and quality of life instruments: attributes and review criteria. Qual Life Res. 2002;11:193–205.
16. Huang H, Grant JA, Miller BS, et al. A systematic review of the psychometric properties of patient-reported outcome instruments for use in patients with rotator cuff disease. Am J Sports Med. 2015;43:2572.
17. Jia Y, Huang H, Gagnier JJ. A systematic review of measurement properties of patient-reported outcome measures for use in patients with foot or ankle diseases. Qual Life Res. 2017;26(8):1969–2010.
18. Calvert M, Blazeby J, Altman DG, et al. Reporting of patient-reported outcomes in randomized trials: the CONSORT PRO extension. JAMA. 2013;309(8):814–22.
19. Terwee CB, Prinsen C, Chiarotto A, De Vet HCW, Westerman MJ, Patrick DL, Alonso J, Bouter LM, Mokkink LB. COSMIN standards and criteria for evaluating the content validity of health-related patient-reported outcome measures: a Delphi study. Qual Life Res. 2018;27(5):1159–70.
20. Reeve BB, Wyrwich KW, Wu AW, et al. ISOQOL recommends minimum standards for patient-reported outcome measures used in patient-centered outcomes and comparative effectiveness research. Qual Life Res. 2013;22:1889–905.
21. Kyte DG, Calvert M, van der Wees PJ, ten Hove R, Tolan S, Hill JC. An introduction to patient-reported outcome measures (PROMs) in physiotherapy. Physiotherapy. 2015;101(2):119–25.
22. Copay AG, Chung AS, Eyberg B, Olmscheid N, Chutkan N, Spangehl MJ. Minimum clinically important difference: current trends in the orthopaedic literature, part I: upper extremity: a systematic review. JBJS Rev. 2018;6(9):e1.

# Length of Follow-Up

# 11

Christopher M. Gibbs, Ryan Murray, Emma Bergerson, Kajsa Persson, Timo Järvelä, and Volker Musahl

## 11.1 Introduction

Merriam-Webster's Dictionary defines "follow-up" in the context of research activities as the "maintenance of contact with or reexamination of a person … to monitor the effects of earlier activities or treatments." [1] Practically speaking, the duration of follow-up is the length of time that contact is maintained with a study participant so that information can be collected to determine the effects of a given intervention initiated during a prospective trial. According to the 2010 Consolidated Standards of Report Trials (CONSORT) statement [2, 3], which was composed to improve the quality of reporting the results of randomized controlled trials (RCTs), the four stages of a trial include enrollment, intervention allocation, follow-up, and analysis. Therefore, follow-up is a fundamental component of all trials (Fig. 11.1).

Over 300,000 clinical trials have been registered since 2000, with 32,000 registered in 2019 alone [4]. However, compared to other medical and surgical subspecialties, the orthopedic field has had a relative paucity of large randomized controlled trials [5] which are considered the study design most likely to yield unbiased, accurate information upon which to base treatment decisions [6]. Thus, there is a need for researchers in the field of orthopedics to be familiar with the process of properly determining length of follow-up.

Adequate reporting of follow-up, which requires allowing for adequate follow-up in the trial design, is necessary to reduce the risk of bias in research, including surgical, trials [7]. As with all elements of a research study, the duration of follow-up should be defined by the study investigators during trial design prior to the initiation of a study. However, given the relative scarcity of resources available to research teams, determining the optimal follow-up duration is often difficult. Failure to determine a proper follow-up period can severely compromise the validity, and subsequently limit the conclusiveness of study results. Therefore, this chapter will discuss considerations relevant for determining duration of follow-up during the study design phase as well as provide an illustration of the use of various follow-up designs from the orthopedic literature.

C. M. Gibbs · R. Murray
Department of Orthopaedic Surgery, University of Pittsburgh, Pittsburgh, PA, USA

E. Bergerson · K. Persson
Department of Orthopaedics, Institute of Clinical Sciences, Sahlgrenska Academy, University of Gothenburg, Gothenburg, Sweden

T. Järvelä
Sports Medicine and Arthroscopic Center, Hospital Mehiläinen, Tampere, Finland

V. Musahl (✉)
Department of Orthopaedic Surgery, University of Pittsburgh, Pittsburgh, PA, USA

Department of Bioengineering, University of Pittsburgh, Pittsburgh, PA, USA


S. Lyman et al. (eds.), *Introduction to Surgical Trials*, https://doi.org/10.1007/978-3-031-77563-5_11

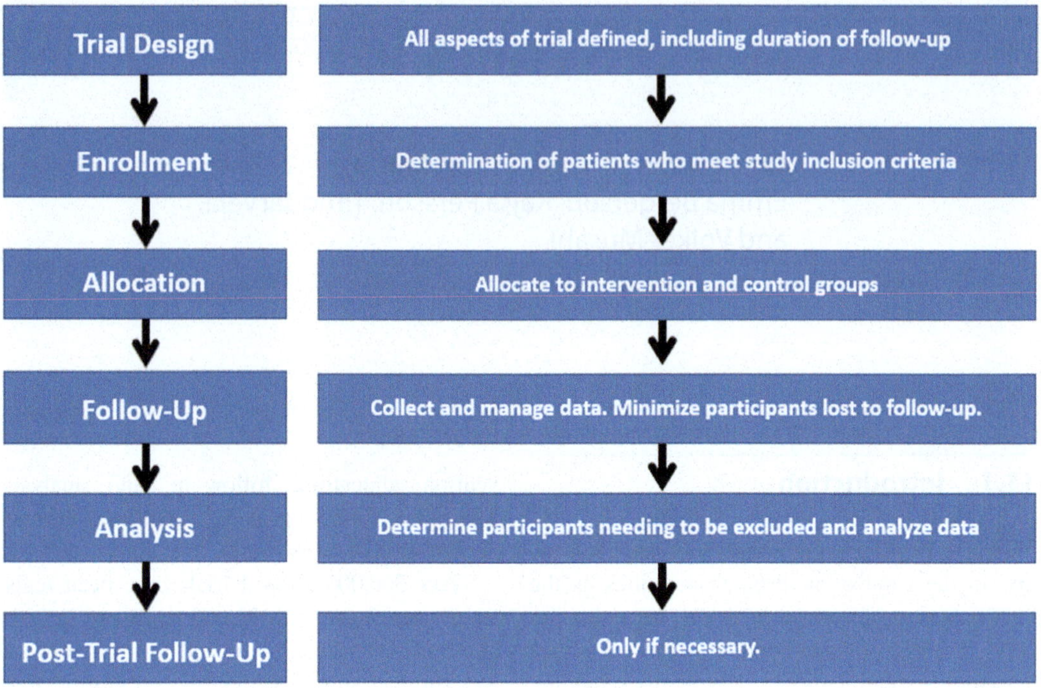


**Fig. 11.1** Critical components of a clinical trial, including follow-up

## 11.2 Determining Proper Duration of Follow-Up

As follow-up involves continuing to collect information for further analysis for a research study, a longer duration of follow-up results in a greater amount of data available for analysis. The treatment of ACL repair is one such example of this. First described in 1905 by Mayo Robson, primary repair of a torn ACL was the most commonly performed surgical treatment for an ACL rupture in the 1970s and 80s [8]. Initial data at 2-year follow-up was promising, however, high failure rates with poor clinical outcomes was found with follow-up of 5 or more years leading to the abandonment of ACL repair in favor of ACL reconstruction [9]. Consequently, additional insights gleaned from the additional data obtained with longer follow-up led to more accurate conclusions regarding the outcomes following ACL repair. Finally, a longer duration of follow-up allows for detection of potential failure of one treatment group as well as cross-over of participants between allocation groups [10].

While a longer duration of follow-up increases the ability of a study to detect effects of an intervention by increasing the amount of time in which to observe an occurrence, it also requires the consumption of resources including money, personnel, and facilities while attempting to minimize the number of participants lost to follow-up. Despite all best intentions and efforts, some loss to follow-up is unavoidable, such as in the case of a research participants' death. This is concerning as the majority of major orthopedic journals with a high impact factor use a minimum standard follow-up percentage of 80% for high-level prospective clinical trials [11]. Therefore, a balance must be achieved to maximize the ability to observe outcomes of interest while responsibly stewarding available resources and preventing an excessive percentage of subjects lost to follow-up.

To achieve such a balance, it is necessary to determine the primary and secondary outcomes of interest for a given research study. Examples of outcomes include survival or mortality rate, degree of recovery such as change in range of motion or pain, return to physical activity or work, rate of complications or adverse events, or the long-term sustainability or unexpected consequences after an intervention [12]. Once the outcomes of interest are defined, the authors must determine through literature review or, if available literature is lacking based on either personal or collective experience, the amount of time that is necessary to capture the occurrences of that particular outcome of interest. For instance, a short-term follow-up would likely be sufficient to effectively determine the rate and time interval of return to activity or work (short-term outcome of interest) following a surgical procedure but the development of degenerative changes will require a longer period of follow-up to allow for the pathology (long-term outcome of interest) to develop.

Another factor to consider is the measurement of a particular outcome at several time intervals in order to measure the sustainability of an intervention's effect. A good example of this can be found in the spine literature. The Spine Patient Outcomes Research Trial (SPORT) which compared surgery vs. nonoperative management of lumbar spinal stenosis showed an advantage of surgery regarding pain and function at 4-year follow-up in an as-treated analysis [13]. However, when studied for a longer period, the advantage in favor of surgery disappeared [14]. Therefore, the time interval studied can affect the results and interpretation of a surgical trial. Authors must therefore carefully consider the question that is intended to be answered and allocate the appropriate follow-up period accordingly. Prospectively evaluating outcomes at different time points allows for the evaluation of short-, mid-, and long-term outcomes in a single cohort. As this can be more challenging in action than in word, we provide an illustration to demonstrate how a well-designed clinical trial can prospectively evaluate different outcomes by varying the follow-up interval post-intervention.

## 11.3 Examples of Follow-Up in Clinical Studies: The Double-Bundle ACL Experience

Few topics in sports medicine, or orthopedic surgery in general, have garnered more attention, and focused research, than double-bundle anterior cruciate ligament (ACL) reconstruction. However, implementing studies on this topic can be challenging because the primary outcome of interest evolves over time. For instance, initially one may be concerned with the rate of failure or return-to-sport, however, in the long term, the purpose of improving this technique is in hopes of preserving the joint and preventing degeneration. As such, a trial of this nature is not simply a "snapshot" in time but a true, prospective, evaluation of an intervention, and the various outcomes over the short and long term. This requires considerable resources in addition to time but is the most reliable way to produce valid results necessary to direct patient care.

Perhaps the most elegant approach to the evaluation of double- versus single-bundle ACL reconstruction was conducted at the Tampere University Hospital in Finland. Using this methodology as a guide for understanding the impact of follow-up, one will hopefully better understand how appropriate follow-up will improve prospective clinical studies.

### 11.3.1 Short-Term Follow-Up

The initial publication on the topic of double- versus single-bundle ACL reconstruction out of Finland was by Suomalainen et al. entitled "Double-Bundle Versus Single-bundle Anterior Cruciate Ligament Reconstruction: Randomized Clinical and Magnetic Resonance Imaging Study With Two Year Follow Up," published in the *American Journal of Sports Medicine* in 2011

[15]. The hypothesis in this study was that double-bundle ACL reconstruction would result in fewer graft failures compared with single-bundle reconstruction. One-hundred fifty-three patients were randomized to single- or double-bundle hamstring autograft ACL reconstruction with interference screw aperture fixation. The patients were followed prospectively for a minimum of 2 years with both clinical and MRI evaluation and 90% of patients were available for final evaluation. There were 8 total graft failures, 7 in the single-bundle group and 1 in the double-bundle group, that subsequently underwent revision surgery. The difference in graft rupture was statistically significant in favor of double-bundle reconstruction. Furthermore, seven patients had an invisible graft at 2 years on MRI follow-up, five in the single-bundle group and two in the double-bundle group. In total, the rate of failure and invisible grafts was significantly higher in the single-bundle group compared with the double-bundle group, 12 patients (15%) versus 3 patients (4%).

This initial 2-year follow-up data illustrates the necessary duration to observe clinical graft failures whereby patients have adequate time to rehabilitate postoperatively and subsequently return to sporting activities with sufficient vigor to place the graft at risk of injury, allowing for graft ruptures to be observed over the time period of the study. These results offered support for the use of a double-bundle technique for ACL reconstruction, however, the authors understood the need to follow these patients for a greater duration of time to validate the durability of this technique over time.

### 11.3.2 Mid-Term Follow-Up

Following the promising results of this initial trial, Suomalainen et al. again published "Double-Bundle Versus Single-Bundle Anterior Cruciate Ligament Reconstruction: A Prospective Randomized Controlled Study With 5-Year Results," in the *American Journal of Sports Medicine* in 2012 [16]. This study followed a similar design whereby 90 patients were randomized equally between three groups; double-bundle hamstring autograft ACL reconstruction with bioabsorbable interference screw fixation, single-bundle hamstring autograft ACL reconstruction with bioabsorbable interference screw fixation and hamstring autograft ACL reconstruction with metal interference screw fixation. The authors hypothesized that double-bundle ACL reconstruction would result in lower rates of graft failure, osteoarthritis, and better stability than single-bundle ACL reconstruction. In this study, 11 patients had a graft failure during the follow-up period and underwent revision, 7 in the single-bundle bioabsorbable screw group, 3 in the single-bundle metal screw group, and 1 in the double-bundle group, which was statistically significant in favor of the double-bundle technique. Of the remaining patients with intact grafts, there were no significant differences in KT-1000 arthrometer or pivot shift tests between the groups at a minimum 5-year follow-up. Furthermore, there was no statistically significant difference in the rate of osteoarthritis between the groups within this follow-up time frame.

These results echoed the previous trial in that the superior failure rates with double-bundle ACL reconstruction were preserved at 5-year follow-up. However, the 5-year duration of follow-up was insufficient to show a difference in the overall "health" of the knee assessed by evaluation of knee stability or radiographic degenerative changes. Therefore, this mid-term follow-up duration was necessary to illustrate longevity of the technique but is inadequate to evaluate for long-term changes to the knee joint, though a more robust sample size may have improved the significance of these results. As such, the study group continued to evaluate these techniques over a longer duration to determine whether knee stability or degeneration are different between double- and single-bundle ACL reconstruction at long-term follow-up.

### 11.3.3 Long-Term Follow-Up

In 2017, the same group published in the *American Journal of Sports Medicine* "Double-Bundle Versus Single-Bundle Anterior Cruciate

Ligament Reconstruction: A Prospective Randomized Study With 10-Year Results." [17] The authors continued to hypothesize in this study that double-bundle ACL reconstruction would result in lower rates of graft failure, osteoarthritis and knee instability. The same cohort from the mid-term evaluation was studied with 90% follow-up at 10 years. There were no new cases of graft rupture in any group with the increased duration of follow-up. No differences in pivot shift testing, KT-1000 arthrometer measurements, or knee scores were observed at long-term follow-up. In addition, there was no difference in osteoarthritis observed between the groups. However, it was noted that the most severe osteoarthritis was observed in patients who had the longest delay to reconstruction and patients who underwent partial meniscectomy at the time of reconstruction.

Therefore, even with longer duration, no differences in clinical or radiographic examination were observed among the groups aside from the previously reported lower graft rupture rates with the double-bundle ACL reconstruction technique. Despite this, the long-term observation of these patients with ACL injuries having undergone reconstruction allowed for an understanding that in general, delayed reconstruction and meniscal resection resulted in higher rates of joint degeneration. This long-term study focused on evaluating the long-term health of the knee joint following ACL reconstruction with anatomic techniques by making this the primary outcome measure. This duration of follow-up is necessary to observe this endpoint of interest but may even be insufficient to observe these changes despite an impressive duration of follow-up.

These nicely designed randomized controlled trials illustrate the power of variable follow-up durations in clinical studies (Fig. 11.2). The short-term study focused on the rate of graft failure at a 2-year duration that allowed for adequate time for rehabilitation and return to sport whereby this endpoint may be observed. In contrast, the mid-term evaluation focused not only on graft rupture, but also on factors associated with the overall well-being of the knee joint including clinical and radiographic parameters. This duration allows for enough time to test the adequacy of the ACL graft under physiologic loading conditions to detect any differences in knee stability or osteoarthritis. Finally, the long-term data at 10 years focused most specifically on osteoarthritis and the detection of risk factors

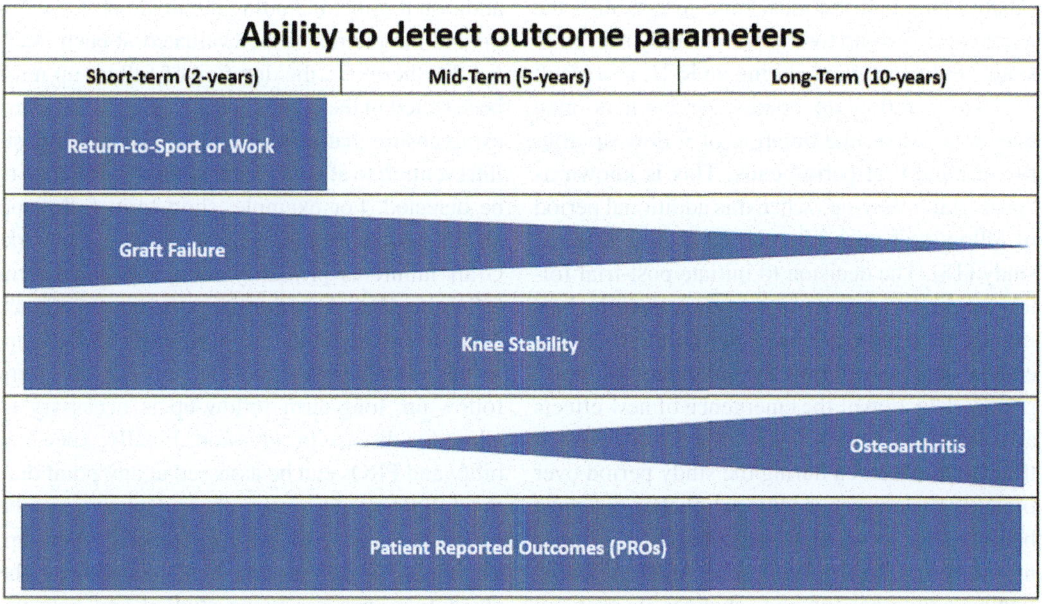


**Fig. 11.2** Ability to detect multiple outcome parameters at various follow-up durations following ACL reconstruction

for degenerative changes following ACL reconstruction. Though no significant difference existed between the techniques, general risk factors for osteoarthritis following ACL reconstruction were identified. Perhaps with even longer follow-up, a difference in osteoarthritis between the two techniques may be observed, though with increasing duration the importance of this outcome diminishes since the importance relates to the prevalence of osteoarthritis of the contralateral side or general population. It is important to note, however, that some outcomes are related; for instance, return to a high-level of activity seen with short-term follow-up may predispose to the development of post-traumatic osteoarthritis in the future observed with long-term follow-up. Thus, in selecting a duration of follow-up, it is important to provide adequate time to observe the primary endpoint with an understanding of the pathophysiologic processes that underlie the recovery from ACL injury to determine the optimal endpoints to be evaluated at variable durations of follow-up.

## 11.4 In-trial vs. Post-trial Follow-Up

Finally, although the ideal time to establish the length of follow-up for a research study is prior to study commencement, during an RCT, as a result of in-trial follow-up results, researchers may decide to extend the duration of follow-up after the original trial period ends. This is known as "post-trial follow-up" when this additional period of follow-up begins after the end of the original study [18]. The decision to initiate post-trial follow-up can be made for numerous reasons including the determination of the duration of any effects observed during the treatment or study period, detection of the emergence of new effects after the study period, and increase or decrease in the effects observed during the study period over time [18]. However, additional challenges must be overcome in order to extend follow-up after the study has already been established including finding additional funding, changes in protocol or data collection, loss of continuity between studies, and obtaining additional consent [19]. Additional funding often needs to be obtained, and when obtained is often less than the funds available for the original study. This may necessitate a change in the protocol or data collected, which may further complicate making comparisons between the in-trial and post-trial follow-up data. Additionally, a gap between the original and post-trial follow-up period may result in the loss of infrastructure or increase the difficulty in retaining prior study participants. Finally, oftentimes additional consent must be obtained to allow for follow-up of study participants past the original study's end date. For these reasons, it is best to carefully consider the outcomes of interest prior to a study's initiation; however, if new or unexpected results are encountered, researchers may consider further extending follow-up after the completion of an RCT.

## 11.5 Conclusion

Follow-up in orthopedic clinical trials is paramount in validating the outcomes of interventions and techniques. When determining follow-up, one must consider several factors in addition to time, including the method of follow-up and the metrics to be evaluated at each interval. Furthermore, the duration of follow-up must be selected in the context of the outcome of interest to ensure that adequate time has passed post-intervention to allow for an outcome difference to be detected. For example, short-term follow-up allows assessment of return-to-sport or work. Graft failure is primarily seen with short-term follow-up, but detection of occurrences can be enhanced with mid- to long-term follow-up. While osteoarthritis may be seen at mid-term follow-up, long-term follow-up is necessary to allow for disease progression. Finally, knee stability and PROs can be assessed at any point during follow-up. However, these factors must be weighed against the costs of extended follow-up. Therefore, it is important to understand the physiologic process being studied and how the experimental intervention intends to alter various outcome measures to allow the investigator to select an appropriate time point for follow-up evaluation. Failure to employ an adequate duration of follow-up may undermine the validity of the study and decrease the perceived value of the experimental intervention of interest.

## References


1. “Follow up.” In The Merriam-Webster.com Dictionary (Merrian-Webster Inc).
2. Schulz KF, Altman DG, Moher D. CONSORT 2010 statement: updated guidelines for reporting parallel group randomised trials. BMJ. 2010;340:c332. https://doi.org/10.1136/bmj.c332.
3. Moher D, et al. CONSORT 2010 explanation and elaboration: updated guidelines for reporting parallel group randomised trials. Int J Surg. 2012;10:28–55. https://doi.org/10.1016/j.ijsu.2011.10.001.
4. ClinicalTrials.gov. https://clinicaltrials.gov/ct2/resources/trends. 2020.
5. Hilibrand AS, Spindler K, O’Keefe RJ. Demonstrating the value of orthopaedic surgery through multicenter trials: AOA critical issues. J Bone Joint Surg Am. 2015;97:e35. https://doi.org/10.2106/jbjs.N.00159.
6. Sprague S, et al. Are large clinical trials in orthopaedic trauma justified? BMC Musculoskelet Disord. 2018;19:124. https://doi.org/10.1186/s12891-018-2029-3.
7. Moher D, Schulz KF, Altman DG. The CONSORT statement: revised recommendations for improving the quality of reports of parallel-group randomised trials. Lancet. 2001;357:1191–4. https://doi.org/10.1016/S0140-6736(00)04337-3.
8. van der List J, DiFelice GS. Primary repair of the anterior cruciate ligament: a paradigm shift. Surgeon. 2017;15:161–8.
9. Taylor SA, Khair MM, Roberts TR, DiFelice GS. Primary repair of the anterior cruciate ligament: a systematic review. Arthroscopy. 2015;31:2233–47. https://doi.org/10.1016/j.arthro.2015.05.007.
10. Katz JN, et al. Surgery versus physical therapy for a meniscal tear and osteoarthritis. N Engl J Med. 2013;368:1675–84. https://doi.org/10.1056/NEJMoa1301408.
11. Musahl V, et al. Basic methods handbook for clinical orthopaedic research: a practical guide and case based research approach. Berlin/Heidelberg: Springer; 2019.
12. Lübbeke A. Research methodology for orthopaedic surgeons, with a focus on outcome. EFORT Open Rev. 2018;3:160–7. https://doi.org/10.1302/2058-5241.3.170064.
13. Weinstein JN, et al. Surgical versus nonoperative treatment for lumbar spinal stenosis four-year results of the Spine Patient Outcomes Research Trial. Spine (Phila Pa 1976). 2010;35:1329–38. https://doi.org/10.1097/BRS.0b013e3181e0f04d.
14. Lurie JD, et al. Long-term outcomes of lumbar spinal stenosis: eight-year results of the Spine Patient Outcomes Research Trial (SPORT). Spine (Phila Pa 1976). 2015;40:63–76. https://doi.org/10.1097/BRS.0000000000000731.
15. Suomalainen P, Moisala AS, Paakkala A, Kannus P, Jarvela T. Double-bundle versus single-bundle anterior cruciate ligament reconstruction: randomized clinical and magnetic resonance imaging study with 2-year follow-up. Am J Sports Med. 2011;39:1615–22. https://doi.org/10.1177/0363546511405024.
16. Suomalainen P, Jarvela T, Paakkala A, Kannus P, Jarvinen M. Double-bundle versus single-bundle anterior cruciate ligament reconstruction: a prospective randomized study with 5-year results. Am J Sports Med. 2012;40:1511–8. https://doi.org/10.1177/0363546512448177.
17. Jarvela S, Kiekara T, Suomalainen P, Jarvela T. Double-bundle versus single-bundle anterior cruciate ligament reconstruction: a prospective randomized study with 10-year results. Am J Sports Med. 2017;45:2578–85. https://doi.org/10.1177/0363546517712231.
18. Llewellyn-Bennett R, et al. Post-trial follow-up methodology in large randomised controlled trials: a systematic review. Trials. 2018;19:298. https://doi.org/10.1186/s13063-018-2653-0.
19. Drye LT, et al. The transitioning from trials to extended follow-up studies. Clin Trials. 2014;11:635–47. https://doi.org/10.1177/1740774514547396.

# Part II

# Conducting a Trial

# Ethics Considerations and Approval in Human Research and Orthopedics

12

Caroline Mouton and Romain Seil

## 12.1 Introduction

Anyone involved in a human subjects research project should adhere according to appropriate ethical standards and understand the importance of not knowingly doing harm during the conduct of a clinical trial.

Ethical approval has become a mandatory step in the conduct of trials involving human subjects. Although obtaining approval from an institutional review board (IRB) or an Independent Ethic Committee (IEC) may seem as an administrative burden, it provides public assurance that the rights, safety, and well-being of trial subjects are protected. Furthermore, it provides reassurance to trial participants and can protect investigators, colleagues, and institutions from public criticism or legal consequences if individual study participants claim inappropriate behavior. Finally, it has become an inevitable requirement from research institutions for conduct of trials in their facilities, funding authorities when considering approval of grant funding, and scientific journals as a condition of publication.

Ethics in research must furthermore not be limited to the conduct of the study itself. Institutions, funding agencies, and scientific journals are also concerned with the professional integrity in all aspects of the conduct of clinical research.

This chapter is designed to discuss a large range of ethical issues, with a specific focus on orthopedic surgical trials research. We aim to increase the awareness of the reader on several major ethical issues that might arise when undertaking such studies.

## 12.2 Research Integrity

All personnel involved in the conduct of scientific inquiry should follow the fundamental principles of research integrity regardless of whether

C. Mouton
Department of Orthopaedic Surgery, Centre Hospitalier de Luxembourg-Clinique d'Eich, Luxembourg City, Luxembourg

Luxembourg Institute of Research in Orthopaedics, Sports Medicine and Science, Luxembourg City, Luxembourg

R. Seil (✉)
Department of Orthopaedic Surgery, Centre Hospitalier de Luxembourg-Clinique d'Eich, Luxembourg City, Luxembourg

Luxembourg Institute of Research in Orthopaedics, Sports Medicine and Science, Luxembourg City, Luxembourg

Human Motion, Orthopaedics, Sports Medicine and Digital Methods, Luxembourg Institute of Health, Luxembourg City, Luxembourg


S. Lyman et al. (eds.), *Introduction to Surgical Trials*,
https://doi.org/10.1007/978-3-031-77563-5_12

the project involves human subjects or not [1]. The four principles include:

1. Reliability in ensuring the quality of research
2. Honesty in developing, undertaking, reviewing, reporting, and communicating research outcomes in a transparent, fair, full, and unbiased way
3. Respect for colleagues, research participants, society, ecosystems, cultural heritage, and the environment
4. Accountability for the research project from idea to publication.

In other words, research projects should be designed, reviewed, and undertaken to ensure that recognized standards of integrity are met, and that quality and transparency are assured. Failing to follow these principles may damage the quality of research, undermine its credibility, and expose research participants or society at large to unnecessary harm. For example, in case of scientific misconduct, trust between researchers and funding agencies may be impacted, making it more difficult to justify continued grant funding. More importantly, the public may lose confidence in research more generally.

In orthopedic research, the retraction of papers due to fraud, plagiarism, or data duplication has been shown to have increased precipitously between 1995 and 2015 [2]. Examples of unacceptable practices in research usually include *fabrication, falsification, plagiarism, and research misconduct*. However, many other questionable research practices exist [3] and seem to be influenced by the stage of a researcher's career with a higher likelihood of misbehavior in mid-career compared to early career. As academic careers become increasingly dependent on acquiring grants and publishing peer-reviewed research, rigorous scientific and ethical principles may be considered an additional time-consuming or even unnecessary burden when added to the competing priorities of trainee education and surgical practice [4]. In this respect, investigators should bear in mind that if fraud or misconduct are uncovered, the investigators themselves would face the most harm due to irreparable damage to their professional careers. However, such unethical activities may also place harm on their own patients as well as the wider academic, scientific, and clinical communities. In fact, scientific misconduct is the responsibility of all collaborators in a research project whether only one or several collaborators were involved in the actions constituting scientific misconduct, encouraged misconduct, were aware of misconduct, or even simply suspected misconduct without taking appropriate action [5].

## 12.3 Independence of Research

In a comparison of the 100 most and 100 least cited articles published between 2000 and 2004 in the *Journal of Bone and Joint Surgery*, Farshad et al. demonstrated that beside scientific factors (e.g., level of evidence), nonscientific factors (e.g., industry support) were also associated with a higher citation rate [6].

Industry relationships may be beneficial for continuing surgical training and developing improved surgical techniques, so is not necessarily unethical. In orthopedic research, financial support from industry is consistently increasing with clear support to individual orthopedic surgeons [7]. However, a large discrepancy has been identified between the self-declared conflict of interest from physicians receiving support from the medical device industry compared to conflicts of interest identified in their publications and available public databases [8]. The orthopedic field has not been spared by this observation [9].

While, cultural differences may exist in the perception of conflicts of interest [10], a generalized universal consensus about what reflects a conflict of interest has been agreed upon within the scientific community. In theory, anything that may be perceived by others as a potential conflict of interest should be explicitly disclosed by each author of a publication regardless of whether there is a direct or indirect conflict of interest. Conflicts of interest arise if an author has obligations toward a private or public funding organization which may directly influence the ability to conduct the research independently. The conflict may be financial or not, direct or indirect, actual or perceived, and may not necessarily have a negative connotation if displayed transparently and if the research results are presented in a neutral and unbiased fashion.

## 12.4 Basic Principles of Research Ethics in Human Subjects

The need for ethical principles for trials on human subjects first arose as a result of the atrocities inflicted during World War II as a result of discovery during the Nuremburg Trials [11]. This resulted in the Nuremberg Code of 1947, a list of ten principles of ethical human subjects research. This was further expanded by the Declaration of Helsinki, first published by the World Medical Association in 1964 and is now in its seventh revision, which was agreed upon in 2013. This now represents the basic ethical principles for medical research. This list of 32 principles is essential reading for anyone involved in human subjects research, particularly those conducting experimental clinical trials [12].

To understand the basic ethical principles in a broader context, which might apply to every situation, the Belmont Report [13] proposed the following three main principles:

1. *Respect for Persons*: Requirement to acknowledge autonomy and to protect those with diminished autonomy. Persons should enter into research voluntarily and with adequate information. One should make sure that the participants are not coerced or influenced into participating in the research to protect their autonomy.
2. *Beneficence*: Do not harm and risk–benefit ratio. The purpose of research is to bring new and helpful information to society. The purpose of research should never be to harm humans or make discovery at the expense of harm to study participants. Human subjects should be treated in an ethical manner by respecting their decisions and protecting them from harm. Researchers should understand it is their responsibility to secure the well-being of their research subjects.
3. *Justice*: Equal opportunity to participate or not. This principle raises the question of how the participants are selected within a clinical trial. One should ensure that underage populations, pregnant women, economically disadvantaged, racial and ethnic minorities, persons confined to institutions, or other vulnerable persons are included or excluded from a study based on their eligibility to participate in the research. These subjects should not be included or excluded due to other barriers (e.g., financial burden) or for their easy availability (e.g., prisoners).

## 12.5 Application of Research Ethics in Human Research

### 12.5.1 Informed Consent: Information, Comprehension, and Voluntariness

Human subjects should enter into research voluntarily, with adequate information, and after a reasonable amount has been given for them to understand information on the purpose of the project, their involvement, and the risks and benefits of participation. They must be given the opportunity to ask questions and should be able to give fully informed consent.

The most effective way to address informed consent is through the use of an information sheet, provided to all persons who are invited to participate in a trial. Ideally, this should be presented on official institutional letterhead to increase awareness of the official nature of the information and also to inform the potential subject that the organization (e.g., hospital, academic center) has approved the research project. Videos or presentations may also be used as an effective way to share information with potential subjects. The manner and context in which information is presented are just important as its content. It is necessary to adapt it to the participant's capacities (e.g., children). Information should thus also be shared orally to allow the participant to ask questions.

The consent process should include a description of: the purpose of the study, the procedures and data collection (including tissue samples and/or videotaping and how this data will be processed during and after the research period), potential risks and discomforts, the procedure to follow in case emergency care is needed, anticipated benefits to participants and society, alternative procedures, alternatives to participation, and the ability to withdraw from the project at any time. The informed consent process should also address: rights of research participants, privacy and confidentiality, and any financial aspects of participation [14].

A consent is considered valid only if voluntarily given. It should be free of coercion and influence. The subject should know that there is no penalty for not participating. In some situations (e.g., prisoners), the application of this principle may not be obvious and so in those circumstances extra caution must be used to assure noncoercive informed consent is obtained.

### 12.5.2 Assessment of Risks and Benefits

When deciding whether or not to participate in a research study, many possible harms and benefits should be considered. These include psychological, physical, legal, social, and economic risks as well as possible benefits. Particular attention should be given to vulnerable groups of human subjects, particularly pregnant women, captive populations (e.g., prisoners, institutionalized, students), mentally ill persons, the elderly, children, the critically ill or dying, impoverished, those with learning disabilities, and those who are sedated or unconscious at the time of recruitment.

The issue of confidentiality and anonymity is closely connected to the risk of participating in a trial, as being identified as a trial participant could have negative ramifications. Protecting the anonymity and confidentiality of participants has grown in importance over the last decade with the development of online databases to house research data. Anonymity is best protected when the participant's identity cannot be linked with personal responses. If anonymity cannot be assured (e.g., audio or video recordings, images), confidentiality should be prioritized. The investigators should ensure that private information is managed securely in order to protect the participant's identity. If researchers plan to share study data with a third party, they should explicitly provide this information during the consent process and specify how data will be shared and whether it will be anonymized. Autonomy should be given to study participants to determine the time, extent, and circumstances under which their information may be shared with others. Likewise, participants need to be informed about the purpose of the collected data and the identity of the stakeholders who will be given access. Participants should be informed as to whether their data will only be used for scientific purposes or if other stakeholders will be granted access for non-research purposes (e.g., product regulatory approval).

### 12.5.3 Selection of Subjects

Injustice may arise from social, racial, sexual, or cultural biases, and unjust social patterns may arise despite an a priori fair selection plan in the study protocol. Trial participants should not only be included simply because they belong to a group that is easily accessible, available, or perhaps vulnerable and less able to decline participation. They should be included because they are invested in the outcomes of the study, hoping to help ensure that it is safe, effective, and acceptable for all potential recipients. This altruistic motivation may help improve compliance and assure complete patient follow-up until the end of the trial. Of course, this is not a requirement for participation. Anyone who is eligible and willing to provide informed consent should be permitted to participate if they so choose.

## 12.6 Approval in Human Research

Currently, peer-reviewed scientific journals are likely to reject a manuscript if there is a failure to meet ethical standards. Nearly any study involving research on human beings must be evaluated for acceptable human subjects' protections by an institutional review board (IRB) or Independent Ethical Committee (IEC), heretofore "ethics panels." This type of research may include studies which are conducted on normal individuals or on persons with a specific condition, review of data from large or selected populations, epidemiological studies, study of human tissue (fresh or from a repository), and, of course, interventional studies.

There are specific ethical exceptions based on the study location, intent of the research, and the characteristics of the study. In general, any study that does not require the subject to be identified (e.g., anonymous survey) may not require prior ethics panel approval. In these cases, depending upon the jurisdiction, only subject verbal assent or employer notification or approval may be required. For any prospective study where identifiers linked to the subject may be used to follow a subject, the ethics panel approval is mandatory. Some countries, such as France, have adapted their regulations (Jardé Law, enacted in 2012) to simplify the approval process [15]. For example, in case of a non-interventional study, written informed consent is no longer required under French law. However, the investigators still have the obligation to inform the patient about the study prior to enrollment.

Regardless of the location of the study, the recruitment of patients in a clinical trial should only start after ensuring that all authorizations and approvals have been given. This may include notification or authorizations from: ethics panels, local health authorities, data protection authorities, insurance companies, or employers. For studies, not requiring prior approval, one may request an official letter from the approving ethics panel to confirm that the study is being conducted according to accepted community standards.

### 12.6.1 Responsibility of the Principal Investigator

In any research involving human subjects, it is the responsibility of the principal investigator (PI) to comply with international and community ethical, legal, and regulatory rules and standards. Ultimately, the PI bears full responsibility for the study, even if delegating trial-related duties to other study personnel. The PI is responsible for study preparation, conduct, and completion and is expected to ensure compliance with the study protocol as written. The study protocol, as approved, may be thought of as a written agreement between the study team and the ethics panel that approved the project. The PI is further responsible for the administrative aspects of the trial (e.g., data use agreements, contracts) in compliance with applicable laws and regulations. In relation to approving ethics panel, the PI should provide period summaries of the trial status, report any meaningful changes to the trial protocol which may increase risk to the subjects, and also report any serious adverse events.

### 12.6.2 Role of Ethics Panels

The role of ethics panels is to oversee human subjects research and help ensure ethical practices. These panels are typically made up of peer clinicians, scientists, and in the case of US-based IRBs, at least one legal representative and one patient representative. These ethics panels are authorized to request clarification on aspects of the study prior to approval and may either reject the submission as unethical or require revisions to the study protocol before approval. While their focus is on the ethical aspects of the study, they often also serve as research peer reviewers as well since poorly designed research could be deemed unethical, because it may not yield useful information. Rejection may occur if the panel determines that the study negatively impacts the protection of the rights, safety, and/or well-being of the research subjects. Continuing reviews, typically annual, are required to monitor the trial progress and, if necessary, prematurely stop the trial if serious unexpected adverse events occur with higher frequency than anticipated. This monitoring process is sometimes done by a Data Safety Monitoring Board (see Chap. 13).

In summary, ethics panels ensure the rights, safety, and well-being of all trial subjects by taking into consideration the following aspects:

- The social and/or clinical value of the research questions: importance for society, patients, and the clinical community.
- The scientific validity: Design, methodology, feasibility.
- Subject recruitment: Fair selection of participants based on the scientific goals rather than on vulnerability, privilege, or other factors.
- Informed consent: Accurate, comprehensive, understandable, and voluntary.
- Privacy and confidentiality: Subject participation status and data are being prioritized for protestation against discovery.
- Autonomy: Subject retains right to withdraw from the study without penalty.
- Risk–benefit ratio: Do benefits of study completion outweigh the risk and inconvenience caused to the study subjects? Are risks being minimized as much as possible?
- Risk monitoring: Determining that appropriate reporting methods are in place for adverse events and that these adverse events will be quickly and appropriately treated when they occur.

### 12.6.3 Documents to Submit to the Ethics Panel

Good clinical practice (GCP) guidelines [14] report the international ethical and scientific standard for designing, conducting, recording, and reporting trials involving human subjects. Compliance with these guidelines provides public assurance that the rights, safety, and well-being of trial subjects are protected in accordance with the principles in the Declaration of Helsinki and that the clinical trial data are credible.

GCP guidelines provide the exhaustive list of essential documents for the conduct of a clinical trial. When preparing these documents, one should keep in mind that (1) participant's needs come first: explicitly mentioning all aspects related to the subject protection, safety, and well-being can help to obtain a favorable decision from the ethics panel and (2) common reasons for rejection are scientific merit, improper consent form, poor study design, unacceptable risk to subjects, or other ethical or legal reasons [16].

The study *protocol* must be exhaustive and consistent. Items are explained in greater detail in GCP guidelines or SPIRIT [7] checklists. For RCTs, the CONSORT checklist [17, 18] may be used to ensure that all methodological aspects are addressed in the protocol. To increase the chances of developing a successful research project, we recommend investigators follow the FINER (Feasible, Interesting, Novel, Ethical, and Relevant) criteria [19] and describe the objectives using the PICOT (Patients, Intervention, Comparison group, Outcomes, Time) criteria [20]. The primary objective should be clearly described. The sample size calculation should be based on this objective. Secondary objectives, number of visits, selection criteria, and other aspects of the design that may infringe on subjects' time or effort should be limited to the minimum justified by the project. Multiplying objectives within the same study is time-consuming and may increase the risk of a lack of compliance with the protocol. A high number of visits may increase the dropout rate and the amount of missing data. Finally, restrictive selection criteria may critically slow down recruitment and influence the external validity of the study. The right balance is critical. Anticipating all these difficulties while writing the protocol is key to a successful study. This extra effort may prevent the need for amendment requests from the ethics panel, which are estimated to be required in approximately two-thirds of clinical protocols [21, 22].

The *Case Report Form (CRF)* is a printed or electronic document designed to record all information to be reported for each trial participant at each trial visit. The CRF should not include any information that can identify the participant. Only a study identification code unique to each patient should be recorded on this document. To avoid missing data, no field should be left blank. For example, provide the options of "not applicable" or "unknown" so that you can be assured that an attempt was made to capture the data even if that effort was unsuccessful. Missed visits or clinical exams that could not be performed should be clearly documented. To improve data consistency and accuracy, text fields should be avoided with discrete response options preferred. If the CRF is electronic, formulas or informatics codes should be implemented to prevent conflicting information and real-time identification of outlier values (e.g., a keystroke error reporting a BMI of 352 rather than 35.2).

The *information to the participant* should be written in a non-technical language. Subjects are less likely to enter studies that they find difficult to understand and that require multiple follow-ups [23]. An appropriate information should explain the following:

- Purpose, duration of the study, total number of subjects, and how they are selected.
- Participation duration, visits and windows, procedures, and whether these are part of the daily clinical practice or experimental.
- Potential side effects, risks, and benefits of participation.
- Volunteer aspect of the participation: Refusal or withdrawal is possible without penalty or loss of benefits.
- Compensation and amount if applicable.
- Reasons for possible early termination of participation/study (e.g., new medical condition interfering with study protocol).
- Communication in case of new information during the study (e.g., participants will be informed if new findings become available during the study that may be relevant to their willingness to continue).
- Data protection: How personal information are recorded, whether records are confidential (identification numbers), and whether third parties have access to data.
- Approval of the trial by an ethics panel.
- Principal investigator, sponsor, and contact person regarding the trial and the rights of subjects, and whom to contact in case of adverse event.
- Medical attention that may be given if the participant requires one (e.g., adverse event) and insurance to cover this care.

## 12.7 Ethical Considerations in Surgical Trials in Orthopedics

Several ethical issues have been raised in orthopedic surgical trials, especially for randomized controlled trials (RCTs). These issues usually concern the learning curve of a surgeon for a new procedure, the blinding of the trial, or the use of sham surgery, all potentially having a significant impact on the validity of the trial.

Individual surgeons tend to primarily use a single surgical approach for a specific problem. This may compromise a conventional RCT where two surgical techniques are compared and for which different surgeons may have different levels of expertise [24, 25]. In order to reduce both bias and ethical concerns, an expertise-based RCT may be considered in which participants are randomized to clinicians according to their specific level of expertise rather than to the surgical treatment itself [24]. Another alternative may be cluster randomization in which orthopedic departments are randomized to exclusively perform one of the surgical interventions being compared.

Practically, blinding surgeons in a surgical intervention trial is impossible. However, it may still be possible to blind outcomes assessors, statisticians, and patients. However, a few RCTs clearly document blinding status [26] which may be of concern as lack of blinding is known to exaggerate treatment effect size [27]. This is especially the case if the outcomes are subjective (e.g., pain, function, quality of life) as they may be more sensitive to the placebo effect influenced by the patient's expectation rather than related to the treatment itself.

Some surgical RCTs have used sham surgery. The ethical concern here is that sham surgeries offer no therapeutic benefit while potentially exposing patients to unnecessary risks. Furthermore, they may compromise the physician–patient relationship, as patients must be kept unaware of their surgery to preserve blinding. However, when the sham surgery is performed in a manner that sufficiently minimizes risks to the patients and truly informed consent is given by the participant, sham surgery may be an acceptable placebo in surgical trials. However, in order to justify the use of sham surgery, it should be reserved for cases in which no standard treatment exists, the intervention being studied has questionable benefits, and any benefits seen previously may be due to a placebo effect of having surgery [28, 29].

## 12.8 Conclusion

Research ethics are the responsibility of everyone involved in trials that involve human subjects. Any study involving research on human beings must go through an ethics panel in order to ensure the rights, safety, and well-being of all trial subjects are adequately protected. In order to maintain public trust, investigators should follow ethical clinical practices to ensure that the participants' needs come first. The selection of participants should be fair and based on the scientific goals. Information provided to potential participants should be comprehensible and individual written consent should be freely given on a voluntary basis. The participants' risks should be acceptable for the value of the potential discovery, and measures should be taken to avoid both the compromise of patient privacy and any potential adverse events. In case of a randomized controlled trial, care should also be taken to address the surgeons' surgical acumen, blinding when possible to assure validity of the results, and the judicious use of sham surgery when appropriate.

## References


1. The European Code of Conduct for research integrity revised edition; 2017.
2. Yan J, MacDonald A, Baisi LP, Evaniew N, Bhandari M, Ghert M. Retractions in orthopaedic research: a systematic review. Bone Joint Res. 2016;5(6):263–8.
3. Martinson BC, Anderson MS, de Vries R. Scientists behaving badly. Nature. 2005;435(7043):737–8.
4. de Girolamo L, Dejour D, Lind M, Karlsson J, Seil R. Surgical competence, research and evidence-based medicine (EBM) in orthopaedic surgery: what the ESSKA is doing to bring it all together. Knee Surg Sports Traumatol Arthrosc. 2020;28(2):335–8.
5. Helgesson G, Eriksson S. Responsibility for scientific misconduct in collaborative papers. Med Health Care Philos. 2018;21(3):423–30.
6. Farshad M, Sidler C, Gerber C. Association of scientific and nonscientific factors to citation rates of articles of renowned orthopedic journals. Eur Orthop Traumatol. 2013;4(3):125–30.
7. Zuckerman JD, Prasarn M, Kubiak EN, Koval KJ. Conflict of interest in orthopaedic research. JBJS. 2004;86(2):423.
8. Ziai K, Pigazzi A, Smith BR, Nouri-Nikbakht R, Nepomuceno H, Carmichael JC, et al. Association of compensation from the surgical and medical device industry to physicians and self-declared conflict of interest. JAMA Surg. 2018;153(11):997–1002.
9. Okike K, Kocher MS, Wei EX, Mehlman CT, Bhandari M. Accuracy of conflict-of-interest disclosures reported by physicians. N Engl J Med. 2009;361(15):1466–74.
10. Grundy Q, Habibi R, Shnier A, Mayes C, Lipworth W. Decoding disclosure: comparing conflict of interest policy among the United States, France, and Australia. Health Policy. 2018;122(5):509–18.
11. Code N. The Nuremberg code. Trials of war criminals before the Nuremberg military tribunals under control council law. 1949;10(1949):181–2.
12. World Medical Association. World Medical Association Declaration of Helsinki: ethical principles for medical research involving human subjects. JAMA. 2013;310(20):2191–4.
13. U.S. Department of Health and Human Services. The Belmont report: ethical principles and guidelines for the protection of human subjects of research. Washington, DC: Author; 1979.
14. Committee for Human Medicinal Products, European Medicines Agency. Guideline for good clinical practice E6(R2). 2016.
15. Lemaire F. La loi Jardé: ce qui change. Presse Med. 2019;48(3, Part 1):238–42.
16. Jones JS, White LJ, Pool LC, Dougherty JM. Structure and practice of institutional review boards in the United States. Acad Emerg Med. 1996;3(8):804–9.
17. Schulz KF, Altman DG, Moher D, CONSORT Group. CONSORT 2010 statement: updated guidelines for reporting parallel group randomised trials. BMC Med. 2010;8(1):18.
18. Moher D, Hopewell S, Schulz KF, Montori V, Gøtzsche PC, Devereaux PJ, et al. CONSORT 2010 explanation and elaboration: updated guidelines for reporting parallel group randomised trials. J Clin Epidemiol. 2010;63(8):e1–37.
19. Hulley SB. Designing clinical research. Philadelphia: Lippincott Williams & Wilkins; 2007.

20. Guyatt G, Drummond R, Meade M, Cook D. The evidence based-medicine working group users' guides to the medical literature. Essentials of evidence-based clinical practice. 2008.
21. Decullier E, Lhéritier V, Chapuis F. The activity of French Research Ethics Committees and characteristics of biomedical research protocols involving humans: a retrospective cohort study. BMC Med Ethics. 2005;6(1):9.
22. Getz KA, Stergiopoulos S, Short M, Surgeon L, Krauss R, Pretorius S, et al. The impact of protocol amendments on clinical trial performance and cost. Ther Innov Regul Sci. 2016;50(4):436–41.
23. Thoma A, Farrokhyar F, McKnight L, Bhandari M. Practical tips for surgical research: how to optimize patient recruitment. Can J Surg. 2010;53(3):205–10.
24. Devereaux PJ, Bhandari M, Clarke M, Montori VM, Cook DJ, Yusuf S, et al. Need for expertise based randomised controlled trials. BMJ. 2005;330(7482):88.
25. Seil R. In high tibial osteotomy, closing and opening wedges did not differ for clinical outcomes at up to two years. J Bone Joint Surg Am. 2018;100(10):882.
26. Bhandari M, Richards RR, Sprague S, Schemitsch EH. The quality of reporting of randomized trials in the Journal of Bone and Joint Surgery from 1988 through 2000. J Bone Joint Surg Am. 2002;84(3):388–96.
27. Savović J, Jones HE, Altman DG, Harris RJ, Jüni P, Pildal J, et al. Influence of reported study design characteristics on intervention effect estimates from randomized, controlled trials. Ann Intern Med. 2012;157(6):429–38.
28. Mehta S, Myers TG, Lonner JH, Huffman GR, Sennett BJ. The ethics of sham surgery in clinical orthopaedic research. J Bone Joint Surg Am. 2007;89(7):1650–3.
29. Bannuru RR, McAlindon TE, Sullivan MC, et al. Effectiveness and implications of alternative placebo treatments: a systematic review and network meta-analysis of osteoarthritis trials. Ann Intern Med. 2015;163:365–72. https://doi.org/10.7326/M15-0623.

# Trial Start-Up Considerations: Budget, Staffing, Logistics

# 13

Antonino Cantivalli, Halah Kutaish, and Jacques Menetrey

## 13.1 Introduction

Clinical trials are research studies on human participants designed to evaluate a medical, surgical, or behavioral intervention. They are the primary way that researchers determine if a new treatment (e.g., surgical technique) is safe and effective for the patient [1]. There are two main types of studies: interventional and observational studies, depending on the exposure to a particular treatment, drug, or device. In interventional studies, perhaps better known as randomized controlled trials (RCTs), researchers assign interventions and study outcomes in a carefully planned and systematic way. Conversely, for observational studies, researcher simply observes what happens during the course of standard clinical care [2, 3]. Regardless of whether a study is interventional or observational, they may involve only one center (e.g., clinic, hospital) or more centers (multicenter study) in the same city or even in different countries [4].

These considerations are essential because planning a surgical interventional trial is much more time-consuming and demanding than the planning phase for observational studies, requiring extensive preparation and careful analysis. For a successful project, all scientific, bureaucratic, and logistical phases should be well planned and described from the beginning in a precise written protocol. This document should describe the study type, specific aims, research questions, interventions, number and groups of patients, data collection methods, outcomes measures (e.g., questionnaires, objective examination tests), informed consent process, follow-up procedures, and ultimate study goals. Failure to plan all these steps may lead to rejection by the ethics committee or data loss (if collected by direct interview or objective examination). A careful analysis of the resource during the planning phase is mandatory to avoid the interruption of the study due to the lack of personnel (e.g., study coordinators, nurses statisticians), research subjects, or resources (e.g., funding). In the event of study interruption, the investigators must redesign the study or re-collect the data with a significant loss of time and money. This chapter aims to describe the practical development of a surgical trial by focusing on three key points: budget,

A. Cantivalli
Department of Orthopaedics and Traumatology, AO Ordine Mauriziano Hospital, University of Torino, Torino, Italy

Centre for Sports Medicine and Exercise, Swiss Olympic Medical Center, Hirslanden Clinique La Colline, Geneva, Switzerland

H. Kutaish · J. Menetrey (✉)
Centre for Sports Medicine and Exercise, Swiss Olympic Medical Center, Hirslanden Clinique La Colline, Geneva, Switzerland

Orthopaedic Surgery Service, University Hospital of Geneva, Geneva, Switzerland
e-mail: jacques.menetrey@hirslanden.ch


S. Lyman et al. (eds.), *Introduction to Surgical Trials*,
https://doi.org/10.1007/978-3-031-77563-5_13

staffing, and logistics, which may vary depending on the country of the study, the design, the number of centers involved, and the intended goals.

## 13.2 Budget

Modern trials are human resource-intensive and adequate funding is necessary to assure high quality data capture, analysis, and reporting of trial results [5]. The final cost varies according to the planned type of study: RCTs are much more expensive than open label trials or prospective cohort studies [6].

**How does the type of study have an impact on the budget?** RCTs have higher expenses because establishing new indications for drugs or surgical interventions have regulatory standards requiring a high degree of safety monitoring and quality control assurances. As such, patient contact is more in-depth and more frequent and greater attention must be paid to optimizing enrollment and maximizing follow-up, which increases costs. Moreover, RCTs usually take longer to complete and include both a randomization process and often blinding of patients and/or observers [6], making these trials more challenging to conduct and requiring a large team of highly qualified investigators. Both the duration of the study and the number of people involved are factors that influence the final cost of the study.

In addition, other expenses must be considered in the initial planning. First, the manufacturing cost the implantable devices and/or instruments (including the operating room) if a new surgical technique is studied. Similarly, funds are needed to pay for the study insurance (in some regions), the ethics committee, trial management (there are for-profit companies that manage trials), communications solutions (particularly vital for multicenter studies), data collection solutions, management of patient communication, conference travel to present results, and publication fees (if any). Employee benefits, such as retirement pensions, health insurance, maternity/paternity leave, and vacation time must also be considered in the budget. Even the costs of paper, telephones, travel, computers, software, and other consumables can be significant [5].

Procuring funds is often a major hurdle in clinical research, and for the most expensive trials, shared funding from more than one source may be necessary. There are different types of sources: private for-profit funding (e.g., medical device manufacturers), private non-profit (e.g., foundations or institutes), and public funding (e.g., government grants). Universities and hospitals have funds available for research, but usually, they contribute by providing clinical spaces, researchers (e.g., methodologists, statisticians, administrative support staff), and nursing staff. However, it is becoming increasingly difficult to conduct RCTs without external funding. Regardless of the funding source targeted, the trial planning and protocol development should be complete before approaching the funding entity [4, 5].

Some efficiency measures should be considered to avoid budget overruns. First, in the case of multicenter studies, choosing a geographic area centrally positioned for all collaborating centers is ideal. Secondly, all phases should be carried out in the shortest possible time according to "good clinical practice". And of course, the budget must be precisely calculated and confirmed prior to the start of the study [4].

## 13.3 Staffing

An essential aspect of surgical trial planning is the fluidity whereby all collaborators work together toward a common goal. The philosophy among collaborators should be compliance and partnership. The recruitment of centers and co-investigators who are dedicated, collaborative, and selfless is essential to achieve the goals and appropriately develop all the planned phases. The number of people involved in a trial is widely variable, depending on the aim of the study, the number of participating centers, and the number of subjects to be enrolled. However, some staff members are constant and critical for the implementation of the study [4].

The *principal investigator (PI)* is usually the team member who conceived the study idea whose role is to bring together the key elements of the process, lead the research team, and assure proper conduct of the trial, and sees the trial through to its proper conclusion. The PI manages all collaborations, clinical care processes, scientific integrity, financial support or sponsorship, and ethical committee approvals.

In addition to the principal investigator, there are other types of investigators [2]:

- *Deputy principal investigator* who can serve as a surrogate for the PI when needed and may have the same level of responsibility, particularly in multicenter trials.
- *Co-investigator or sub-investigator* (there can be more than one per trial) has secondary responsibility, usually reporting to the PI.
- If multiple centers are involved, each center needs a "*responsible investigator*" to coordinate the trial at their institution.

Despite the hierarchy, all of these investigators have extensive responsibilities relating to identifying and allocating resources, ethical subject enrollment, safe trial participation, appropriate handling of study materials, and final disposition of the trial information [2, 4, 5].

The *study coordinator* (often a senior researcher or other appropriately experienced healthcare professional) works closely with the investigators and is usually responsible for the day to day management of the trial by coordinating scheduling, personnel, data, and other managerial responsibilities as needed [2].

The *steering committee* typically comprises of the *principal investigator* and *the study coordinator,* along with clinical co-investigators, and experts in study design, data management, and statistical analysis. This steering committee serves a vital role in trial oversight by advising the PI on protocol modifications necessary when problems nearly invariably arise during study implementation and execution [5].

The *ethics committee* is a crucial component of clinical trial development. These committees are typically comprised of medical professionals and non-medical members tasked with ensure the safety and welfare of participants in human subjects' research. These committees are independent of individual trial study teams and are typically organized by either the medical institution where the trial is scheduled to take place (coordinating center in a multicenter trial, though local ethics committee approval is often necessary as well) or by an independent private ethics committee. Approval from this committee is mandatory before undertaking any research involving human subjects [5].

In some cases, an *endpoint adjudication committee* may be set up to judge clinical endpoints when there are subjective elements of decision-making or when decisions are complex or error-prone. It should include people not involved in the trial and be blinded to the participants' intervention [5].

A *data safety and monitoring committee* is required for interventional trials. This committee is responsible for determining whether a trial should continue or be stopped early due to safety or efficacy findings during pre-planned periodic interim analyses. This committee, similar to the previous one, should be blinded to the intervention groups and made up of experts who are not involved in the trial, including at least one statistician and other relevant specialists depending on the study subject (e.g., orthopedist, radiologist). Typically this committee will allow a trial to continue through to its planned conclusion unless: A) a substantial safety risk is identified in one of the intervention arms (e.g., a very high rate of a serious adverse event with an experimental treatment) or overwhelming evidence of superiority for one trial arm over the other [5].

Universities and academic hospitals play a central role in international research, and the personnel involved in high quality interventional trials are often employed by these institutions. In particular, statisticians and clinical epidemiologists are critical during the planning phase to avoid pitfalls in methods, data collection, sample size determination, and statistical analysis plans. Before drafting the protocol, it is vital to discuss with the statistician the design options and calculate the possible number of patients (power analysis). Moreover, the study statistician is responsible for determining the correct data format, selecting the correct statistical tests, performing stratification (if scheduled), and finally conducting the analyses in order to assist the study team in interpreting the results. The epidemiologists' role is slightly different because, even if they collaborate with the statistician, they also have methodological and medical knowledge and can help greatly in reducing biases introduced during the study design phase and in helping interpret the results.

Researchers, surgical residents, doctoral students, and administrative staff are crucial for data and space management, appointments, transportation, and paperwork. Research nurses (nurses trained in trial conduct) can help in patient identification, application of inclusion and exclusion criteria, patient recruitment, obtaining informed consent from patients, managing clinical paperwork, and drug administration (if any).

Finally, the study subjects play a fundamental role. Patients can be enrolled only by medical staff involved in the study and then assigned their treatment through systematic or random allocation [6]. However, enrollment is only the beginning of their journey. Their continued participation and trial completion is vital to its success.

## 13.4 Logistics

Conducting a clinical trial requires practical necessities that should be considered for a successful study outcome. These are paperwork management, pre-trial training, patient recruitment, appropriate space (e.g., private consultation rooms), materials management (e.g., medical supply chains), computer devices, and software solutions.

| Checklist: Logistics | | | | | |
|---|---|---|---|---|---|
| Paperworks management | Pre-trial training | Patient management | Finding appropriate spaces | Materials management and transportation | Computer devices and programs |
| *Drugs*<br>– Local drug agency approval<br>– Suspected Unexpected Serious Adverse Reaction (SUSAR)<br>– Serious adverse event module<br>*Imaging*<br>– Description of the machine used (X-ray, MRI, etc.)<br>– Location for the imaging<br>*Patients*<br>– Informed consent<br>– Scores used to evaluate patients<br>*Ethics Committee*<br>– The document can vary according to country, they usually include:<br>  – Protocol<br>  – Information module for GP and patients<br>  – CV Principal investigator<br>  – Informed consent<br>  – Scores used<br>  – Centers involved (if multi-center) | All the staff members<br>Data safety and monitoring committee should be present | *Advertising*<br>– Patient organizations<br>– Registries<br>– Hospitals<br>– Pharmacies<br>– GPs<br>*Enrolling patients*<br>– Only MD can enroll patients | Offices<br>Laboratories<br>Operating rooms (ORs)<br>Consulting rooms<br>Archives | Correct quantity of medication<br>Not external differences between the real medicine and placebo<br>Medical supplies (sphygmomanometers, ECG, stethoscopes, syringes, sanitizers)<br>OR instruments<br>Organized transportations (companies, timelines)<br>Adequate and approved (local drug agency) boxes (if needed) | Computer devices<br>Storage method (USB key, archives, hard disks, etc.)<br>Specific software to register and ensure data |

### 13.4.1 Paperwork Management

The bureaucratic burden before starting a trial is enormous and consists of all the documents needed to coordinate each phase of the trial. If the trial involves drug administration, approval by the local and/or national drug control agency is often required as well as the development of the forms that will be used to record adverse reactions. If the trial is based on radiological images, the researchers should describe the imaging modality and associated risks as well as plans for risk mitigation. In addition, there are many other documents required for ethics committee approval including those needed to enroll patients (informed consent) or forms used to collect data by medical evaluation or self-assessment (questionnaires, diaries, self-evaluation tools). The PI and study coordinator must create and manage all these documents to submit to the ethics committee for approval. Therefore, it is essential for the study developers to get familiar with the local ethics committee requirements, as they usually have checklists for each study type and they may have templates for each needed form.

### 13.4.2 Pre-Trial Training

Staff members should be familiar with the study design and the established protocol, their roles, the different phases, the study's goals, and endpoints.

Usually, there is a training session prior to the first patient recruitment at the recruiting site. This training session should include the study developers, the local investigators, all site staff, and members from the local monitoring committees. The aim of this session is to familiarize all involved researchers with the study protocol, inclusion/exclusion criteria, the role of each staff member, serious adverse event reporting mechanism, and contact persons. The principal investigator is usually responsible for holding meetings to illustrate (through slides, graphs, and tables) all the trial details to educate the staff. A question and answer session should also be conducted to clarify any confusing topics.

### 13.4.3 Patient Management

Recruitment and screening of patients for a clinical trial needs meticulous organization. Trial organizers may use available structures like patient advocacy organizations, hospitals waiting rooms, pharmacies, or general practitioner (GPs) offices to reach target patient populations via printed flyers, pamphlets, or posters. Recently, print-based advertising methods have been replaced by digital tools such as clinical trial recruitment websites (e.g., the EU Clinical Trials Registries, social media sites, or smartphone apps. However, this requires collaboration with GPs, graphic designers, printers, and computer experts. Finally, physicians participating in the trial are expected to work with research nurses to screen patients, assess eligibility, collect relevant medical history on study specific forms, and possibly register them in a database to be enrolled [7].

### 13.4.4 Appropriate Space

An essential factor in the practical organization is the availability of adequate space such as offices, laboratories, operating rooms (ORs), or consulting rooms. The offices are crucial for the administrative management of a clinical trial where an employee (hired for the study or, most of the time, already working for the institute) will organize and store the administrative paperwork required for trial documentation. In addition, this is where the necessary documents for the clinical practice (medical records, informed consent) are usually prepared and where confidential patient lists are managed. Depending on the type of study, researchers may need consulting rooms, ORs, laboratories, or some combination of these places.

Dedicated trial consulting rooms may be where patients get screened and informed about the study and where periodical physical examinations are performed. Some interventions might need to be undertaken in the physician's consultation office such as intra-articular injection or at a treatment room for intravenous drug administration. However, if a new surgical technique is studied, then OR will be used and the OR staff must be trained on the new technique or material used. Different laboratories may be necessary depending on the goals: cytology, histology, immunology, and blood testing facilities are the most widely used. However, the researchers must be vigilant on how different laboratories run the desired tests as a change in testing methodology or varying machinery might give different results and thus leading to measurement errors [8]. This is especially true for multicenter studies. This also applies to imaging centers where MRI machines or CT scanners might be of different strengths or come from different manufactures and may lead to unreliable results.

### 13.4.5 Materials Management

Another critical aspect is the management of materials, like the surgical hardware under study. A sufficient number of implants and related hardware should be available, and if the study is blinded, the experimental intervention and alternative treatment should not be distinguishable if possible. Depending on the study, other medical supplies may be necessary including appropriate OR instrumentation. Transportation of surgical implants or biological specimens from one site to another should be carefully planned ensuring the safety of the material, cold chain stability, and punctual departure and arrival times. The responsible person on each side of the transportation chain should be identified and provided with all necessary documents regarding the material of the study (e.g., quality control form). An external specialized company can be involved, and depending on the subject of the study, short recovery times or high-speed transportation may be necessary. Moreover, if special containers are needed, they should be tested beforehand by study personnel to ensure accurate handling of the containers and the materials.

### 13.4.6 Computer Hardware and Software

Computer devices have largely replaced the paper equipment used for trial development and implementation. Electronic records (E-Case Report Forms) have often replaced paper records, many laboratory devices have been computerized, and medical records are often electronic as well. Appropriate software is required to randomize patients, schedule appointments and follow-up visits, record data, encrypt and secure data, conduct statistical analysis, and graphically present results. The management of data collection should be defined in the protocol: the methods of collection, where and how all the information will be stored, and how sensitive data will be protected and eliminated at the end of the study by the principal investigator and study coordinator. For a multicenter study, software that can ensure data safety and simultaneous data recording are highly recommended.

## 13.5 Conclusion

Conducting a clinical trial is challenging and requires meticulous planning and execution. The study protocol is the key document where the study's goals, endpoint, and methods should be clearly defined to avoid data loss or increasing study time and costs. Obtaining the necessary funds is often demanding, but necessary. The number of people involved in the study and their tasks are crucial for developing an appropriate budget and for achieving the final study goals. Logistics should be carefully evaluated to conduct the trial according to best practices.

## References


1. What Are Clinical Trials and Studies? [Internet]. National Institute on Aging. 2022. https://www.nia.nih.gov/health/what-are-clinical-trials-and-studies. Accessed 15 Sep 2022.
2. Ray S, Fitzpatrick S, Golubic R, Fisher S, curatori. Oxford handbook of clinical and healthcare research. 1st ed. Oxford: Oxford University Press; 2016. p. 580. (Oxford medical handbooks).
3. Mouton C. Clinical Research Tool Kit. ESSKA; 2018.
4. Chung KC, Song JW. A guide on organizing a multicenter clinical trial: the WRIST Study Group. Plast Reconstr Surg. 2010;126(2):515–23.
5. Curtis BM, Barrett BJ, Parfrey PS. How to design a clinical trial. Methods Mol Med. 2003;86:475–89.
6. Evans SR. Fundamentals of clinical trial design. J Exp Stroke Transl Med. 2010;3(1):19–27.
7. European Medicines Agency. Note for Guidance on Good Clinical Practice (CPMP/ICH/135/95). London: EMEA; 2015. http://www.ema.europa.eu/docs/en_GB/document_library/Scientific_guideline/2009/09/WC500002874.pdf.
8. Banerjee A, Chitnis UB, Jadhav SL, Bhawalkar JS, Chaudhury S. Hypothesis testing, type I and type II errors. Ind Psychiatry J. 2009;18(2):127–31.

# Introduction to Surgical Trials: Adverse Events Reporting and Data and Safety Monitoring

14

Kathleen M. Poploski, Alexandra B. Gil, Charity G. Patterson, Volker Musahl, and James J. Irrgang

## 14.1 Introduction

Most clinical trials assess efficacy and effectiveness outcomes with few specifically designed to assess potential harms [1]. Reporting on potential harms is necessary to evaluate the safety of procedures, devices, and other interventions and balance harms with the potential benefits [2]. Assessing harms can be challenging due to confusing and inconsistent terminology, variability in patient populations and settings, and varying methods of ascertainment across research studies or study sites. To best overcome such barriers and protect study participants, safety should be prioritized during each stage of study planning, conduct, analysis, and reporting.

K. M. Poploski (✉) · A. B. Gil · C. G. Patterson
Department of Physical Therapy, School of Health and Rehabilitation Sciences, University of Pittsburgh, Pittsburgh, PA, USA
e-mail: kmp174@pitt.edu; agil@pitt.edu; cgp22@pitt.edu

V. Musahl
Department of Orthopaedic Surgery, UPMC Freddie Fu Sports Medicine Center, University of Pittsburgh, Pittsburgh, PA, USA
e-mail: musahlv@upmc.edu

J. J. Irrgang
Department of Physical Therapy, School of Health and Rehabilitation Sciences, University of Pittsburgh, Pittsburgh, PA, USA

Department of Orthopaedic Surgery, UPMC Freddie Fu Sports Medicine Center, University of Pittsburgh, Pittsburgh, PA, USA
e-mail: jirrgang@pitt.edu

### 14.1.1 Adverse Events

Several terms are used to define harms (adverse events, adverse reactions, adverse effects, complications, incidents, side effects), but many regulatory bodies, including the Office for Human Research Protections (OHRP)/Department of Health and Human Services (DHSS), the FDA (Food and Drug Administration), IRB (Institutional Review Board), ClinicalTrials.gov, and sponsor/funding agencies, mandate monitoring and reporting of **adverse events (AEs)**. Definitions of adverse event vary across government and non-government entities and often focus on drug or medical device interventions. Information specific to adverse events in drug or device trials is available in other resources [3].

The OHRP's definition of adverse events, modified from the 1996 International Conference on Harmonization (ICH) E-6 Guidelines for Good Clinical Practice definition, is applicable to surgical trials:

**An adverse event** is "any untoward or unfavorable medical occurrence in a human subject, including any abnormal sign (for example, abnormal physical exam or laboratory finding), symptom, or disease, temporally associated with the subject's participation in the research, whether or


S. Lyman et al. (eds.), *Introduction to Surgical Trials*,
https://doi.org/10.1007/978-3-031-77563-5_14

not considered related to the subject's participation in the research" (modified from the definition of adverse events in the 1996 International Conference on Harmonization E-6 Guidelines for Good Clinical Practice) [4].

Adapted from an outline by Liu and Davis [3], an adverse event may be:

- Physical sign or symptom.
- Abnormal laboratory values.
- Change in vital signs, physical examination, imaging, or test.
- An increase in the severity or frequency of a pre-existing symptom or condition.
- Complications from surgery or procedure.
- Device malfunction or failure.
- Device user error.
- Psychological event.

AEs are not:

- Procedures or surgeries (the medical condition that caused the need for the procedure or surgery is the AE).
- Pre-existing events or illnesses that do not worsen during the study period [3].

### 14.1.2 Serious Adverse Event

An adverse event is considered a **serious adverse event (SAE)** if it meets one or more of the following criteria:

- Results in death.
- Is life-threatening (places the subject at immediate risk of death from the event as it occurred).
- Results inpatient hospitalization or prolongation of existing hospitalization.
- Results in a persistent or significant disability/incapacity.
- Results in a congenital anomaly/birth defect.

An important medical event that may not result in death, be life-threatening, or require hospitalization may be considered an SAE when, based upon appropriate medical judgment, the event may jeopardize the subject and may require medical or surgical intervention to prevent one of the outcomes listed in the above definition.

(Modified from the definition of serious adverse drug experience in FDA regulations at 21 CFR 312.32(a).)

## 14.2 Recording/Documenting Adverse Events

During study planning, all anticipated or potential adverse events should be outlined in the protocol and informed consent form based on existing literature to date. This should include all potential complications that may occur as a result of the surgical procedure, including those that are discussed as potential risks associated with the surgical procedure during the surgical consent process. In planning the study, the expected frequency of each of these expected adverse events should be specified based on a review of the literature and/or experience of the surgeon. Documentation of AEs should include timing, severity, relationship to study intervention, and expectedness. *All* adverse events must be recorded throughout the study regardless of these factors.

Standardized terminology and case report forms should be used for documenting AEs. The National Institute of Neurological Disorders and Stroke (NINDS) of the National Institute of Health (NIH) has developed the Common Data Element (CDE) Project to standardize and streamline data sharing across the neuroscience research community [5]. One sub-domain of the project includes standardized adverse events data elements, which are also applicable to surgical trials and can be used to guide documentation (Appendix) [6].

### 14.2.1 Defining Adverse Events

As with any primary or secondary outcome, expected adverse events specific to the patient population/intervention should be identified and defined during study planning. The use of clear and consistent adverse event definitions is particularly important in multi-center trials as different investigators or institutions may use highly variable language for recording events in clinical practice.

There are both passive and active methods for ascertaining AEs. Often, clinicians may identify AEs based upon observations during examination, test results, or from patient-reported symptoms or events such as falls. Standardized, active methods of surveying participants and clinicians for potential AEs at regular time points should also be considered. Patients and clinicians can complete a yes/no checklist of expected AEs based on previous studies, even if the events are rare. Such methods provide consistency and may promote recall, though some suggest being too specific can bias participants [3]. If interviewing a participant, the clinician/researcher could simply check those items that were endorsed as having occurred rather than listing all items, which could prompt participants to over-report. Systematic use of more open-ended questions such as "Have you had any changes in your medical history since your last visit" allows for identification of unexpected AEs. The method of collecting AEs (checklist vs. open-ended question) can influence reporting [7], so investigators should carefully consider which method or combinations of methods are most appropriate for their study.

Use of established classification and naming systems such as the Medical Directory for Regulatory Activities (MedDRA) or the National Cancer Institute (NCI) Common Terminology Criteria for Adverse Events (CTCAE) should be considered for AE documentation and reporting (Box 14.1). Such terminologies improve consistency across investigators and sites, make reporting easier for clinicatrials.gov, and allow comparison across studies. Standardized classifications also reduce the possibility of missing safety concerns due to different terminologies being used for similar AEs. Researchers should be aware that some AEs associated with orthopedic procedures are not included in the taxonomies for these classification systems and broader or related terms may need to be used. For example, there is no specific CTCAE term for ligament injury. If a participant sustained a medial collateral ligament injury during the study, a broader categorization such as "Musculoskeletal and connective disorder – Other, specify)" may need to be used. The lack of standardized classification specific to orthopedic procedures highlights the need for review and adjudication of all AE documentation (see Sect. 14.5). Acknowledgment of ill-defined AEs or AEs that were not prespecified should be stated in any publications [8].

**Box 14.1 Example Adverse Events Classifications**

- **Medical Dictionary for Regulatory Activities (MedDRA)** is a standardized medical terminology designed for use in registration, documentation, and safety monitoring of medical products developed by the International Conference on Harmonization [9]. Its hierarchical structure includes terms for signs, symptoms, diseases, diagnoses, procedures, and others [8].
- **Common Terminology Criteria for Adverse Events (CTCAE)** is a descriptive terminology and severity grading scale that can be used for AE reporting. It uses some elements of MedDRA [10].

For most studies, recording a*ll "untoward medical occurrences"* throughout the study is necessary to prevent unrecognized bias in adverse event reporting. While investigators may be concerned with overburdening clinicians or inflating the number of adverse events, documenting all adverse events is the only way to determine if an event is truly related or unrelated to the study procedures. Alternatively, in certain populations, such as critically ill patients, compromises may need to be made as to what is deemed an adverse event. It may be appropriate for only serious adverse events to be documented as reporting all adverse events may lead to excessive reporting and workload with little useful safety information in such populations. A surgical trial of congenital heart disease in pediatric patients transitioned from reporting all adverse events to using sentinel events for safety reporting for this reason [11]. The Joint Commission on Accreditation of Healthcare Organizations defines sentinel events as a patient safety event that results in death, permanent harm, or severe, temporary harm [12]. The change from adverse event reporting to only sentinel events allowed the investigators to identify patients at highest risk while decreasing reporting variability and administrative burden. The authors recommend that such methods be used in other surgical or device trials and with critically ill populations [11].

There may be adverse events defined in the protocol that may not meet a clinician investigator's definition of clinical significance [3]. For instance, joint stiffness/limited range of motion after knee ligament surgery in the first 6–12 weeks after surgery or pain upon progression of rehabilitation may be fairly common during the recovery process after orthopedic surgery but should be reported as AEs in a clinical trial to ensure there are no differences between groups or that rates are consistent with expectations.

When comparing to other studies or standard care, the influence of any additional testing for study procedures should be recognized. For example, in a randomized controlled trial comparing single-bundle vs. double-bundle ACL reconstruction using quadriceps tendon autograft, helical computed tomography (CT) was performed 6 months after surgery [13]. The CT scan was part of the research protocol to create 3D models to assess knee joint kinematics. From these scans, two patients were identified to have patellar fractures. As both patients were asymptomatic and progressing through rehabilitation as expected, these fractures likely would have gone undetected under standard clinical care.

### 14.2.2 Timing of Follow-Ups and AE Monitoring

Timing of active AE data collection should also be considered relative to the occurrence of the intervention, length of the follow-up, and other major time points for data collection. For example, the frequency of systematic AE surveillance timepoints and tests could be at clinical visits at 1 week, 1 month, 3 months, 6 months, and 12 months post-surgery. Longer follow-ups allow for increased opportunities to identify adverse events, particularly rare AEs. Many AEs, such as anterior cruciate ligament graft rupture or the development of post-traumatic knee osteoarthritis, would be less common until months or years after the intervention when a patient returns to higher-level activities.

Importantly, AEs occur and can be reported by the participant at any time throughout the study, not only during pre-defined clinical visit timepoints. For instance, the patient or a family member may contact the surgeon after a fall or schedule a for-cause appointment due to increased pain. These AEs must be recorded in an electronic AE form that is not tied to a specific time point (i.e., an event-driven electronic case report form).

The onset and duration of AE (start and stop dates/times) should be recorded as accurately as possible. The incidence of AEs can then be summarized across the duration of follow-up, relative to the timing of the intervention, or at specific time increments. Any treatments provided or changes to the study procedure due to an AE should be documented in a standardized manner [8] (see Box 14.2—Actions Taken with Study Procedure and Other Actions Taken) and with detailed descriptions. AEs that persist from one visit to the next should be documented as one AE and status updated accordingly (Box 14.2—

Outcome Status). The study protocol should state the timeframe for following reported events. Common practice is to follow a patient until the AE has resolved or stabilized or 30 days after the participant's involvement in the study has ended, whichever occurs first [14].

**Box 14.2 Examples of Additional Information to Collect on AEs [6, 15]**

| Actions taken with study procedure | Other actions taken[a] | Outcome status |
|---|---|---|
| • None | • None | • Recovered/resolved |
| • Study intervention interrupted | • Treatment given | • Recovered/resolved with sequelae |
| • Study intervention discontinued | • Discontinued from study | • Recovering/resolving |
| • Study intervention modified | • Hospitalized | • Not recovered/not resolved |
| | | • Fatal |
| | | • Unknown or lost to follow-up |

[a]Other Actions Taken: Categories may need to be tailored to study as shown here. If using NINDS Common Data Elements, 2 categories are included (None, Non-study Treatment Required) [6]

### 14.2.3 Severity

The severity of the AE should be graded based upon input from both the patient and clinician at the point of care whenever possible. There is no universally accepted scale for classifying AE severity, however, the CTCAE includes a 5-level grading scale [10]. Intensity should be graded at its most severe presentation.

- **Grade 1** Mild; asymptomatic or mild symptoms; clinical or diagnostic observations only; intervention not indicated.
- **Grade 2** Moderate; minimal, local, or noninvasive intervention indicated, limiting age-appropriate activities of daily living.
- **Grade 3** Severe or medically significant but not immediately life-threatening; hospitalization or prolongation of hospitalization indicated; disabling; limiting self-care activities of daily living.
- **Grade 4** Life-threatening consequences; urgent intervention indicated.
- **Grade 5** Death related to AE.

Pre-defined grading scales such as the CTCAE improve the consistency of grading, but both participants and clinicians may have varying perceptions of severity. Therefore, other measures such as frequency, duration, and recurrence of AEs can also be used to quantify severity. Constant knee pain lasting for 1 month is likely more severe than intermittent pain 1–2 times per week. Attention to patients who discontinued or withdrew from the trial, were non-adherent, or were lost to follow-up may provide additional insight to patient tolerance of applicable treatments and severity of AEs [16].

It is important to note the difference in the severity and seriousness of an adverse event. Severity defines the intensity of the event, while seriousness refers to the threat to the patient's life or function [14]. For example, loss of joint motion following anterior cruciate ligament reconstruction could be classified as severe without being serious if it was resolved through physical therapy management. If manipulation under anesthesia and/or arthroscopic lysis of adhesions was needed to recover range of motion and prevent permanent impaired motion and disability, the event would be classified as a serious adverse event.

### 14.2.4 Relatedness to Study Procedures

Adverse events may or may not be related to the study intervention or study participation. An AE could be related to research procedures, underlying disease, disorder or patient condition, or other circumstances unrelated to the study or patient condition [4]. If the AE is determined to be solely caused by the disease/condition or other circumstance, then it would be classified as **unrelated** to participation in the research. If the AE is determined to be at least partially caused by the research, then it would be considered **related** to participation in the research. Determining AE relatedness can be challenging to dichotomize as related/unrelated; therefore, scales of relatedness are often used. Although there is no standard relatedness/causality scale [17], there are several commonly used. The NINDS Common Data Elements and ICH guidelines reference categories are outlined in Box 14.3 [15]. The World Health Organization-The Uppsala Monitoring Centre (WHO-UMC) system is a tool for classifying adverse drug reactions but could also be adapted for describing relatedness of AEs for surgical trials [18].

There are several factors to consider when assessing relatedness of the AE to study procedures, including timing between intervention and AE, plausibility based upon signs, symptoms, tests, and mechanism, current knowledge of associated AEs, and exclusion of other causes [17, 19]. Though likely less applicable for surgical trials, for other interventions such as medications or treatments, discontinuation of the intervention to determine if the AE resolves, and reintroduction of the intervention to determine if the AE recurs, may provide additional information on relatedness if appropriate [17].

In surgical trials, it is important to carefully consider whether an AE is related to the study intervention or surgery itself. Consider the Surgical Timing and Rehabilitation (STaR) for Multiple Ligament Knee Injuries trial [20]. The goal of the study is to compare the effects of early versus delayed surgery and early versus delayed postoperative rehabilitation for the treatment of multiple ligament knee injuries. The intervention is the *timing* of surgery and rehabilitation, not the surgery or postoperative rehabilitation itself. A patient may present with painful hardware after surgery, an AE related to the surgery but unlikely to be related to the timing of when surgery is performed. Conversely, postoperative joint stiffness/limited range of motion may be related to the timing of surgery and postoperative rehabilitation. While there is a lack of level 1 evidence currently, some may hypothesize that early surgery, while the knee is still actively inflamed, or the delayed start of postoperative rehabilitation may increase the risk of postoperative joint stiffness/limited range of motion.

**Box 14.3 Examples of Relatedness/Causality Scales**

| NINDS Common Data Elements [21] | ICH E2B | WHO-UMC |
|---|---|---|
| • Unrelated | • Unrelated | • Unlikely |
| • Unlikely | • Unlikely related | • Possible |
| • Reasonable possibility | • Possibly related | • Probably/likely |
| • Definite | • Probably related | • Certain |
| | • Definitely related | • Conditional/unclassified |

### 14.2.5 Expectedness

Significant time, research, and clinical expertise must be dedicated to determining AEs that are expected during the study. AEs are considered unexpected if they are not listed in the study protocol or informed consent document or are not identified prior to the start of the study in terms of nature, severity, or frequency of the event in protocol-related documents taking into account the characteristics of the subject population being studied [14].

**Box 14.4 Characteristics of Adverse Events to Consider in Planning/Reporting**

- Timing.
- Severity including frequency, duration, changes to protocol.
- Relatedness to study protocol.
- Expectedness.

## 14.3 Unanticipated Problems

OHRP defines an unanticipated problem (UAP) as any incident, experience, or outcome that meets all of the following criteria:

1. Unexpected (in terms of nature, severity, or frequency) given (a) the research procedures that are described in the protocol-related documents, such as the IRB-approved research protocol and informed consent document; and (b) the characteristics of the subject population being studied;
2. Related or possibly related to participation in the research (in this guidance document, possibly related means there is a reasonable possibility that the incident, experience, or outcome may have been caused by the procedures involved in the research); and
3. Suggests that the research places subjects or others at a greater risk of harm (including physical, psychological, economic, or social harm) than was previously known or recognized [4].

**Box 14.5 Unanticipated Problems**

If the answer is YES to all three questions, then the event would be considered an unanticipated problem:

1. Is the event unexpected in nature, severity, or frequency?
2. Is the event related or possibly related to participation in the research study?
3. Does the event suggest that the research places subjects or others at a greater risk of physical or psychological harm than was previously known or recognized? Note: If the adverse event is serious, the answer is always YES.

Questions adapted from OHRP flowchart [4].

Only a small subset of AEs meets all three criteria and are also considered UAPs. There are also UAPs that are not classified as AEs, such as a data breach. UAPs may lead to significant changes to the study protocol, monitoring, and/or informed consent, require disclosure to currently enrolled participants, or suspension of the study.

**Case Examples: Adverse Events and Unanticipated Problems**

Consider a surgical trial comparing quadriceps tendon autograft with or without a bone block to bone patellar tendon bone autograft for ACL reconstruction on the incidence of ACL clinical failure in young active individuals at high risk for re-injury.

**Case 1:** At the 3-month postoperative follow-up visit, an 18-year-old male patient presents with effusion in the surgical knee. After evaluation, the surgeon-investigator decides that intervention is needed and aspirates 41 cc of clear fluid. Lab test results on the fluid come back within normal ranges, and effusion resolves within 1 week. This is the fourth reported case of joint effusion in the study of 100 patients, below the expected frequency.

1. **Is this an AE?** Yes, persistent joint effusion at 3-month clinical visit after ACLR is an abnormal (though expected) finding.
2. **Is this a Serious AE?** No, joint effusion with no other abnormal findings does not meet one or more of the criteria for SAE.
3. **Is this an Unanticipated problem? (Yes, if answer yes to all 3 of the following questions)** No, as the answer is “no” to the following questions.
   (a) **Is this event related to or possibly related to participation in the research?** No. While the effusion is likely related to the surgery, it is unlikely related to the use of a patellar or quadriceps tendon autograft (study intervention).
   (b) **Is this an unexpected event in nature, severity, or frequency?** No, joint effusion is common after ACL reconstruction and the overall reported frequency is below the expected rate. The effusion resolved soon after aspiration of fluid.
   (c) **Does the event suggest that the research places subjects or others at a greater risk of physical or psychological harm than was previously known or recognized? Note: If the adverse event is serious, the answer is always YES.** No, no abnormal findings were found from

lab results, and effusion resolved after aspiration.

**Case 2**: At 6-month postoperative follow-up visit, a 21-year-old female patient presents with persistent severe pain secondary to retained tibial fixation hardware impacting self-care ADLs. The patient undergoes surgery to remove the hardware, recovers, and pain subsides. This is the first reported case of painful hardware in the study and is below the expected frequency.

1. **Is this an AE?** Yes, painful hardware is a complication of ACL reconstruction.
2. **Is this a Serious AE?** Yes, this AE required surgical intervention to prevent persistent or significant disability/ incapacity.
3. **Is this an Unanticipated problem? (Yes, if answer yes to all 3 of the following questions)** No, as the answer is "YES" to only 2 of the 3 questions/criteria below.
   (a) **Is this event related to or possibly related to participation in the research?** No, painful fixation should not be related to the use of either a quad or patellar tendon.
   (b) **Is this an unexpected event in nature, severity, or frequency?** Yes, although painful hardware is an expected postoperative complication of ACL reconstruction, the severity of the pain and impact on the participant's ability to perform self-care ADLs is unexpected.
   (c) **Does the event suggest that the research places subjects or others at a greater risk of physical or psychological harm than was previously known or recognized? Note: If the adverse event is serious, the answer is always YES.** Yes, as per OHRP Guidelines, when an adverse event is serious, the answer to this question is always YES. This is a serious adverse event because, based on appropriate medical judgment, surgical intervention was required to prevent persistent or significant disability/incapacity.

**Case 3**: At 6-month postoperative follow-up visit, a 17-year-old male who received a quadriceps tendon graft with bone block felt a pop during maximal isometric quadriceps strength testing. The individual immediately felt pain anteriorly over the patella. Imaging showed an oblique, nondisplaced patellar fracture of the superior pole of the patella. The fracture was treated non-operatively with immobilization in full extension for 8 weeks. This was the third case in the study of 100 participants. The expected rate of patellar fractures was 2% or less.

1. **Is this an AE?** Yes, a patellar fracture is a complication from the ACL surgery.
2. **Is this a Serious AE?** Yes, this AE requires medical intervention to prevent persistent or significant disability/ incapacity.
3. **Is this an Unanticipated Problem?** Yes, as the answer is "Yes" to all 3 of the following questions.
   (a) **Is this event related to or possibly related to participation in the research?** Yes, the participant could have been randomized to receive a quadriceps tendon autograft with bone block or bone patellar tendon bone autograft, either of which may have weakened the structure of the patella and led to the patellar fracture.
   (b) **Is this an unexpected event in nature, severity, or frequency?** Yes, this was the third individual to experience a patellar fracture in the study, higher than the 2% expected rate of patellar fracture.
   (c) **Does the event suggest that the research places subjects or others at a greater risk of physical or psychological harm than was previously known or recognized? Note: If the adverse event is serious, the answer is always YES**. Yes, this event, in conjunction with the other observed patellar fractures, suggests that the risk of patellar fracture is higher than previously expected after ACL reconstruction using a quadriceps or patellar tendon autograft.

## 14.4 Training

Investment in pre-trial and ongoing training for clinicians and research staff is paramount for preventing erroneous data collection or significant burden rectifying adverse event data at the end of the trial. The study Manual of Operating Procedures (MOOP) should provide guidelines for documenting AEs/SAEs. It can also be helpful to have a "cheat sheet" of the most common events or diagnoses. Weekly local meetings and monthly meetings across sites for multi-center studies to discuss data quality, including documentation of AEs and continued training throughout the study, will help to ensure consistency in recognizing, recording, and reporting AEs. All decisions regarding AEs should be documented for easy reference by study personnel.

## 14.5 Adverse Event Adjudication

Adverse events are initially assessed by the treating clinician with input from the patient; however, concerns over inconsistencies and investigator biases in determining specific AE elements suggest the need for independent review of adverse events. In a spinal device surgical trial, an independent committee reclassified the level of severity, relation to surgery, and/or relation to the device in 37.3% of adverse events, with the majority of reclassifications being upgrades in the level of severity or relatedness to the surgery or device [22]. Thus, systematic, unbiased, and independent assessment of event terms, severity, relatedness, seriousness, and expectedness is recommended.

A two-level AE adjudication and review process is proposed. At the first level, an Internal Adjudication Committee, comprised of at least three members of the study team, reviews each event and votes to determine if any changes to event term, severity, relatedness, seriousness, and expectedness are needed. Second-level review is then completed by an External Adjudication Committee, composed of members unaffiliated with the study. Once events have been discussed, amended as necessary, and approved by the external committee, the final classification and status of the AE are recorded. Rationale for all decisions should also be documented. When possible, all parties involved in determining and reviewing relatedness should be blinded to treatment group [16]. The frequency of changes to AE documentation should be monitored, and additional training on AE documentation provided as necessary.

## 14.6 Responsibilities for Reporting

Investigators must be compliant with all applicable institutional, sponsor/funding agency, and federal regulations (OHRP, FDA, etc.) for reporting AEs and UAPs, including the timeframes for reporting. These regulations can be complicated and often vary by organization. The U.S. Code of Federal Regulations (CFR) requires investigators to have written procedures and to promptly report to the IRB, appropriate institutional officials, and the Food and Drug Administration any "unanticipated problems involving risks to subjects or others..." [21 CFR 56.108(b)(1), 21 CFR 312.53(c)(1)(vii), 21 CFR 312.66, and 45 CFR 46.103(b)(5)]. ICH Section 4.11 requires "all serious adverse events should be reported immediately. .. except those that are designated in the protocol or investigator brochure as not needing reporting immediately."

Investigators should work with the research office at their institution and sponsor to understand all applicable regulations for reporting AEs and UAPs. Typically, procedures for identifying, monitoring, and reporting AEs and UAPs must be described in a data and safety monitoring plan (DSMP) and approved by the study's IRB and sponsor. Individual AE/UAP and summary reports should be provided to the IRB regularly as outlined in the DSMP. Generally, investigators report UAPs to the sponsor, DSMB, and IRB. From there, the IRB reports the events to appropriate institutional parties who report the UAPs to OHRP [3]. Similar reporting may be required for AEs.

Some SAEs and UAPs may require expedited reporting, with varying timeframe requirements by regulatory body [23]. These should be defined during study planning and typically include unexpected SAEs determined to be related to the study. Additional documentation for expedited reporting may include detailed description of the event, medical history, laboratory and diagnostic test results, medications, treatment, and outcome as applicable [3].

Multi-center trials require additional considerations for safety monitoring and reporting. As of January 2020, both the NIH and DHSS require the use of a single IRB (sIRB) of record for multi-site studies that are implementing the same protocol to streamline the IRB review process [24]. Reliance agreements are made between institutions allowing the IRB of one institution to rely on the IRB of another institution (IRB of record) for review of human subjects' research. For multi-center trials, recording and reporting of all events is particularly important. An event may appear isolated and unrelated to the trial to an investigator at one site but might be part of a developing pattern of events across sites [3].

Details of Regulatory Standards are covered in detail in Part VI of this book: Chaps. 19, 20 and 21.

## 14.7 Monitoring

Study monitoring should be consistent with the risks of the study, vulnerability of the study population, size and complexity of the trial, and policies of the study sponsor. Studies often require multiple levels of safety monitoring, but all studies must have local monitoring. The study protocol must specify that the site PI and study team will monitor study implementation, recruitment, intervention, data integrity, safety, visit completeness, withdrawals, and any external issues impacting the study on a regular basis. In addition, multi-center trials may have central monitoring by the coordinating center and independent monitoring by an outside committee. An independent group, known as the Data Monitoring Committee (DMC) or Data and Safety Monitoring Board (DSMB), is needed because study teams have an inherent conflict of interest. The DMC/DSMB, as outlined by Ellenberg et al., has three primary responsibilities:

1. "Safeguard the interest of the study participants.
2. Preserve the integrity and credibility of the trial in order that future patients may be treated optimally.
3. Ensure that definitive and reliable results be available in a timely way to the medical community" [25].

Specifically, these data and safety monitoring committees may review study protocol for feasibility and safety, monitor adherence to study procedures, intervention implementation, and participant recruitment, assess safety of outcomes through review of AEs and UAPs, and review data quality and completeness, all to ensure participants in the trial are not unduly harmed and that study results are of high quality and integrity (Table 14.1) [26, 27]. Interim reports reviewed by the committee in a closed session (i.e., without the investigators present to maintain blinding of the investigators) typically identify intervention groups as randomized (unblinded) to ensure appropriate safety recommendations can be made. The committee may be advisory to the investigator, IRB or ethics committee, sponsor of the trial, and regulatory agencies [8].

The DSMB should be a multidisciplinary team of at least three members, often clinical and scientific experts in the field, biostatisticians, epidemiologists, bioethicists, basic scientists, and patient advocates as appropriate [8, 25]. These individuals should have expertise in the field but be independent of institutional, financial, intellectual, professional, or regulatory conflicts of interest [25].

Frequency of committee meetings depends on a number of factors, but for longer-term clinical trials, committees typically meet every 4–6 months or when specific percentages of the primary outcome have been collected (i.e., 10%, 25%, 50%, 75%, 100%) [8]. Meetings entail open sessions with the study team and closed sessions for only the DSMB members, an executive secretary, and an unblinded study statistician. Reports are provided to the board typically 10–14 days prior to the meeting containing

**Table 14.1** Responsibilities of Data Monitoring Committees

| Responsibility | Frequency |
|---|---|
| Review of protocol | Often |
| Approval of protocol | Sometimes |
| Assessment of adequacy of recruitment progress | Always or almost always |
| Assessment of data quality[a] | Always or almost always |
| Assessment of safety outcomes | Always or almost always |
| Assessment of efficacy outcomes[b] | Always or almost always |
| Recommendation regarding trial continuation | Always or almost always |
| Review of trial presentations and manuscripts | Sometimes |
| Approval of presentations and manuscripts | Sometimes |



[a]The data assessed can include the dropout rate, incomplete data, and the time-liness of data

[b]Assessment of efficacy outcomes can be a risk–benefit analysis as well as a consideration of early termination on the basis of efficacy

information on recruitment, enrollment, patient characteristics, visit completeness, adverse events, and protocol deviations. Individual adverse events may be monitored by the committee chairperson or an appointed safety officer, with the authority to convene the entire committee as needed [26]. As the committee reviews the treatment group data multiple times, there can be concerns for repeated testing for significance. This issue should be considered during study planning and data monitoring, but participant safety is paramount [26]. Many resources dedicated solely to the roles and responsibilities of DMC/DSMBs are available for reference [25, 28–30].

Each level of monitoring has a responsibility to ensure patient safety. An appropriate course of action should be determined by reviewing individual and aggregate AE data (Box 14.6). Often, no action will be required. Other times, changes to the study protocol such as adding tests for safety or amendments to the participant consent form may be appropriate. If new potential risks are identified, current participants should be notified. Study suspension or termination of the entire trial for a specific subgroup of patients or one arm of a multi-arm study may be necessary if significant safety concerns arise. For example, enrollment in a surgical trial of single- versus double-bundle ACL reconstruction was terminated by the DSMB due to five patellar fractures related to the harvest of the patellar bone plug [13, 31]. A study may also be terminated due to overwhelming benefit-to-risk, or if there is little or no chance the study question can be answered due to poor recruitment, compliance, or other recently published findings [26].

**Box 14.6 Potential Actions/Changes Due to AE/ UAP**

- No action required.
- Amend protocol.
- Amend consent document.
- Inform current participants.
- Terminate or suspend protocol.
- Extension of trial.
- Other.

## 14.8 Reporting in Literature and Clinicaltrial.Gov

Reporting of adverse events in dissemination of results is described by the CONSORT (Consolidated Standards of Reporting Trials) Statement and is required by clinicaltrials.gov. The CONSORT Statement (see Chap. 18) is a checklist of essential items created to improve transparency and consistency in reporting randomized controlled trials in the literature [16]. The importance of reporting harms is underscored by two items on the CONSORT 2010 Statement with additional reference to the CONSORT extension "Better Reporting of Harms in Randomized Trials " [21]. The extension is a 10-item checklist that includes specific recommendations for proper reporting of harms in randomized controlled trials [21]. Harms are defined as "the totality of possible adverse consequences of an intervention or therapy; they are the direct opposite of benefits, against which they must be compared" [21]. Recommendations specific to harms reporting are outlined for each section of a manuscript, including defining AEs that were addressed, clarifying how harms were collected, describing analysis of harms and participant withdrawals due to harms, and providing a balanced discussion of benefits and harms. For ClinicalTrials.gov, a tabular summary of serious adverse events and adverse events exceeding a specified frequency threshold is required. A checklist and templates for reporting at provided at ClinicaTrials.gov.

## 14.9 Conclusion

In surgical trials, safety monitoring should be prioritized during each stage of the study to ensure potential benefits outweigh harms to patients. Many regulatory bodies require reporting of adverse events (AEs), serious adverse events (SAEs), and unanticipated problems (UAPs). Potential AEs and SAEs should be carefully identified and outlined in study documents using established classification and naming systems. Documentation of AEs should include timing, severity, expectedness, and relationship to study intervention. Regular training and meetings of study personnel to discuss safety monitoring procedures ensures consistent reporting and minimizes risk of unrecognized harm to patients. Internal and external safety monitoring mechanisms, including Data Monitoring Committees or Data and Safety Monitoring Boards, should also be implemented. Investigators can work with the research office at their institution and sponsor to understand all applicable regulations for reporting events and utilize guidance from the CONSORT (Consolidated Standards of Reporting Trials) Statement and ClinicalTrials.gov for dissemination of safety findings.

## Appendix: Adverse Event Form Example

**STUDY NAME**

| | |
|---|---|
| **Visit Date:** ____________________<br>**Site ID:** ____________________<br>**Participant ID:** ____________________ | **Type of report:**<br>☐ Initial report<br>☐ Follow-up report<br>☐ Final report |

**Record diagnoses (if known) or signs/symptoms the participant experienced during the study that qualify as adverse events.**

| Adverse Event | Severity | Date and Time of Onset | Date of Resolution | Relatedness to Study Procedures | Action Taken with Study Procedure | Other Action Taken[1] | Outcome Status | Unexpected event?[2] | Serious Adverse event?[3] |
|---|---|---|---|---|---|---|---|---|---|
| | ☐ Mild<br>☐ Moderate<br>☐ Severe<br>☐ Life-threatening/ Disabling<br>☐ Death | | ☐ Ongoing | ☐ Unrelated<br>☐ Unlikely<br>☐ Reasonable<br>☐ Possibility Definite | ☐ None<br>☐ Study intervention interrupted<br>☐ Study intervention discontinued<br>☐ Study intervention modified | ☐ None<br>☐ Treatment given (describe)<br>☐ Discontinued from study<br>☐ Hospitalized | ☐ Recovered/ resolved<br>☐ Recovered/ resolved with sequelae<br>☐ Recovering/ resolving<br>☐ Not recovered/ not resolved<br>☐ Fatal<br>☐ Unknow or lost to follow-up | ☐ No<br>☐ Yes | ☐ No<br>☐ Yes* |

| **Additional information for serious adverse event** | |
|---|---|
| **Outcome of the serious adverse event (check all that apply):** | |
| ☐ Death | ☐ Congenital anomaly/birth defect |
| ☐ Life-threatening | ☐ Required intervention to prevent permanent impairment |
| ☐ Hospitalization-initial or prolonged | ☐ Disability/incapacity |
| ☐ Other: | |

[1] Other Actions Taken: Categories may need to be tailored to study as shown here. If using NINDS Common Data Elements, 2 categories are included (None, Non-study Treatment Required)
[2] Unexpected: "Yes" should be answered for adverse events that are not listed in the protocol or informed consent, or not identified prior to the start of the study in terms of nature, severity, or frequency of the event in protocol related documents taking into account the characteristics of the subject population
[3] Serious: "Yes" should be answered when the adverse event results in death, is life-threatening, requires in-patient hospitalization or prolongation of existing hospitalization, results in persistent or significant disability/incapacity, or is a congenital anomaly/birth defect.

**Brief description of the nature of the (serious) adverse event. If applicable, include relevant tests, laboratory data, concomitant medications, and history:**

Signature of Principal Investigator: ____________________ Date: ____________________

## References


1. Huang HY, Andrews E, Jones J, Skovron ML, Tilson H. Pitfalls in meta-analyses on adverse events reported from clinical trials. Pharmacoepidemiol Drug Saf. 2011;20(10):1014–20.
2. Goldhahn S, Sawaguchi T, Audigé L, Mundi R, Hanson B, Bhandari M, et al. Complication reporting in orthopaedic trials: a systematic review of randomized controlled trials. J Bone Joint Surg Am. 2009;91(8):1847–53.
3. Lui MB, Davis K. A clinical trials manual from the Duke Clinical Research Institute. Lessons from a horse named Jim. 2nd ed. Hoboken, NJ: Wiley-Blackwell; 2013.
4. U.S. Department of Health and Human Services: Office for Human Research Protections. Reviewing and Reporting Unanticipated Problems Involving Risks to Subjects or Others and Adverse Events: OHRP Guidance (2007). https://www.hhs.gov/ohrp/regulations-and-policy/guidance/reviewing-unanticipated-problems/index.html#:~:text=Adverse%20event%3A%20Any%20untoward%20or,considered%20related%20to%20the%20subject's. Accessed 22 Dec 2021.
5. NINDS Common Data Elements https://www.commondataelements.ninds.nih.gov/. Accessed 29 Dec 2021.
6. NINDS Common Data Elements. Adverse Events Detailed Report. https://www.commondataelements.ninds.nih.gov/cde_detailed_report/22914/

Adverse%20Events/Safety%20Data/General%20%28For%20all%20diseases%29/Adverse%20Events. Accessed 29 Dec 2021.

7. Wallin J, Sjövall J. Detection of adverse drug reactions in a clinical trial using two types of questioning. Clin Ther. 1981;3(6):450–2.
8. Friedman LM, Furberg CD, DeMets DL. Fundamentals of clinical trials. 4th ed. New York: Springer; 2010.
9. MedDRA: Medical Dictionary for Regulatory Activities. https://www.meddra.org/how-to-use/support-documentation/english/welcome. Accessed 22 Dec 2021.
10. U.S. Department Of Health And Human Services, National Institutes of Health and National Cancer Institute. Common Terminology Criteria for Adverse Events (CTCAE) Version 5.0. https://ctep.cancer.gov/protocoldevelopment/electronic_applications/ctc.htm#ctc_60. Accessed 22 Dec 2021.
11. Virzi L, Pemberton V, Ohye RG, Tabbutt S, Lu M, Atz TC, et al. Reporting adverse events in a surgical trial for complex congenital heart disease: the pediatric heart network experience. J Thorac Cardiovasc Surg. 2011;142(3):531–7. https://doi.org/10.1016/j.jtcvs.2010.11.052.
12. The joint commission. Sentinel Event Alert. https://www.jointcommission.org/en/resources/patient-safety-topics/sentinel-event/. Accessed 22 Dec 2021.
13. Fu FH, Rabuck SJ, West RV, Tashman S, Irrgang JJ. Patellar fractures after the harvest of a quadriceps tendon autograft with a bone block: a case series. Orthop J Sports Med. 2019;7(3):2325967119829051. https://doi.org/10.1177/2325967119829051.
14. National Drug Abuse Treatment Clinical Trials Network. Good clinical practice: patient safety and adverse events module. https://gcp.nidatraining.org/. Accessed 22 Dec 2021.
15. ICH Harmonised Tripartite Guideline. Maintenance Of The ICH Guideline On Clinical Safety Data Management: Data Elements For Transmission Of Individual Case Safety Reports E2b(R2). https://admin.ich.org/sites/default/files/inline-files/E2B_R2_Guideline.pdf. Accessed 22 Dec 2021.
16. Moher D, Hopewell S, Schulz KF, Montori V, Gøtzsche PC, Devereaux P, et al. CONSORT 2010 explanation and elaboration: updated guidelines for reporting parallel group randomised trials. Int J Surg. 2012;10(1):28–55.
17. Gliklich RE, Dreyer NA, Leavy MB, editors. Registries for evaluating patient outcomes: a User's guide. (Prepared by Outcome DEcIDE Center [Outcome Sciences, Inc. dba Outcome] under Contract No. HHSA29020050035ITO1.) AHRQ Publication No. 07-EHC001-1. 3rd ed. Rockville, MD: Agency for Healthcare Research and Quality; 2014.
18. Edwards IR, Biriell C. Harmonisation in pharmacovigilance. Drug Saf. 1994;10(2):93–102. https://doi.org/10.2165/00002018-199410020-00001.
19. World Health Organization. Safety monitoring of medicinal products: reporting system for the general public. Geneva: Switzerland; 2012.
20. National Library of Medicine (US). STaR Trial: Multiple ligament knee injuries. Identifier: NCT03543098. 2018. https://clinicaltrials.gov/ct2/show/NCT03543098. Accessed 3 Jan 2022.
21. Ioannidis JP, Evans SJ, Gøtzsche PC, et al. Better reporting of harms in randomized trials: an extension of the CONSORT statement. Ann Intern Med. 2004;141(10):781–8. https://doi.org/10.7326/0003-4819-141-10-200411160-00009.
22. Auerbach JD, McGowan KB, Halevi M, Gerling MC, Sharan AD, Whang PG, et al. Mitigating adverse event reporting bias in spine surgery. J Bone Joint Surg Am. 2013;95(16):1450–6. https://doi.org/10.2106/jbjs.L.00251.
23. NHLBI Adverse Event and Unanticipated Problem Reporting Policy. http://nhlbi.nih.gov/grants-and-training/policies-and-guidelines/nhlbi-adverse-event-and-unanticipated-problem-reporting-policy. Accessed 22 Dec 2021.
24. U.S. Department of Health & Human Services: National Institute of Health. Single IRB Policy for Multi-Site or Cooperative Research. https://grants.nih.gov/policy/humansubjects/single-irb-policy-multi-site-research.htm. Accessed 22 Dec 2021.
25. Ellenberg SF, Thomas R, DeMets DL. Data monitoring committees in clinical trials: a practical perspective Wiley encyclopedia of clinical trials. Chichester: Wiley; 2002.
26. DeMets D, Furberg C, Friedman L. Data monitoring in clinical trials: a case studies approach. New York, NY: Springer; 2006.
27. DeMets DL, Ellenberg SS. Data monitoring committees—expect the unexpected. N Engl J Med. 2016;375(14):1365–71. https://doi.org/10.1056/NEJMra1510066.
28. Herson J. Data and safety monitoring committees in clinical trials. 2nd ed. Boca Raton, FL: CRC Press; 2016.
29. Fleming TR, Ellenberg SS, DeMets DL. Data monitoring committees: current issues. Clin Trials. 2018;15(4):321–8. https://doi.org/10.1177/1740774518764855.
30. Ellenberg SS, Ellenberg JH. Proceedings of the University of Pennsylvania 10th annual conference on statistical issues in clinical trials: current issues regarding Data and safety monitoring committees in clinical trials. Clin Trials. 2018;15(4):319–20. https://doi.org/10.1177/1740774518781817.
31. Irrgang JJ, Tashman S, Patterson CG, Musahl V, West R, Oostdyk A, et al. Anatomic single vs. double-bundle ACL reconstruction: a randomized clinical trial-part 1: clinical outcomes. Knee Surg Sports Traumatol Arthrosc. 2021;29:2665. https://doi.org/10.1007/s00167-021-06585-w.

# 15 Trial Closeout

Iain R. Murray, Andrew D. Duckworth, and Marc R. Safran

## 15.1 Introduction

The closeout of a clinical trial is usually a complex process requiring careful planning [1]. Like the recruitment and implementation phase, the closeout phase of clinical trials may bring a myriad of challenges. Although the whole protocol of a clinical trial is subject to external ethical and regulatory review, the recruitment phase tends to be where most attention is focused, with trial closeout receiving less attention [2]. Although some details of the closeout period will depend on factors that only become known once the trial is underway or enrollment is completed, planning for both expected and contingency actions should nevertheless begin early.

## 15.2 Defining Trial Closeout

Study closeout concerns the termination of a study at participating sites once all subjects have completed the study. Depending upon the length of follow-up, this be a long time after the trial ceases recruiting subjects. The sponsor, funder, ethics committee, and other stakeholders should be aware of the planned end of trial date, which in most cases will be the date of the last visit of the last participant or the completion of any follow-up monitoring and data collection described in the protocol. Final data analysis and report writing is routinely commenced after formal completion of the trial. Trial closeout is defined as the act of ensuring that all research study related activities are appropriately reconciled, recorded, and reported at the end of a trial in accordance with the protocol, standard operating procedures (SOPs), good clinical practice (GCP), and the applicable regulatory requirements [3]. Closeout is vital to the quality control of a clinical trial and is intended to safeguard study quality according to the requirements set by regulators and the sponsor. It also serves to ensure that all necessary documents are in place should trial information need to be retrieved in the future.

Most clinical trials have a predefined expected endpoint. For various reasons, including funding, the plan for a clinical trial usually includes this date by which the trial must end, regardless of outcome [4]. However, provisions should be made for monitoring the trial (often through designated trial Steering and Data Monitoring Committees) and terminating either the entire trial or an intervention early for speci-

I. R. Murray · A. D. Duckworth
Edinburgh Orthopaedics, The University of Edinburgh, Edinburgh, UK
e-mail: Iain.murray@ed.ac.uk; Andrew.Duckworth@ed.ac.uk

M. R. Safran (✉)
Orthopaedic Surgery and Sports Medicine, Stanford University, Stanford, CA, USA
e-mail: msafran@stanford.edu; Marc.safran@stanford.edu


S. Lyman et al. (eds.), *Introduction to Surgical Trials*,
https://doi.org/10.1007/978-3-031-77563-5_15

fied reasons, including clear evidence of benefit or harm. Unexpected early closeout is not rare [1]. Montori et al. identified 143 randomized controlled trials that were stopped for benefit [5] with multiple other trials having been stopped for other reasons [6–8]. Evaluation of the orthopedic literature reveals many trials stopped earlier than initially planned [9, 10]. It is likely that even more trials have been terminated early but not reported [11]. The problems encountered during closeout in these trials are not well reported [1, 12].

## 15.3 Early Planning Pays off

During planning, the investigators, sponsor, and coordinating center staff are understandably focused on the details of setup and day-to-day running of the clinical trial. Aspects of the closeout period may depend on elements that only become clear once the trial has started or enrollment is complete. Therefore and there is often an inclination to leave the details of closeout for later consideration. However, the practical details of closeout are often more complex than anticipated and are easy to underestimate. If planning is delayed, the condensed planning can be disruptive for those involved and important details may be overlooked [13].

There are substantial advantages of early contingency planning for clinical trial closeout. Firstly, the time spent planning is less restricted and all available expertise can be rallied with fewer logistical barriers. The complexities of study closeout require detailed planning, and the close coordination can be time-consuming between various stakeholders including sponsor, regulators, coordinating center staff, and personnel at other participating centers. Secondly, early contingency planning also means that termination protocols are already established should early stopping criteria be triggered. Thirdly, planning early for a variety of closeout scenarios would be made considering interim trial results, negating misinterpretation of reasons for closeout by participating patients and trial staff.

While literature to guide trial closeout is relatively scant, early planning for closeout is now widely recommended [13, 14]. The closeout phase needs its own written operating procedures and should include plans for major contingencies depending on the nature of the trial and condition or procedure under investigation. Problematic closeout issues should be anticipated and addressed before the study begins [15]. At least three basic contingencies should be considered and planned for: (a) marked evidence of harm with one treatment mandating that one arm or the entire trial must be discontinued immediately, (b) one intervention shows clear and steady benefit over another necessitating early closeout in an orderly fashion, and (c) trends that validate planned trial completion.

## 15.4 Closeout Procedures

In multicenter studies, closeout occurs in two ways—firstly, at the individual sites (site closeout) and subsequently at the coordinating center (study closeout). There is considerable overlap in many of the concepts and tasks required to ensure effective site and study closeout. There are also geographic and sponsor and regulatory variation in the specific tasks required at closeout. Therefore, local guidelines should be followed. The principal concepts of site and study closeout are outlined below.

### 15.4.1 Data Cleanup and Verification

The cleanup and verification of data can take considerable time and may conflict with internal or external pressure to rapidly publish findings. While publication of important information should not be withheld unnecessarily, results should not be disseminated before data are verified [16]. Despite attempts to collect complete data, some data deficiencies are nearly inevitable. Cleanup and verification can reveal missing forms, unanswered items on forms, and conflicting data. In rare cases, they may also uncover falsification of individual data [17, 18] or even worse, fabrication of all data on fictitious participants [19, 20]. While data cleanup and verification typically continue for several months after completion of closeout visits, the use of electronic records has provided opportunities to flag incomplete data early, and has the potential to significantly streamline this process [21]. Within a reasonable time frame, the data must be cleaned and locked (i.e., frozen as the official dataset for reporting purposes), even if some data remains incomplete. Efforts during cleanup should therefore be directed toward the most critical areas—those crucial to answering the primary research questions and evaluation of serious adverse effects. Continuous monitoring of study data as the trial proceeds is best practice not only to facilitate timely closure but to reveal systematic problems that can be addressed early. Approaches for statistical process control audits are now available and have been shown to significantly reduce overall database error rates [22]. This process of data verification, cleanup, and locking is best performed by the trial statistical team.

Any clinical trial should be prepared to have its results reviewed, questioned, and audited. Traditionally, this review has been to confirm scientific accuracy. However, regulators and special interest groups may also want to interrogate the data. Therefore, key results should be properly verified, documented, and, filed in an intuitive and easily retrievable manner. The extent of this additional documentation of important data will depend on the design of each trial but is greatly aided by modern electronic databases.

Procedures for data cleanup and verification in trials conducted for regulatory approval can add substantially to the trial cost and complexity. Many trials collect a large quantity of data and final verification is both time-consuming and costly [23]. As such, investigators should consider collecting only essential data when designing such trials [24].

### 15.4.2 Management of Study Related Materials

In planning for trial closeout, an agreement should be made as to whether and how any trial supplies or equipment should be returned at the end of the trial. This may include kits or equipment such as centrifuges or outcome testing equipment such as or ultrasound or functional testing machines. Unused trial supplies may need to be returned directly to the organization that sent the supplies initially, or to the coordinating center, or the agreement may state that the sites are allowed to keep the supplies for their own use once the trial has finished. The trial manager should ensure that sites are aware of the requirements for the end of trial and that any evidence for return of supplies is received and recorded by the coordinating center in a timely manner.

### 15.4.3 Archiving of Records and Specimens

#### 15.4.3.1 Records

Research records should be retained following trial completion in conformance with the applicable regulatory requirements of the geographical region or as described in the protocol. The EU Clinical Trials Regulation (EU) 536/2014 requires that the clinical trial master file be stored for at least 25 years after the completion of the clinical trial [25]. In the USA, there are a number of different regulatory bodies each of which has different requirements. As a result, researchers must comply with the longest applicable standard according to institutional policies. Research records must be maintained a minimum of 3 years after the research is completed and the study closed with the Institutional IRB. The United States Food and Drug Administration (FDA) has determined that information should be stored until 2 years after the investigation is discontinued and FDA is notified. The Health Information Portability and Accountability Act (HIPAA) requirements dictate that adult records must be retained for a minimum of 6 years after subjects have signed a HIPAA authorization. Therefore, it is good practice to have a standard operating procedure (SOP) describing the archiving process based on the coordinating center's jurisdiction.

The documents that individually and collectively permit evaluation of the conduct of a trial and the quality of the data produced are defined as essential documents according to International Council for Harmonization (ICH) GCP guidelines [26]. These include but are not limited to the trial master file, source documents, and individual case report forms. All essential documents should be archived, including essential documents held by investigators, sponsors, and others involved. Documents may be paper, electronic or, both. In addition, a list containing identifying information for all participants who enrolled in a trial should be stored at the institution where the investigation took place. In multicenter trials, complete patient lists should be maintained at the coordinating center, and lists of those patients recruited from each participating site should also be maintained at the site of recruitment [26]. Some local regulations require that individual participant data such as copies of study forms, laboratory reports, and radiographs be stored for a stated period of time within the patient's medical records. Storage of these data electronically clearly eases most concerns about adequate storage space. Essential documents must be archived for sufficient time to allow audit and inspection by regulators and should be freely available when requested. Funders, sponsors, scientific journals, and institutions where the research is being conducted will also have local policies and requirements relating to the archiving and storage process that must be considered.

The trial master file (TMF) should be archived in a way that access can be appropriately supervised. It is good practice to designate a named archivist and, in many jurisdictions, this is a legal requirement. This role can be combined with other roles, for example, if the records are being retained electronically this may be a member of the information technology staff. An archivist is responsible for assuring that the archiving facilities are appropriate as well as controlling and keeping a record of access to the archive. Access to archives should be restricted to authorized personnel and any change in the ownership or location should be clearly documented.

Electronic data should be stored in a format that permits viewing in standard software, avoiding the need for dependence upon specific proprietary software programs that may not be available in the future. Many large multi-center trials now use bespoke electronic data capture, so data can be is uploaded in real-time as the trial is being carried out. Appropriate back up of electronic data must be planned for should there be a failure of storage media, and copies of all data must be made and kept in a separate location. For more information, *A Guide to Archiving of Electronic Records by the Scientific Archivists Group* is available online [27].

There is no requirement to delete research data if it is being held for research purposes and even personal data can be stored indefinitely if it is in the "public interest", subject to safeguards, transparency, and fairness [28]. If the decision is made to delete some or all of the essential documents, reasons for this should be explicitly documented and approved by persons or committees with appropriate authority. This record should be retained for a further defined period as appropriate. A certification of destruction should be obtained if using an outside contractor.

#### 15.4.3.2 Biomaterials

The storage of biological material is becoming increasingly relevant in orthopedic surgery [29]. The rapid expansion in clinical trials evaluating biological products as stand-alone therapies and as surgical adjuncts has highlighted the need for comprehensive characterization of the products delivered [30, 31]. Analysis can range from simple histological staining to sophisticated genetic analysis. The availability of these specimens for analyses depends on the wording of the informed consent and use out with this is not permitted. Patient privacy must always be considered. Storage of biomaterials generates unique challenges including storage conditions that maintain integrity of the samples, labeling and retrieving samples or aliquots, and the associated costs, which can be substantial. Unlike with retrieval and distribution of data, many specimens may only be used once. Therefore, investigators need to develop a system for deciding when and how to distribute or use biospecimens. The cost, benefit, and duration of storage must be considered. Central specimen repositories have been created to which investigators may be able to send their materials [32].

### 15.4.4 Site Closure Meeting and Report

Once the trial is completed at a site and the database is locked, the study monitor will arrange a closeout meeting with the principal investigator and study team. Individual sites should have been well informed of closeout procedures early in the trial process and the closeout meeting serves to confirm that all aspects of this agreed upon plan have been completed. This includes completion of the site delegation log, return of equipment where necessary, transfer of all biological samples, and appropriate archiving of study documents. A study closure report should then be formulated to include the following details as a minimum requirement:

- The number of participants enrolled at the site.
- The number of participants who have completed the study.
- The number of participants who have been lost to follow-up, including the reason for this.
- A list of serious adverse events (SAEs)/adverse events.
- Information about the final ethics report including date submitted.

### 15.4.5 Reporting Study Closure/Updating Study Status

Before a study is declared complete, the principal investigator should review the plans approved by the ethics committee and local regulators with regard to the use of data and tissue collected, expectations for reporting study results to participants, and the formal public dissemination of study results. If changes to these approved arrangements are required or anticipated, the study team should determine whether this would be considered a substantial amendment, which may require notification of the sponsor or regulators before the end of study notification is submitted. The trial manager should ensure that the sponsor, the research ethics committee that approved the trial, any relevant clinical trials registries, and any other stakeholders are informed in writing that the study has reached its defined end date. There may be different reporting requirements based on the jurisdiction in which the trial was conducted so local requirements should be identified and followed.

## 15.5 Recording the Study Closure Process

Documentation of the study closure process is important [15]. It is the responsibility of the study coordinating center and the principal investigator to ensure that all the approvals, notifications, and documentation required as part of study closure are signed and completed. The data management plan will be useful in successfully completing this process, and archived documents are to be listed on the study specific archives register, SOP, or checklist.

## 15.6 Reporting and Dissemination of Results

The results of a trial must be published, irrespective of the outcome and it is widely considered scientific misconduct not to plan to publish trial results [33]. It is good practice to establish a publication and dissemination plan early in the trial process and ensure this is appropriately resourced. This plan should consider how best to ensure that the trial results impact clinical practice and policy most appropriately, and how all stakeholders are best informed about the trial results. This should include participating patients, trial staff, clinicians involved in the ongoing care of patients, sponsors, and the wider scientific community. Investigators should carefully consider the order in which the various interested parties are informed. This plan must be adjusted to the specific nature and sensitivities of the trial. This is particularly true in multicenter studies where the participants may be referred by clinicians or surgeons not involved in the trial. In this case, the investigators have an obligation to report the trial conclusions to these physicians, preferably before they learn about them from their patients or public reporting. Study sponsors may want to make the findings known publicly through a press conference or press release. While an early press release may be strategic to the sponsor, it may not be in the best interests of the participants, referring physicians, or medical community at large. These stakeholders may feel that they should have been informed before the results were reported in the mainstream press [16]. These challenges all highlight the importance of reaching an agreement on the dissemination plan early in the trial.

A good practice to set up a writing committee who work with the trial scientific committee (TSC) and trial monitoring groups (TMGs) to produce initial drafts of documents at each step of the dissemination process. Numerous guidelines and checklists now exist that provide minimum reporting criteria for clinical trials including the Consolidated Standards of Reporting Trials (CONSORT) [34]. The Equator Network (Enhancing the Quality and Transparency of Health Research) provides a centralized source of minimum standards of reporting with many relevant to orthopedics including orthobiologics [30]. The use of minimum reporting standards has led to improvements in the quality of the reporting of study design in clinical studies [35, 36].

Prior to disseminating any trial results that may have Intellectual Property Rights, the sponsor, and any local intellectual property representatives should be consulted. Trial registries and relevant research databases should also be updated with the results. The exact requirements for final reports and deadlines for submission vary and the guidance given by sponsors and funders should be followed. Some funders may require a separate report or a detailed account of the trial. A summary of the final research report should be sent to the ethics committee who granted permission for the study within 12 months of the end of the trial. At a minimum, this should include whether or not the trial achieved its objectives, the main findings, and arrangements for publication or dissemination of the research, including any feedback to participants.

Patients should be given the opportunity to learn about the results of the studies to which they have contributed. This information could be delivered by printed letter or email, a lay language summary on the trial website, or a newsletter to study participants. Toolkits that help ensure that lay information is delivered in an understandable manner should be resourced into trial planning [37].

Most public funders of research have a Public Access Policy including the National Institute for Health (NIH), Medical Research Council (MRC), and The Wellcome Trust, that mandates Open Access publication [38]. In addition, public funders generally require notification of any manuscripts or other research outputs, such as conference presentations or press releases, prior to publication, sent cognizant of the funder's timescale for review. Funders or sponsors must be acknowledged appropriately with a statement of support or disclaimer and their policy on copyright should also be considered before journal copyright waivers are signed.

## 15.7 Conclusions

The closeout phase of clinical trials typically receives less attention in the planning of clinical trials than earlier phases including recruitment. While, aspects of the closeout will depend on factors that only become known once the trial is underway, planning for both expected and contingency actions should begin early to ensure that it is accomplished in an orderly and effective fashion. Involvement and clear communication from all stakeholders will minimize delays and enable the research team to focus on ensuring the results of trials are most effectively disseminated.

## References

1. Shepherd R, Macer JL, Grady D. Planning for closeout—from Day One. Contemp Clin Trials. 2008;29(2):136–9. https://doi.org/10.1016/j.cct.2007.06.001.
2. Petryna A. When experiments travel: clinical trials and the global search for human subjects. Princeton, NJ: Princeton University Press; 2009.
3. The King's Health Partners Clinical Trials Office. Investigator Site Close-Out Procedure (KHP-CTO/CT/SOP16.0) Finalv5.0. 2019. https://khpcto.co.uk/SOPs/16_siteCloseOutSOP.php. 2019.

4. Committee on Strategies for Responsible Sharing of Clinical Trial Data; Board on Health Sciences Policy; Institute of Medicine. Sharing clinical trial data: maximizing benefits, minimizing risk. The clinical trial life cycle and when to share data. Washington, DC: National Academies Press (US); 2015. p. 4. https://www.ncbi.nlm.nih.gov/books/NBK286004/.
5. Montori VM, Devereaux PJ, Adhikari NK, et al. Randomized trials stopped early for benefit: a systematic review. JAMA. 2005;294(17):2203–9. [published Online First: 2005/11/03]. https://doi.org/10.1001/jama.294.17.2203.
6. Agodoa LY, Appel L, Bakris GL, et al. Effect of ramipril vs amlodipine on renal outcomes in hypertensive nephrosclerosis: a randomized controlled trial. JAMA. 2001;285(21):2719–28. [published Online First: 2001/06/21]. https://doi.org/10.1001/jama.285.21.2719.
7. Black HR, Elliott WJ, Grandits G, et al. Results of the controlled ONset verapamil INvestigation of cardiovascular endpoints (CONVINCE) trial by geographical region. J Hypertens. 2005;23(5):1099–106. [published Online First: 2005/04/19]. https://doi.org/10.1097/01.hjh.0000166853.26087.22.
8. Rossouw JE, Anderson GL, Prentice RL, et al. Risks and benefits of estrogen plus progestin in healthy postmenopausal women: principal results from the Women's Health Initiative randomized controlled trial. JAMA. 2002;288(3):321–33. [published Online First: 2002/07/19]. https://doi.org/10.1001/jama.288.3.321.
9. Hamid N, Ashraf N, Bosse MJ, et al. Radiation therapy for heterotopic ossification prophylaxis acutely after elbow trauma: a prospective randomized study. J Bone Joint Surg Am. 2010;92(11):2032–8. [published Online First: 2010/09/03]. https://doi.org/10.2106/jbjs.I.01435.
10. Duckworth AD, Clement ND, McEachan JE, et al. Prospective randomised trial of non-operative versus operative management of olecranon fractures in the elderly. Bone Joint J. 2017;99-b(7):964–72. [published Online First: 2017/07/01]. https://doi.org/10.1302/0301-620x.99b7.Bjj-2016-1112.R2.
11. European Society of Cardiology. The early termination of clinical trials: causes, consequences, and control. With special reference to trials in the field of arrhythmias and sudden death. Task force of the working group on arrhythmias of the European Society of Cardiology. Circulation. 1994;89(6):2892–907. [published Online First: 1994/06/01]. https://doi.org/10.1161/01.cir.89.6.2892.
12. Walter SD, Han H, Guyatt GH, et al. A systematic survey of randomised trials that stopped early for reasons of futility. BMC Med Res Methodol. 2020;20(1):10. [published Online First: 2020/01/18]. https://doi.org/10.1186/s12874-020-0899-1.
13. Pressel SL, Davis BR, Wright JT, et al. Operational aspects of terminating the doxazosin arm of the antihypertensive and lipid lowering treatment to prevent heart attack trial (ALLHAT). Control Clin Trials. 2001;22(1):29–41. [published Online First: 2001/02/13]. https://doi.org/10.1016/s0197-2456(00)00109-4.
14. Bell RL, Curb JD, Friedman LM, et al. Termination of clinical trials: the beta-blocker heart attack trial and the hypertension detection and follow-up program experience. Control Clin Trials. 1985;6(2):102–11. [published Online First: 1985/06/01]. https://doi.org/10.1016/0197-2456(85)90115-1.
15. Muth K, Yu E, Alston B, et al. The closeout process for a clinical trial terminated early for lagging enrollment and inadequate follow-up. Control Clin Trials. 2001;22(1):49–55. [published Online First: 2001/02/13]. https://doi.org/10.1016/s0197-2456(00)00111-2.
16. Friedman LM, Furberg CD, Demets DL. Closeout. Fundamentals of clinical trials. Berlin: Springer Science and Business Media; 2010. p. 463–75.
17. Fisher B, Redmond CK. Fraud in breast-cancer trials. N Engl J Med. 1994;330(20):1458–60. [published Online First: 1994/05/19]. https://doi.org/10.1056/nejm199405193302015.
18. Buyse M, George SL, Evans S, et al. The role of biostatistics in the prevention, detection and treatment of fraud in clinical trials. Stat Med. 1999;18(24):3435–51. [published Online First: 1999/12/28]. https://doi.org/10.1002/(sici)1097-0258(19991230)18:24<3435::aid-sim365>3.0.co;2-o.
19. Ross DB. The FDA and the case of Ketek. N Engl J Med. 2007;356(16):1601–4. [published Online First: 2007/04/20]. https://doi.org/10.1056/NEJMp078032.
20. George SL, Buyse M. Data fraud in clinical trials. Clin Investig (Lond). 2015;5(2):161–73. [published Online First: 2015/03/03]. https://doi.org/10.4155/cli.14.116.
21. Cowie MR, Blomster JI, Curtis LH, et al. Electronic health records to facilitate clinical research. Clin Res Cardiol. 2017;106(1):1–9. [published Online First: 2016/08/26]. https://doi.org/10.1007/s00392-016-1025-6.
22. Rostami R, Nahm M, Pieper CF. What can we learn from a decade of database audits? The Duke Clinical Research Institute experience, 1997–2006. Clin Trials. 2009;6(2):141–50. [published Online First: 2009/04/04]. https://doi.org/10.1177/1740774509102590.
23. Zarin DA, Tse T, Williams RJ, et al. The ClinicalTrials.gov results database—update and key issues. N Engl J Med. 2011;364(9):852–60. [published Online First: 2011/03/04]. https://doi.org/10.1056/NEJMsa1012065.
24. Krishnankutty B, Bellary S, Kumar NB, et al. Data management in clinical research: an overview. Indian J Pharm. 2012;44(2):168–72. [published Online First: 2012/04/25]. https://doi.org/10.4103/0253-7613.93842.
25. Regulation (EU) No 536/2014 of the European Parliament and of the council of 16 April 2014 on clinical trials on medicinal products for human use, and repealing directive 2001/20/EC, OJ L 158, 27.5.2014, p. 1.

26. Guideline for good clinical practice. Committee for Human Medicinal Products. European Medicines Agency. 1995. www.ema.europa.eu/docs/en_GB/document_library/Scientific_guideline/2009/09/WC500002874.pdf.
27. A guide to archiving of electronic records. Health Sciences Records and Archives Association. https://the-hsraa.org/resources/publications/guide-archiving-electronic-records. Accessed 12 Jul 2020.
28. Data Protection Act 2018. www.legislation.gov.uk/ukpga/2018/12/contents/enacted.
29. Chu CR, Rodeo S, Bhutani N, et al. Optimizing clinical use of biologics in orthopaedic surgery: consensus recommendations from the 2018 AAOS/NIH U-13 conference. J Am Acad Orthop Surg. 2019;27(2):e50–63. [published Online First: 2018/10/10]. https://doi.org/10.5435/jaaos-d-18-00305.
30. Murray IR, Geeslin AG, Goudie EB, et al. Minimum information for studies evaluating biologics in orthopaedics (MIBO): platelet-rich plasma and mesenchymal stem cells. J Bone Joint Surg Am. 2017;99:809.
31. Murray IR, Chahla J, Safran MR, et al. International expert consensus on a cell therapy communication tool: DOSES. J Bone Joint Surg Am. 2019;101(10):904–11. [published Online First: 2019/05/17]. https://doi.org/10.2106/jbjs.18.00915.
32. Belden SE, Uppalapati CK, Pascual AS, et al. Establishment of a clinic-based biorepository. J Vis Exp. 2017;(123):55583. [published Online First: 2017/06/13]. https://doi.org/10.3791/55583.
33. Duley L, Farrell B, editors. Clinical trials. London: BMJ Books; 2002.
34. Begg C, Cho M, Eastwood S, et al. Improving the quality of reporting of randomized controlled trials. The CONSORT statement. JAMA. 1996;276(8):637–9. [published Online First: 1996/08/28].
35. Moher D, Schulz KF, Altman DG. The CONSORT statement: revised recommendations for improving the quality of reports of parallel-group randomised trials. Lancet. 2001;357(9263):1191–4. [published Online First: 2001/04/27].
36. Plint AC, Moher D, Morrison A, et al. Does the CONSORT checklist improve the quality of reports of randomised controlled trials? A systematic review. Med J Aust. 2006;185(5):263–7. [published Online First: 2006/09/05].
37. Barnes A, Patrick S. Lay summaries of clinical study results: an overview. Pharmaceut Med. 2019;33(4):261–8. https://doi.org/10.1007/s40290-019-00285-0.
38. Mayor S. Opening the lid on open access. BMJ (Clin Res Ed). 2008;336(7646):688–9. DB [published Online First: 2008/03/29]. https://doi.org/10.1136/bmj.39526.467951.

# Part III

# Trial Completion

# Missing Data and Imputation

# 16

Gianluca Camillieri

## 16.1 Introduction

When you conceive, design, and implement an orthopedic surgical trial, there are many steps to follow to reduce the risk of bias that may occur during the process. One of the biggest enemies of the validity of any clinical research from a simple case series to the most sophisticated meta-analysis is missing data. Statistical power and the validity of a study are based on having complete information for all study subjects at all study time points. If data is not captured completely or patients miss follow-up visits, the integrity of the study begins to be compromised. Missing data, or missing values, occur when no data value is stored for the variable in an observation. Missing data is a common occurrence and can have a significant effect on the conclusions that can be drawn from a study. Often, especially in orthopedic research, a lot of time and resources are needed to accomplish a complete and well-designed study, but missing data and/or patients lost to follow-up for studies with long follow-up in particular, may corrode the validity of the study findings to a point that the results cannot be trusted.

In this eventuality, we can choose to exclude observations or even entire patients with missing data or turn toward a mathematical method to save our effort. Statistics comes to help us with Imputation, the process of replacing missing data with substituted values. These techniques are used because removing the data from the dataset every time is not feasible and can lead to a reduction in the size of the dataset to a large extent, which not only raises concerns for biasing the dataset but also may lead to incorrect conclusions. Simple and/or complex imputation algorithms have been developed up to and including deep neural networks (Fig. 16.1).

G. Camillieri (✉)
University of Pittsburgh Medical Center Italy, Salvator Mundi Hospital, Rome, Italy
e-mail: camillierig@upmc.it


S. Lyman et al. (eds.), *Introduction to Surgical Trials*,
https://doi.org/10.1007/978-3-031-77563-5_16

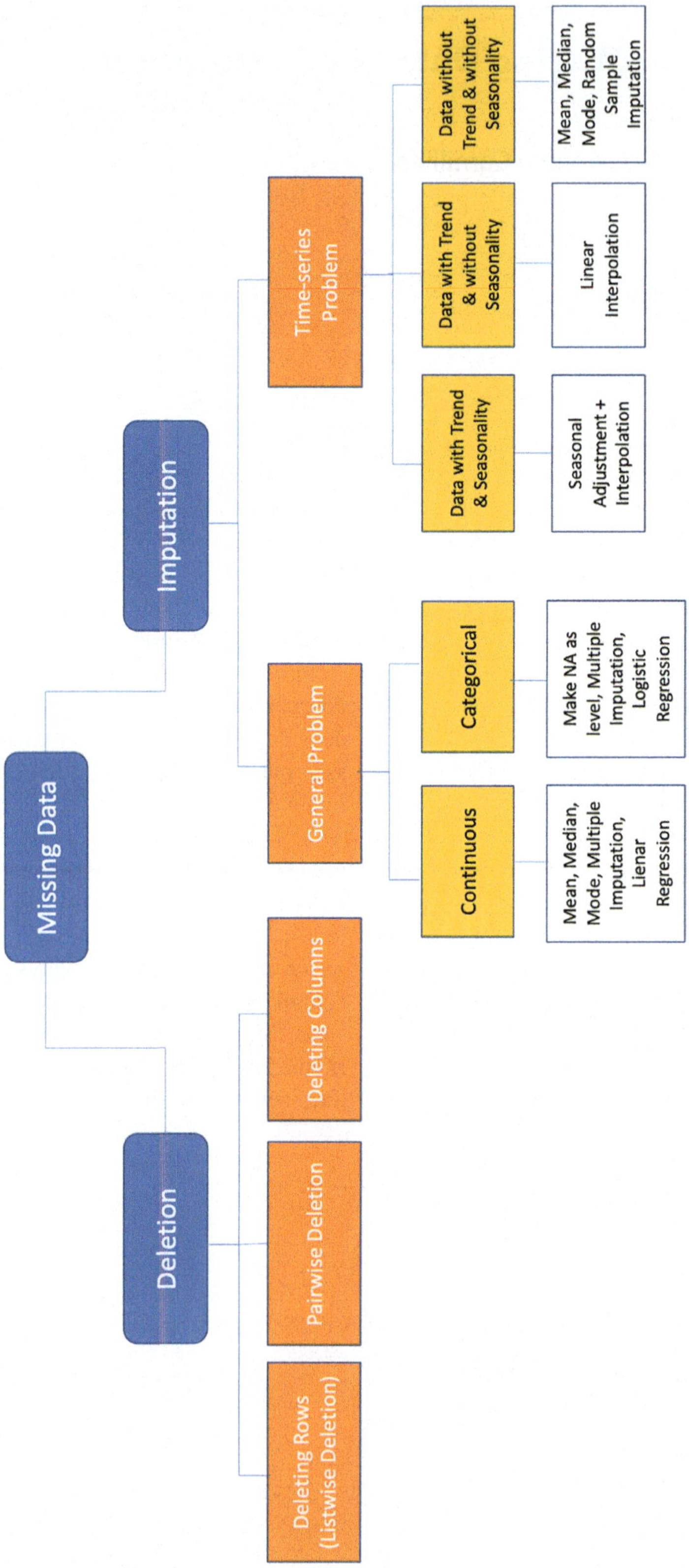


**Fig. 16.1** Shows an example on how to move in case of missing data

## 16.2 Missing Data

Despite implementation of standardized data collection forms, missing data is nearly ubiquitous in clinical research. Missing data can occur in various data sources (databases, medical records, and patient reported data), data collection methods (paper-based and online registration forms), registration time (e.g., pretreatment and post-treatment), and registration frequency (e.g., one postoperative outcome measurement and several follow-up measurements). Missing data can occur for many reasons: loss to follow-up, failure to attend medical appointments, lack of measurements, failure to send or retrieve questionnaires, health literacy limitations, inaccurate transfer of data from paper registration to an electronic database, among others.

There are many ways to minimize the extent of missing data. It may be helpful to incorporate standardized rules to optimize data collection, such as training staff to collect and coordinate data collection, using well-defined data definitions, and incorporating logic and range checks for each data element. Pilot studies can help to identify variables particularly susceptible to missing values, and steps can be taken to improve completeness [1]. Regular monitoring of data quality and completeness provides essential feedback to clinicians and researchers on the extent of missing data [2].

Furthermore, when collecting information about the quality of life or other sensitive issues, patients may be asked to provide reasons for refusing to answer, such as a lack of time, problems understanding language, length of survey, or too intimate questionnaires. This information can be used in the analyses of data and interpretation of the results to evaluate the likelihood of bias due to this missing information.

Missing data represents a big challenge to orthopedic researchers. The central enigma of missing data is to produce estimates that mimic the non-existent or missing data, while keeping the uncertainty inherent in missing values [3]. For researchers with the resources and time, the solution is to work with a biostatistician to identify the pattern (if any) for the missing data and provide a model for the "missingness" of the data, which will provide suitable estimates accounting for possible biases. Typically, in a large clinical trial, the observations with missing values will simply be deleted (listwise deletion) to avoid bias, unless there is evidence that there is some observable pattern to the "missingness" of the data that is relevant to the drug or procedure under investigation (a non-ignorable pattern).

Missing data in smaller studies can be more problematic. These studies include pilot studies, research that is done by medical students, or unfunded research by house staff or attending physicians. Typically, these missing observations will be dealt with by eliminating them, as this is the default in most statistical programs. Listwise deletion in this setting may still be a reliable method as it is relatively unbiased provided the data are missing completely at random (MCAR). However, if the study is small, or the amount of missing data is above 5 to 10% of the total data set, significant loss of power is possible [4].

Fortunately, there are a few accessible methods for those with limited resources or those who do not have a statistician available. These methods in general are easily applicable, but rely on basic assumptions that are illustrated below.

Many real-world datasets may contain missing values for various reasons. They are often encoded as NaNs (Not Numbers), blanks, or any other predetermined placeholder that is intended to reflect missing data. However, a word of caution is necessary. Many statistical programs assume that all values are numerical and hold meaningful value so you should understand your software program's limitations.

One way to handle this problem is to get rid of the observations that have missing data. However, you will risk losing data with valuable information. An alternative strategy would be to impute the missing values. In other words, we need to infer those missing values from the existing part of the data. Before we can do that, we need to consider the missing data pattern.

There are three main types of missing data:

1. Missing completely at random (MCAR).
2. Missing at random (MAR).
3. Not missing at random (NMAR).

**Missing Completely at Random (MCAR)** The fact that a certain value is missing has nothing to do with its hypothetical value and with the values of other variables. This is the most powerful assumption. Suppose there are two variables X and Y. Consider values for Y. The values if missing is MCAR if the probability of missing data on Y is unrelated to the value of Y and unrelated to the value of any other variable in the data set.

**Missing at Random (MAR)** Missing at random means that the propensity for a data point to be missing is not related to the missing data, but it is related to some of the observed data. This assumption is that the probability of missing a variable Y is unrelated to the value of Y but may be related to the value of one or more variables in the data set. This assumption is weaker, and impossible to test (because the data are missing) [4]. For example, consider a case where it was desired to determine if hospital X treated more patients daily than hospital Y. If the probability of missing data on the number of patients treated depended on which hospital they were in, but within each hospital, the probability of missing data on number of patients was unrelated to the number of patients treated, MAR would be satisfied. In this case, the missing data is a result of poor hospital record keeping that is unrelated to the true values for the patients treated.

Ignorable missing data: This condition is satisfied if first, the data is MAR or MCAR and second, the mechanism governing the pattern of missing data is unrelated to the mechanism of effect to be measured (in the case illustrated above, the probability of missing a case is unrelated to the number of patients treated).

**Missing Not at Random** Usually this occurs in cases where the missing data are not MAR (NMAR). The mechanism of missing the data must be modeled. In the previous example, if it was discovered that hospital Y systematically underreported low census days, this would be an example of non-ignorable missing data [4]. If a non-ignorable mechanism for missing data is suspected, a biostatistician (preferably one with interest in this area) should be consulted.

## 16.3 Deletion

When dealing with missing data, researchers can use two primary methods to solve the error: imputation or the removal of data. The imputation method develops reasonable guesses for missing data. It is most useful when the percentage of missing data is low. If the portion of missing data is too high, the risk of bias increases to the point of futility. The resulting analysis is very unlikely to reveal trustworthy results.

The other option is to remove data. When dealing with data that is missing at random, related data can be deleted without risk of bias. Removing data may not be the best option if there are not enough observations to result in a reliable analysis. This is especially true when you are interested in a binary outcome that occurs relatively infrequently (e.g., dislocation). Losing even a few events may compromise the ability of your study to draw reliable conclusions.

Before deciding which approach to employ, researchers must understand why the data is missing and if are dealing with MAR, MCAR, or NMAR.

There are two primary methods for deleting data when dealing with missing data: listwise and dropping variables [5].

### 16.3.1 Listwise

Listwise deletion (complete-case analysis) removes all data for an observation that has one or more missing values. Particularly if the missing data is limited to a small number of observations, you may just opt to eliminate those cases from the analysis [6]. However, in most cases, it is often disadvantageous to use listwise deletion. This is because the assumptions of MCAR (Missing Completely at Random) are typically hard to justify. As a result, listwise deletion methods are more likely to produce biased parameters estimates. This method is popular because it is easy to implement, and it is the default option in most statistical packages. However, the results of such analyses may yield biased estimates of associations, because complete cases are assumed to be a random sample of the whole population, i.e., data are MCAR. That is not always the case, as often individuals with complete data are different from those with missing data, and missingness can depend on either observed data or unobserved data. By comparing data in a UK Primary Care Database with a population survey, Marston et al. [7] showed that the distributions of alcohol consumption and smoking were different in the two data sources. This may suggest that data in these two variables are not MCAR. Complete-case analyses in this case may have serious consequences if the aim of a future study is to investigate an association between alcohol and postoperative complications. Another issue with complete-case analysis is that a large proportion of valuable research data are discarded, which affects the statistical power and precision of the estimates. In some cases, it may be reasonable to use complete-case analyses, such as when working with large datasets with few missing observations, because the risk of bias is minimal and the precision is still good [8].

### 16.3.2 Pairwise

Pairwise deletion analyses all cases in which the variables of interest are present and thus maximizes all data available for each analysis. A strength to this technique is that it increases power in your analysis but it has many disadvantages. It assumes that the missing data are MCAR. If you delete pairwise then you will end up with different numbers of observations contributing to different parts of your model, which can make interpretation difficult.

This method is mentioned briefly here, because it can produce some confusing situations when attempting to determine an appropriate model in regression analysis, in addition to producing problems with bias. Pairwise deletion is an enticing option because it allows one to use more of the data from the initial data set than does listwise deletion. In listwise deletion, if one parameter is missing, that entire observation (all variables) is deleted. In pairwise deletion, all of the data are used for all of the analyses for which they can be used. So for computation of a covariance matrix, all cases of X and Y are considered; whereas for listwise deletion, only the cases with full data would have been considered [9]. The problem with this method is that if there is any violation of MCAR, there can be serious problems with bias. So the decreased standard errors that are observed with pairwise deletion (because more information is used) may not be worth the price that is paid in terms of biased estimates. As a result, if any deletion is used, listwise deletion is recommended because of the aforementioned reasons, in addition to the decrease in confusion when using automated mechanisms of model building. In addition, pairwise deletion can make selection of linear models with computer programs confusing.

Another method concerns Dropping Variables. It is always better to keep data than to discard it. Sometimes you can drop variables if the data is missing for more than 60% observations but only if that variable is not considered particularly important for your study. Having said that, imputation is always a preferred choice over dropping variables.

Finally, before transition to into imputation, we should mention weighting techniques for missing data. This method is commonly used when unit non-response exists. Unit non-response is said to occur when, for some reason, some individual fails to return a survey, answer a research question, or in some other way is recruited, but does not participate. This method assumes that there is demographic information present about the subject that would allow for comparison with others. Then, a subject with similar demographic characteristics is assigned a weight of 2 to account for the fact that a demographically similar subject's data were missing. This method eliminates all variability between demographically similar data points, which can affect standard errors adversely [10]. In addition, this technique does not account for stratification of samples, which could make weighting cumbersome.

## 16.4 Imputation

Imputation is one of the key strategies that researchers use to fill in missing data in a dataset. By using various calculations to find the most probable answer, imputed data is used in place of actual data in order to allow for more accurate analyses [11].

When substituting for a data point, it is known as "unit imputation"; when substituting for a component of a data point, it is known as "item imputation". There are three main problems that missing data causes: missing data can introduce a substantial amount of bias, make the handling and analysis of the data more arduous, and create reductions in efficiency.

There are two main categories of imputation:

1. Single Imputation.
2. Multiple Imputation.

Single imputation involves less computation and provides the dataset with a specific number in place of the missing data. While there is more than one type of single imputation, in general the process involves analyzing the other responses and looking for the most likely (or a set of the most likely) responses the individual would have answered, and then picks one of those possible responses at random and places it in the dataset.

When the amount of missing data is small, single imputation provides an simple and efficient tool. It fills in the data points well and the variance between the results of your analyses is unlikely to be altered by any significant margin. But when you are dealing with a considerable amount of missing data, single imputation models can cause a serious problem—once the imputed number has been added to the dataset, it is treated as equal to data that was not imputed, allowing for potentially misleading analysis.

Multiple imputation seeks to solve that problem [12]. Multiple imputation uses simulation models that take from a set of possible responses and impute in succession to try to come up with a variance/confidence interval that one can use to better understand the differences between imputed datasets, depending on the numbers that the simulation chooses to use for the missing data.

Recall that different types of computations are used to discover what data is most likely to have been placed in the missing responses, so studies where the results of the research are more uniform (where people with similar responses to the person with the missing data tended to change fairly evenly throughout), the imputed datasets should have much less variance. If, however, the results of those with similar attributes had varying responses themselves, then the imputed sets will likely vary as well.

The greatest drawback of multiple imputation is the complex nature of performing these imputations. You will need to be familiar with how to not only run analyses, but also combine the results. Similarly, if very little data is missing, single imputation may be simpler and solve the problem without much risk of serious errors. But otherwise, multiple imputation seeks to introduce the variability of imputed data in order to find a range of possible responses from which to work from.

### 16.4.1 Simple Imputation

Under single value imputation, missing data are replaced by a single value, such as the mean score of the complete cases in the study sample (i.e., mean imputation).

In longitudinal studies where some variables are measured repeatedly, for example, yearly controls of glycated hemoglobin(HbA1c), the "last observation carried forward" approach can be used where missing values are replaced with the most recently observed value for a given variable. Another single imputation approach is regression-based single imputation of missing values (also known as predicted mean imputation), in which values of the missing observations are predicted using a regression model based on the complete cases.

In general, single imputation methods do not account for the uncertainty of missing data, and as a result, standard errors of the estimates are likely to be too small (thereby overestimating the precision of the results). This can potentially lead to Type 1 error (i.e., identifying an association when none exists) [6]. Mean imputation also does not preserve the relationships between variables; it only preserves the mean of the observed data. Therefore, if the data are MCAR, the estimate of the mean remains unbiased [13, 14]. Under MCAR, if our aim is to estimate means (which is rarely the focus of research studies), mean imputation will not bias the estimates; it will only bias the standard errors as mentioned earlier. Since most of the research studies are interested in the relationship between variables and not just the mean, mean imputation should be avoided in general. It has been pointed out previously that last observation carried forward method can produce biased estimates in both directions even under MCAR and have warned against using this method as the first or only choice for handling missing data [15]. Computing the overall mean, median or mode is a very basic imputation method, it is the only tested function that takes no advantage of the time series characteristics or relationship between the variables. It is very fast but has clear disadvantages. One disadvantage is that mean imputation reduces variance in the dataset.

When we have to deal with missing data in time-series, specific methods have been developed to improve the data set after imputation.

#### 16.4.1.1 Last Observation Carried Forward (LOCF) and Next Observation Carried Backward (NOCB)

This is a common statistical approach to the analysis of longitudinal repeated measures data where some follow-up observations may be missing. Longitudinal data track the same sample at different points in time. Both these methods can introduce bias in analysis and perform poorly when data has a visible trend.

#### 16.4.1.2 Linear Interpolation

This method works well for a time series with some trend but is not suitable for seasonal data. Linear interpolation is often used to approximate a value of some function by using two known values of that function at other points. This formula can also be understood as a weighted average. The weights are inversely related to the distance from the end points to the unknown point. The closer point has more influence than the farther point.

When dealing with missing data, you should consider using this method in a time series that exhibits a clear trend.

#### 16.4.1.3 Seasonal Adjustment + Linear Interpolation

When dealing with data that exhibits both trend and seasonality characteristics, use seasonal adjustment with linear interpolation. First you would perform the seasonal adjustment by computing a centered moving average or taking the average of multiple averages—say, two 1-year averages—that are offset by one period relative to another. You can then complete data smoothing with linear interpolation as discussed above.

#### 16.4.1.4 Sensitivity Analyses with Worst-Case and Best-Case Scenarios

This method involves the replacement of missing values with the worst or best value in the observed data. For example, analyses can be performed by replacing missing data with the highest or lowest observed value and running regression models afterward in order to examine the association of interest. The results of these two regression analyses can then be compared. When both analyses produce similar estimates of an association, it is rather straightforward to draw conclusions about the effect of missing data. However, analyses yielding opposing results can be difficult to interpret. If we have information on exposure but lack outcome data on some patients, we can replace missing data with the worst case (e.g., death at the end of follow-up) or best case (patient is alive at the end of follow-up) and compare the results afterward. The usual procedure in smoking cessation studies is to assume that nonrespondents (missing smoking data) have resumed smoking [16]. Thus, the data are analyzed as if all nonrespondents have returned to active smoking, which might not be a correct assumption. Barnes et al. [16] showed in a simulation study that this method yields biased estimates.

### 16.4.2 Multiple Imputation

Multiple imputation is considered a good approach for data sets with a large amount of missing data. Instead of substituting a single value for each missing data point, the missing values are exchanged for values that encompass the natural variability and uncertainty of the right values. Using the imputed data, the process is repeated to make multiple imputed data sets. Each set is then analyzed using the standard analytical procedures, and the multiple analysis results are combined to produce an overall result.

The various imputations incorporate natural variability into the missing values, which creates a valid statistical inference. Multiple imputations can produce statistically valid results even when there is a relatively small sample size or a large amount of missing data [17].

Furthermore, it solves the problem of "too small or too large" standard errors obtained using traditional methods of dealing with missing data (Table 16.1). The aim of multiple imputation is to provide unbiased and valid estimates of associations based on information from the available data, i.e., yielding estimates similar to those calculated from full data [15].

Missing data and hence multiple imputation may affect not only the coefficient estimates for variables with missing data but also the estimates for other variables with no missing data.

Multiple imputation is widely recognized as the standard method to deal with missing data in many areas of research, and the method has become more popular with the increasing availability of software. Rubin [18], in 1987, developed a method for averaging the outcomes across multiple imputed data sets to account the problem of increased noise due to imputation. Carpenter and Kenward [19], and Buuren [15].

The multiple imputation procedure in most statistical software builds on the MAR assumption [20], but the method can handle both MCAR and MNAR.(3Pedersen) Although we cannot prove whether data are MAR, it is likely that in many situations, the MAR assumption is more plausible when more variables are included in the multiple imputation model [21].

Furthermore, as happens for single imputation, multiple imputation supports multiple meth-

**Table 16.1** Advantages and limitations of multiple imputation respect other methods

| Methods | Presuption to achieve unbiased estimates | Advantages | Limitations |
|---|---|---|---|
| Complete case analysis | MCAR | Simplicity<br>Comparability across analyses | – Low representativeness<br>– Minimize the sample size<br>– Low statistical power<br>– Standard error too large |
| Missing indicator method | None | Considers the whole package of information regarding to missing observation and recollects the full dataset | – Dimension and direction of bias difficult to predict<br>– Standard error too small<br>– Confounding factors may create a bias |
| Single value imputation | MCAR, when estimating mean only | Analysis computed as if data are complete<br>Keeps full dataset | – Standard error too small<br>– Potentially biased results<br>– Lowers the validity of covariance and correlation |
| Sensitivity analysis (worst- and best-case) | MCAR | Simplicity<br>Evaluates full dataset | – Standard error too small and overestimation of precision<br>– Difficult to interpret opposite results |
| Multiple imputation | MAR (MCAR and MNAR together) | Variability more precise for single missing values until it includes variability due to sampling and imputation | – Possibility of error when specifying models |

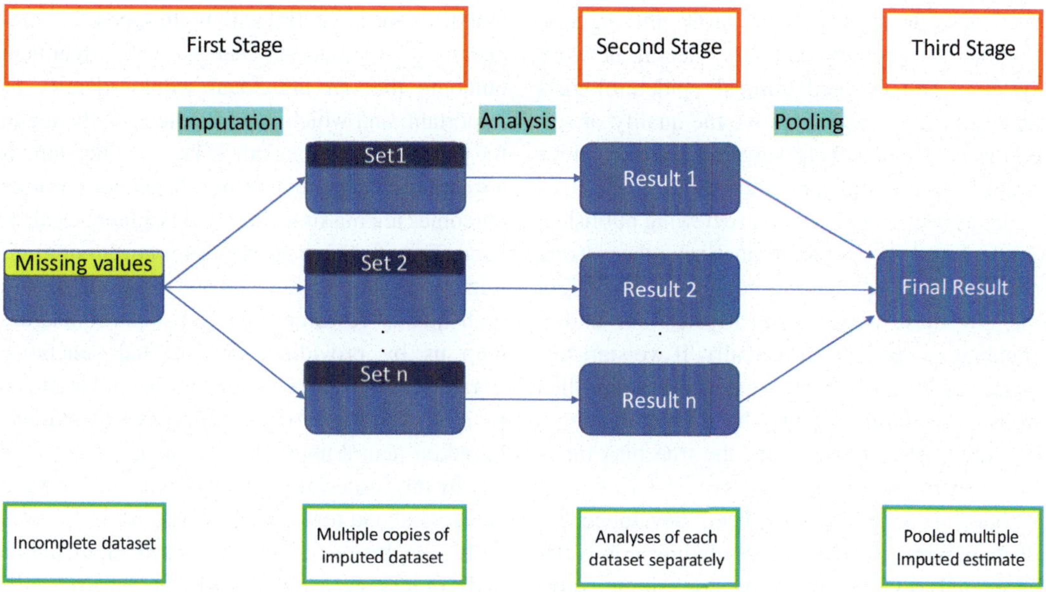


**Fig. 16.2** The multiple imputation (MI) process. In the first step, missing data (shown in white) are imputed (shown in dark blue) to create n complete data sets. Then each complete imputed data set is analyzed using standard methods such as linear regression. Finally, the results are pooled using Rubin's rules

ods to estimate missing data values. Most of these methods follows three steps (Fig. 16.2).

Imputation—Missing values are imputed. However, the imputed values are drawn n times from a distribution rather than just once. At the end of this step, there should be m completed datasets.

Analysis—Each of the m datasets is analyzed. At the end of this step, there should be m analyses.

Pooling—The m results are consolidated into one result by calculating the mean, variance, and confidence interval of the variable of concern or by combining simulations from each separate model [22, 23].

Sometimes we can apply different methods to solve a problem of missing data, a typical example is when we have to deal with categorial variables:

Mode imputation is one method but it will definitely introduce bias.

Missing values can be treated as a separate category by itself. We can create another category for the missing values and use them as a different level. This is the simplest method.

Prediction models: Here, we create a predictive model to estimate values that will substitute the missing data. In this case, we divide our data set into two sets: One set with no missing values for the variable (training) and another one with missing values (test). We can then use regression equations to predict the imputed values.

## 16.5 Discussion

Missing data seem to be "epidemic" in orthopedic clinical research. A study by Ondeck et al. [24] on missing data in a large national data (National Surgical Quality Improvement Program, USA) showed how data interpretation, even though obtained from an evolved and apparently complete database, may be misunderstood if a process of seeking missing data and relative correction by imputation is not executed. Rheumatology researchers consider missing data and use imputation more often than orthopedic researchers. This may be due to a lack of awareness of a lack of concern over missingness. Fortunately, modern software, neural network systems, and devoted clinical epidemiologists and statisticians may improve the quality of scientific research to help surgical research move toward "real" significant outcomes.

It has been suggested that reviewing published surgical trial papers and re-analyzing them using alternative missing data strategies may shed light on how these biases have affected our understanding of our field historically. If we start this process with prospective randomized controlled trials, in the future, we may have a meta-analysis providing greater context to the true bias introduced by missing data.

Several methods have been developed for dealing with missing data including complete-case analyses, missing indicator, single value imputation, and sensitivity analyses incorporating worst- and best-case scenarios.

If applied under the MCAR assumption, these methods can provide unbiased estimates. If MCAR is not fulfilled, estimates may be biased. In addition, these methods are characterized by too large standard errors due to the lack of precision of the results or by too small standard errors due to the overestimation of the precision of results.

On the other hand, multiple imputation is an advanced method to deal with missing data. Standard imputation programs build on the MAR assumption, but the method can handle both MCAR and MNAR, although imputation is considerably more complex under MNAR. Multiple imputation provides unbiased and valid estimates of associations based on information from the available data—i.e., yielding estimates similar to those calculated from full data. The method affects not only the coefficient estimates for variables with missing data but also the estimates for other variables with no missing data.

In order to increase the transparency and understanding of the research results, the use of extended STROBE guidelines [25, 26] for reporting of multiple imputation analyses is recommend.

Much modern patient focused research attempts to detect the minimally clinically important difference (MCID) with highest possible precision. The smallest change in a treatment outcome that an individual would identify as important, and which would indicate a change in the patient's state of health, is key to understand if a treatment is effective or not. If patient reported outcomes are missing, the MCID cannot be calculated. Therefore, our strategies to prevent or minimize missing data is fundamental to accomplishing high quality research. Our statistical colleagues help us by providing sophisticated functions, libraries, and macros for imputation and methods to correct missing data. Complex calculations based on neural networks became more accurate day by day, especially for solving missing data of categorical and non-numerical features.

In conclusion, as for the world of medicine and surgery as for the world of statistics, the same citation is valid:" To prevent is better than to treat" but if prevention has not been successful, the treatment with imputation methods may solve the problem.

## References


1. Cappelleri JC, Zou KH, Bushmakin A, Alvir MJM, Symonds T. Patient-reported outcomes: measurement, implementation and interpretation. Boca Raton, FL: CRC Press; 2013.
2. Wisniewski SR, Leon AC, Otto MW, Trivedi MH. Prevention of missing data in clinical research studies. Biol Psychiatry. 2006;59(11):997–1000.
3. Schafer J. Analysis of incomplete multivariate data. Boca Raton, FL: Chapman & Hall/CRC; 2002.
4. Allison P. Missing data. Thousand Oaks, CA: SAGE; 2002.
5. Graham JW. Missing data analysis: making it work in the real world. Annu Rev Psychol. 2009;60:549–76.
6. Little RJA. Regression with missing X's: a review. J Am Stat Assoc. 1992;87(420):1227–37.
7. Donders AR, van der Heijden GJ, Stijnen T, Moons KG. Review: a gentle introduction to imputation of missing values. J Clin Epidemiol. 2006;59(10):1087–91.
8. Apold H, Meyer HE, Espehaug B, Nordsletten L, Havelin LI, Flugsrud GB. Weight gain and the risk of total hip replacement a populationbased prospective cohort study of 265,725 individuals. Osteoarthr Cartil. 2011;19(7):809–15.
9. Allison P. Missing data techniques for structural equation modeling. J Abnorm Psychol. 2003;112(4):545–57.

10. Patrician P. Multiple imputation for missing data. Res Nurs Health. 2002;38:76–84.
11. Rogier A, Donders T, van der Heijden GJMG, Stijnen T, Moons KGM. Review: a gentle introduction to imputation of missing values. J Clin Epidemiol. 2006;59(10):1087–91.
12. Pedersen AB, Mikkelsen EM, Cronin-Fenton D, Kristensen NR, Pham TM, Pedersen L, Petersen I. Missing data and multiple imputation in clinical epidemiological research. Clin Epidemiol. 2017;9:157–66.
13. Jones M. Indicator and stratification methods for missing explanatory variables in multiple linear regression. J Am Stat Assoc. 1996;91:222–30.
14. Vach W. Logistic regression with missing values in covariates. New York: Springer-Verlag; 1994.
15. Buuren SV. Flexible imputation of missing data. Interdisciplinary statistics series. Boca Raton, FL: Chapman & Hall/CRC; 2012.
16. Barnes SA, Larsen MD, Schroeder D, Hanson A, Decker PA. Missing data assumptions and methods in a smoking cessation study. Addiction. 2010;105(3):431–7.
17. Sterne JA, White IR, Carlin JB, et al. Multiple imputation for missing data in epidemiological and clinical research: potential and pitfalls. BMJ. 2009;338:b2393.
18. Rubin DB. Multiple imputation for nonresponse in surveys. New York: Wiley; 1987.
19. Carpenter J, Kenward M. Multiple imputation and its application. New York, NY: Wiley; 2013.
20. Schafer JL, Graham JW. Missing data: our view of the state of the art. Psychol Methods. 2002;7(2):147–77.
21. Moons KG, Donders RA, Stijnen T, Harrell FE Jr. Using the outcome for imputation of missing predictor values was preferred. J Clin Epidemiol. 2006;59(10):1092–101.
22. Yuan YC. Multiple imputation for missing data: concepts and new development, vol. 49. Rockville, MD: SAS Institute; 2010. p. 1–11.
23. Van Buuren S. 2. Multiple Imputation. In: Flexible imputation of missing data. Interdisciplinary statistics series, vol. 5. Boca Raton, FL: Chapman & Hall/CRC; 2012. p. 24–5.
24. Ondeck NT, Fu MC, Skrip LA, McLynn RP, Su EP, Grauer JN. Treatments of missing values in large National Data Affect Conclusions: the impact of multiple imputation on arthroplasty research. J Arthroplasty. 2018;33(3):661–7.
25. Vandenbroucke JP, von Elm E, Altman DG, Gøtzsche PC, Mulrow CD, Pocock SJ, et al. Strengthening the reporting of observational studies in epidemiology (STROBE): explanation and elaboration. PLoS Med. 2007;4:e297.
26. Von Elm E, Altman DG, Egger M, Pocock SJ, Gøtzsche PC, Vandenbroucke JP, et al. Strengthening the reporting of observational studies in epidemiology (STROBE) statement: guidelines for reporting observational studies. BMJ. 2007;335:806–8.

# Statistical Analysis for Surgical Trials

# 17

Emily Leary and Jinpu Li

## 17.1 A Note on Statistical Software

Throughout this chapter, code examples are referenced which can be used to perform each of these concepts, these are provided in appendices. All code utilizes R, which is free to download and use (available from https://www.r-project.org/). The RStudio development environment (available from https://rstudio.com/) is recommended and the required R packages are *'GMMBoost'*, *'ggplot2'*, *'GGally'*, *'ggcorrplot'*, and *'dslabs'*. A knee data set from '*GMMBoost*' is used for examples (available from https://cran.r-project.org/package=GMMBoost). Note that R code is annotated using "#" as the first character for lines containing annotations. The required packages can be installed using the R code in Appendix 1.

## 17.2 Preparation for Analysis: Data Pre-Processing

Data for clinical trials are intended to be uniformly collected, complete, and without error. However, in reality and throughout the trial process, data may be incomplete, inconsistently formatted, or contain unintended errors. Therefore, data pre-processing is a critical step to identify and remedy such issues to ensure data quality and the confidence of subsequent conclusions.

### 17.2.1 Harmonization

Data harmonization refers to the process of combining data together from various sources. In the context of a clinical trial, this may reflect a summary data pull from hospital electronic records being combined with data collected specifically for the trial, or perhaps data from different sites, in a multi-center trial. Prior to trial implementation, a detailed data collection protocol and staff training should be provided to ensure uniform data collection and data storage (see Chap. 13 for more details) [1]. A detailed understanding of how data are collected and stored is important to assess data quality and detect potential issues that could impact analyses and interpretations. If data are not directly entered into a standardized collection system, data should be checked against the original data obtained. This can be done either by checking all data or by comparing distributions (frequencies for nominal/categorical variables or measures of center and spread for continuous variables). Furthermore, checks should be completed to ensure that data have acceptable or biologically plausible values. For example, an ASA score of

E. Leary (✉) · J. Li
Department of Orthopaedic Surgery, School of Medicine, University of Missouri, Columbia, MO, USA
e-mail: learye@health.missouri.edu; lijinp@health.missouri.edu


S. Lyman et al. (eds.), *Introduction to Surgical Trials*,
https://doi.org/10.1007/978-3-031-77563-5_17

"10" where the largest possible value is ASA "VI" or "6" [2]. Furthermore, given that we are referring specifically to surgical trials, ASA over "IV" or "4" may indicate a potential protocol violation for elective orthopedic surgery. Alternatively, there may be inconsistency in data recording between study personnel or study sites. For example, VAS Pain scores at one site ranging from 1 to 10, but other sites range from 0 to 100 [3]. These discrepancies or inconsistencies must be identified and re-coded for analysis, where possible, so that bias is minimized and valuable information is not lost. The code in Appendix 2 uses this process with an example with the knee dataset.

## 17.2.2 Data Visualization

Once all the data are combined, and all formats and values have been aligned across sites or clinical teams, the next step is to assess the data visually. Data visualization is the graphical representation of data and provides a visual summary of information. This may display unknown or unanticipated patterns or trends. Effective visualization contributes to internal quality checks required for rigorous clinical trial planning and analyses. To appropriately visualize data, the type of variable is first considered. Visualization is typically an iterative process with data cleaning processes (see next section), such that there may be multiple versions of visualizations as additional items for data cleaning are identified. More advanced skills can be found in *Data Visualization with R* [4]. For a deeper exploration into the field of visual excellence, consider Edward Tufte's seminal *The Visual Display of Quantitative Data* or his more recent works expanding on various aspects of data visualization to improve human perception [5–7].

### 17.2.2.1 Continuous Variables

Continuous variables are typically visualized using a histogram or density curve, encoded with dots, bars, or lines, while categorical variables may be visualized with a bar chart or balloon plot. These visualizations can also be expanded to look at pairwise relationships between continuous variables or to color code data with respect to separate categorical variables. Scatter plots are one of the most common visualizations and use dots or other symbols to represent the values of two numerical variables such that the linear relationship between the variables can be observed. A box plot figure could be considered for visualization when one variable is categorical and another is continuous (Fig. 17.1). See Appendix 3 for an example with corresponding R code.

### 17.2.2.2 Categorical Variables

Researchers often must report the frequencies and proportions for categorical variables, such as sex. To visualize these variables, a bar chart is commonly used. Additionally, pairs of categorical variables can be evaluated together using a frequency table or bar graphs representing a contingency table. These visualizations may help identify areas to investigate further for data checking and, later, the analysis itself (Fig. 17.2). See Appendix 4 for an example with corresponding R code.

## 17.2.3 Data Cleaning

To avoid the unintentional impact of extreme values, which are used to denote other information, data cleaning should be completed before analysis. In addition to data harmonization and visualization to check for validity, reasonability, and formatting, additional data cleaning may be required. Sometimes missing data are denoted by ".", "_", "NA", "NaN", "-99", "9999" or some other "extreme" or "unrealistic" value. Alternatively, sometimes data might be entered or recorded incorrectly, for example, a negative weight or a weight for a person that is considered biologically implausible (e.g., 9999 kg). Such values should be checked prior to calculation of any summary statistics. Recoding or excluding these values may be necessary, but all decisions should be appropriately documented and justified. Note that data cleaning is not falsifying data, it is only conducting quality checks using multiple considerations to ensure that the data reflect the measured values as accurately as possible. See Appendix 5 for an example with corresponding R code.

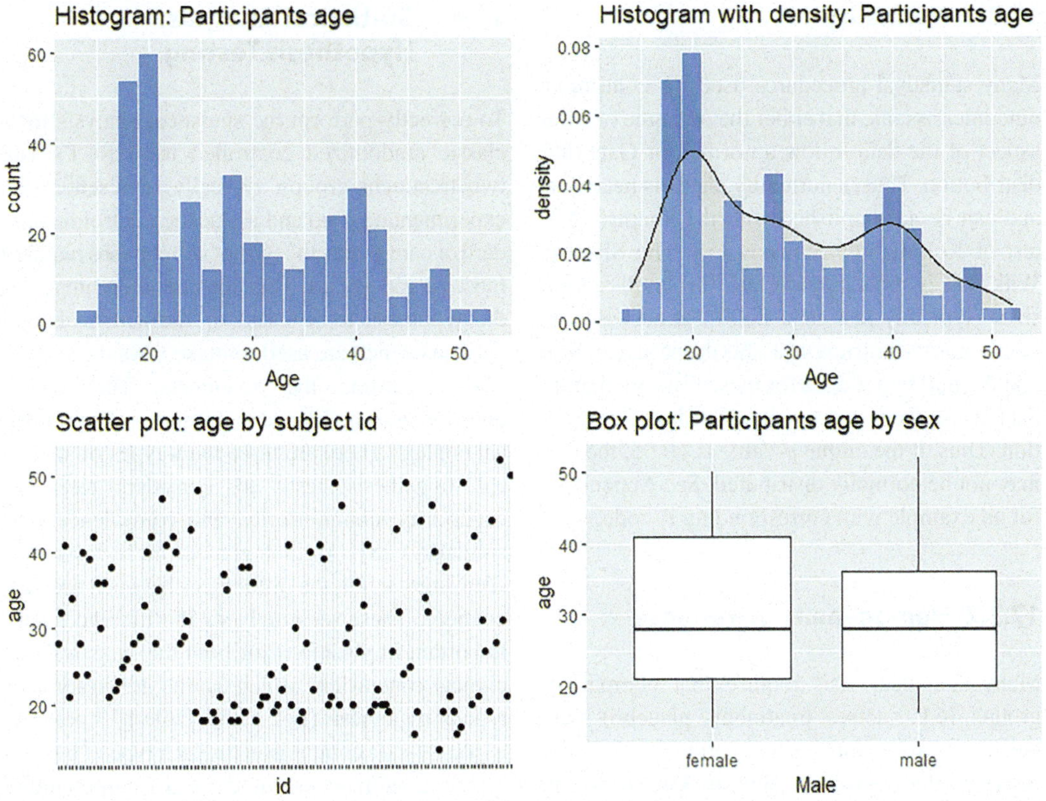


**Fig. 17.1** Figures which visualize continuous data: from top histograms; bottom left, a scatter plot; and bottom right, a boxplot

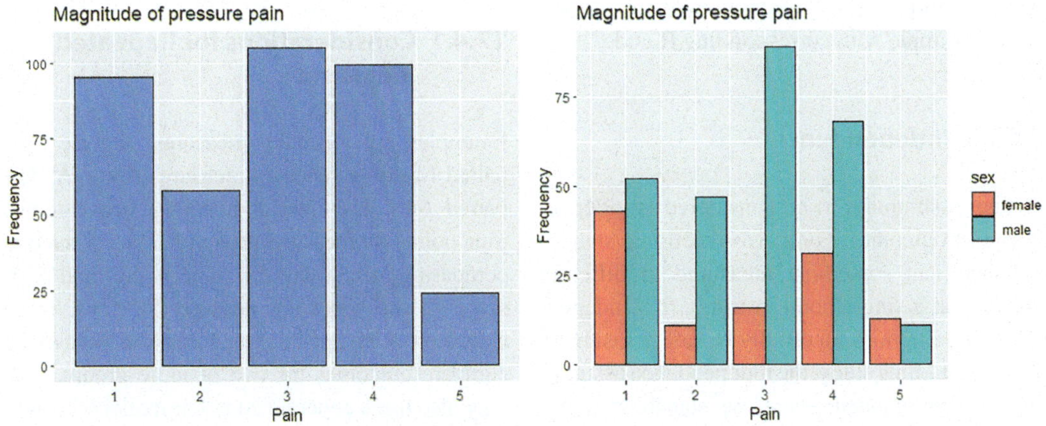


**Fig. 17.2** Bar graphs which visualize categorical data: left, pain; and right, pain by sex

## 17.3 Statistical Analysis: Checking Assumptions

All statistical tests make assumptions of some type, typically of the data distributions for each variable. Statistical results and conclusions (i.e., statistical inference) from these tests may not be valid when the respective assumptions are violated. Therefore, checking the assumptions for any statistical test is a critical step.

### 17.3.1 Normality

Many statistical procedures used for continuous outcomes assume that either the outcome or some aspect of the data follow a normal, or Gaussian, distribution. Thus, a normality check is necessary and can be accomplished with the Shapiro-Wilk test or Kolmogorov-Smirnov test. The Shapiro-Wilk test is more appropriate for small sample sizes (typically less than 2000). Otherwise, the Kolmogorov-Smirnov test should be used. Note that the null hypotheses for these tests are that the data come from a normally distributed population. Thus, if the output $p$-value is <0.05, the data may not be normally distributed. See Appendix 6 for an example with corresponding R code.

### 17.3.2 Homogeneity of Variance

Many statistical tests require that comparison groups (e.g., active treatment, placebo) have equal variance for each continuous variable between these groups. This is known as the homogeneity of variances. The equal variance assumption can be tested with the $F$-test to compare variances between two groups or the Bartlett test for more than two groups. See Appendix 7 for an example with corresponding R code.

### 17.3.3 Independence

A final assumption to be considered is independence of outcomes. For a cross sectional statistical test (i.e., something measured in different subjects at a single point in time), this independence assumption can usually be safely assumed. In a longitudinal study, the independence assumption may be violated. Therefore, statistical analyses should incorporate the potential for this dependency, or covariance, structure. In this scenario, repeated measures analyses which incorporate the time component or "repeated" nature of the observations should be considered. See section on Considerations for Repeated Measures Analyses for more details.

## 17.4 Statistical Analysis: Hypothesis Testing

To correctly perform the statistical analysis for a classic randomized controlled trial (RCT) with two treatment groups, typically representing an experimental group and a placebo control or standard of care group, the type of conclusions required must be considered. This consideration hinges on the hypothesis to be tested, or, the statistical comparisons which are used to make formalized decisions regarding the treatments. The clinical question must be framed in the appropriate statistical context. There are three main types of statistical hypothesis tests to consider: tests for superiority, noninferiority, and equivalence (i.e., similarity) [8]. At first glance, these tests may seem similar, but the differences between each are nuanced. These seemingly small differences have important implications for both the statistical and clinical conclusions which can be drawn for each type of hypothesis (Fig. 17.3). Table 17.1 provides a side-by-side comparison for each type of hypothesis test, with notes for clinical interpretations, how to code the statistics for each, assumptions for each test, and possible conclusions.

### 17.4.1 Considerations for Repeated Measures

Examples of repeated measures analyses are paired t-tests or repeated measures ANOVA. The paired $t$-test tests mean outcomes between two time points for the same group of subjects, such as comparing pain scores for subjects pre- and post-surgery. The repeated measures ANOVA is an extension of the paired $t$-test and can be used to compare outcomes for two or more groups. One may also use a generalized linear model with subject effect to account for the dependency or a specified covariance structure. Repeated measure analysis using a noninferiority and an equivalence hypothesis is beyond the scope of this chapter but please refer to Mascha and Sessler (2011) for more details [11]. See Appendix 8 for examples of the paired $t$-test and repeated measures ANOVA in R.

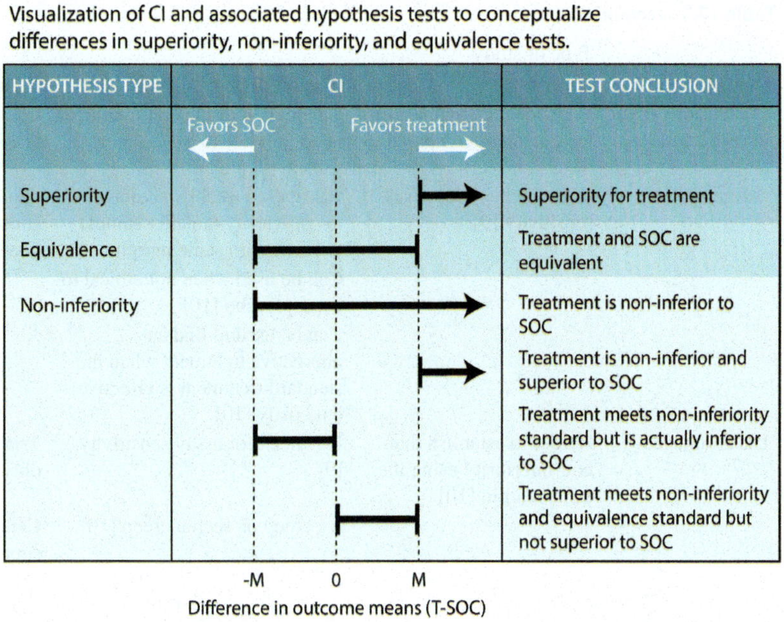


**Fig. 17.3** Difference in Statistical and Clinical Conclusions with Possible Results (Point Estimate and $(1-\alpha)\%$ CI, Assuming Margin as M). Figure authors Emily Leary, Jinpu Li, and Stacy Cheavens

**Table 17.1** Side-by-side comparison for superiority, noninferiority, and equivalence studies considering one experimental group and one control group or standard of care (SOC)

| | Type of study | | |
|---|---|---|---|
| Considerations | Superiority | Noninferiority | Equivalence |
| Study goal | Show experimental surgical treatment is better than SOC surgery | Show experimental surgical treatment is as good as the SOC surgery | Show experimental |
| Translate study goal to type of hypothesis | Response to experimental surgical treatment is superior to a SOC surgery | Response to experimental surgical treatment is no worse or not clinically inferior to a SOC surgery | Response to the experimental surgical treatment or SOC surgery differs by an amount that is clinically unimportant |
| Write statistical hypothesis | $H_0: \mu_t - \mu_{SOC} \leq \delta$<br>$H_1: \mu_t - \mu_{SOC} > \delta$ | $H_0: \mu_t - \mu_{SOC} \leq -\delta$<br>$H_1: \mu_t - \mu_{SOC} > -\delta$ | $H_0: \lvert \mu_t - \mu_{SOC} \rvert \geq \delta$<br>$H_1: \lvert \mu_t - \mu_{SOC} \rvert < \delta$ |
| Delta definition | $\delta \geq 0$, clinical importance (which can be 0) | $\delta \geq 0$, margin of clinical significance (usually small) | $\delta \geq 0$, tolerance margin |
| Assumptions | Constancy assumption: the effect of the SOC surgery in the trial is consistent with the effect that was observed in previous trials<br>Assay sensitivity: the clinical trial has the ability to demonstrate a difference between treatments if such a difference truly exists | | |
| Basic R code for analysis | # nc : sample size of SOC group<br># nt : sample size of treatment group<br># M : margin of clinical significance<br># Cbar : mean for SOC group (average outcome value for SOC group)<br># Tbar : mean for treatment group (average outcome value for treatment group<br># sigma2bar : pooled variance (variance for both treatment and control groups) | | |
| | ## p-value<br>1 - pnorm(abs(Tbar – Cbar - M) / sqrt(sigma2bar * (1/nc + 1/nt))) | ## p-value<br>1 - pnorm(abs(Tbar – Cbar - (-M)) / sqrt(sigma2bar * (1/nc + 1/nt))) | ## p-value<br>1 - pnorm((M - abs(Tbar - Cbar)) / sqrt(sigma2bar * (1/nc + 1/nt))) |
| Conclusions if reject null | Superiority for treatment t | Treatment is noninferior to SOC | Treatment and SOC are equivalent |

(continued)

**Table 17.1** (continued)

| | Type of study | | |
|---|---|---|---|
| Considerations | Superiority | Noninferiority | Equivalence |
| Conclusions if fail to reject null | No evidence of superiority for treatment compared to SOC | Cannot determine that treatment is noninferior to SOC | Cannot determine that treatment is equivalent to SOC |
| Advantages | Internal check for assay sensitivity [9] | "Easier" to establish compared to superiority (smaller sample needed) with same margin | "Easier" to establish compared to superiority (smaller sample needed) with the same margin |
| | | Can be used when not ethical to use a placebo [10] | |
| | | Can be used to find an alternative treatment when the standard treatment is effective but costly [10] | |
| Disadvantages | Harder to establish than non-inferiority using the same margin [10] | No check for assay sensitivity [9] | Trials cannot be conducted with only placebo group. |
| | | Biocreep or Technocreep [10] | Cannot be used to determine superiority or one treatment is better than other |
| | | Anti-conservative [10] | |

It is assumed that treatment means are compared and that larger mean values indicate a better outcome

### 17.4.2 Considerations for Non-Parametric Statistics

Non-parametric statistics do not require a normality assumption. In fact, these statistics have no distributional assumptions. However, these statistics are less efficient than their parametric (i.e., statistics requiring normal distribution), counterparts [12]. For this reason, consider using data transformations before resorting to the use of non-parametric statistics. For a detailed discussion of transformations, please see the seminal work from Box and Cox (1964) as well as more recent extensions [13–15].

### 17.4.3 Translation into Clinical Interpretations

Statistical results should always be framed for the clinical application and given appropriate clinical consideration. Statistical significance does not equate to clinical importance. Statistical inference is a formalized process for decision-making based on data and it is up to the study investigators to translate that quantitative information into meaningful conclusions for the clinical and scientific community. For ease of interpretation, it is best practice to report the outcome variable's 95% confidence intervals (CI) in addition to *p*-values for any hypothesis tests. Once the statistics are reported, then the results can be framed in terms of clinical importance, for example, if the statistical difference exceeded the minimum clinically important difference for an outcome (e.g., the smallest difference which can be perceived by patient or clinician) [16]. Please refer to the following references for a detailed discussion of these concepts [17–23].

## 17.5 Statistical Analysis: Potential Pitfalls to Avoid

### 17.5.1 "Intention to Treat" and "Per Protocol"

The "intention to treat" population defines subjects who were randomized to one treatment group but may not have actually received the assigned treatment or adhered to the post-treatment protocol. The "per protocol" or "as treated" population defines subjects who were randomized to the surgical treatment, received that treatment and were adherent to the post-surgical protocol. In many high-quality clinical trials, multiple patient populations are considered for analyses to provide internal quality control; however, for randomized studies, the intention to treat analysis should be the primary analysis [24]. These analyses use the same analytical techniques or hypothesis tests but consider different study populations to determine if the conclusions change. The following references provide a detailed discussion on intention to treat analyses and Losina et al. provides a similar discussion for per protocol analyses [24–26].

### 17.5.2 "Interim Analyses" and "Multiple Comparisons"

Interim analyses and multiple comparisons should be planned, if considered essential for the trial. Unambiguous and complete instructions should be included in the study operations manual so that an independent statistician could perform the analyses. A Data and Safety Monitoring Board (DSMB) is an independent group of experts that monitor, review, and evaluate the study data for participant safety, study conduct and progress, and efficacy when appropriate. To fulfill their responsibilities, it is within the purview of the DSMB to request additional analyses or analyses to assess the need to stop a study early or continue recruitment or follow-up; however, this process should be explicitly outlined in the DSMB's charter, which provides a detailed list of the responsibilities and duties for the DSMB [27, 28]. Interim analyses for recruitment or early stopping differ from other, planned interim analyses in both intention and implications [29–31]. However, interim analysis and multiple comparisons for any reason must be "adjusted" for the final analyses as these types of analyses impact the Type I error of the final analysis; these are considered adjustments for the false discovery rate. Most have heard of, or read studies, which utilize the Bonferonni adjustment; however, more efficient adjustments exist and are recommended, such as the Benjamini-Hochberg method. Chen et al. provide an excellent overview of these different methods [32, 33].

### 17.5.3 "Post-Hoc Power Analyses"

An a priori power analysis should be conducted prior to trial initiation for both sample size target and site planning. The result of this a priori power analysis reflects the smallest sample size that is suitable to detect the minimally clinically important effect size for a given statistical test at a desired level of significance. The power analysis is therefore defined by the analysis framework planned and the proposed detectable effect, both of which should be stated as part of any power analysis description. Post-hoc power analysis, or a power analysis conducted after the study is conducted, is inappropriate for any clinical trial. Powering the surgical trial should be completed in the planning stage of the trial and should use a predetermined clinically significant difference [34]. Assuming a normal distribution and known variance, performing a post-hoc power analysis using the *observed* difference from a clinical trial will always result in power less than 0.50 [35]. Appropriate post-hoc power analyses must consider a specific, clinically significant difference which is *not the observed difference* for the trial performed.

## 17.6 Summary

In this chapter, we reviewed the concepts required to successfully analyze the main hypothesis for a surgical randomized controlled trial and provided examples with corresponding R code. Prior to any analysis, we reviewed the importance of data checking, harmonization, and processing to ensure the highest quality and complete data. Common statistical assumptions for inferential tests were reviewed, as well as what to do when these assumptions are not met. Three hypothesis frameworks useful for surgical trials were considered and the advantages and disadvantages of each were outlined, while highlighting the importance of clinical meaning for any statistical result.

**Table 17.2** Additional information for superiority, noninferiority, and equivalence studies considering one experimental group and one control group or standard of care (SOC) for a *dichotomous (yes/no)* outcome

| Considerations | Type of study<br>Superiority | Noninferiority | Equivalence |
|---|---|---|---|
| Statistical hypothesis | $H_0: p_t - p_{SOC} \leq \delta$<br>$H_1: p_t - p_{SOC} > \delta$ | $H_0: p_t - p_{SOC} \leq -\delta$<br>$H_1: p_t - p_{SOC} > -\delta$ | $H_0: \lvert p_t - p_{SOC}\rvert \geq \delta$<br>$H_1: \lvert p_t - p_{SOC}\rvert < \delta$ |
| Basic R code for analysis | # nc : sample size of SOC group<br># nt : sample size of treatment group<br># pC : proportion control group<br># qC : 1 - pC<br># pT : proportion of treatment group<br># qT : 1 - pT | | |
| | ## p-value of categorical outcome<br>1 - pnorm(abs(pT – pC - M) / sqrt(pC*qC/nC + pT*qT/nT)) | ## p-value of categorical outcome<br>1 - pnorm(abs(pT – pC – (-M)) / sqrt(pC*qC/nC + pT*qT/nT)) | ## p-value of categorical outcome<br>1 - pnorm((M - abs(pT – pC)) / sqrt(pC*qC/nC + pT*qT/nT)) |

## Glossary

**ANOVA** Analysis of Variance—this is a test to determine differences in mean outcome values across three or more groups.

**Anticonservative** A poorly designed and conducted noninferiority study has a greater chance of a false positive outcome, a Type I error. This is the opposite situation for a superiority study which has an internal check for assay sensitivity.

**Assay sensitivity** If the trial had included a placebo, then the difference between the outcome for the placebo and control would be at least as large as the margin of clinical significance [9, 37].

**Biocreep/Technocreep** The iterative process of establishing noninferiority to the current gold standard of a slightly less effective, new treatment, followed by the use of this new treatment as a gold standard for an even newer, noninferior but again slightly less effective treatment, and so on [10].

**Categorical variables** These are variables with descriptive outcomes rather than numerical. Generally, these can be nominal, or variables with no inherent order (e.g., male and female), or ordinal, or variables that are still descriptive with an inherent order (e.g., less than high school education, high school education, and greater than high school education).

**Continuous variables** Are numeric variables that can take on an infinite number of values, e.g., weight or height of a person.

## Additional Resources

Thoma et al.: Users' guide to the surgical literature [36].

## Supplementary Material

Understanding differences in the analysis used for dichotomous outcomes in surgical trials, e.g., failure/success, may be useful.

Table 17.2 provides a summary of these differences.

## Appendix 1

R code to install the required packages for the functions described in this chapter.

```
#install packages.
install.packages("GMMBoost")
install.packages("ggplot2")
install.packages("GGally")
install.packages("ggcorrplot")
install.packages("dslabs")
```

```
# load in packages
library(ggplot2)
library(GMMBoost)
library(GGally)
library(ggcorrplot)
library(dslabs)

# load in the data
data(knee)
```

## Appendix 2

R code to demonstrate a scenario in which the data are incomplete and must be harmonized from two separate datasets, dataset 1 and dataset 2. In this example, each participant has three measurements corresponding to three different time points for the trial. Assume the first two measurements, corresponding to the first and second time point of the trial, collected from site 1 and saved as dataset 1 while the last measurement, corresponding to the third time point of the trial, was from site 2 and saved in dataset 2. We will create a scenario in which sex is not documented at site 2 and the scaling of pain scores are different across sites—these must be added and harmonized for complete data for later analysis.

```
# In this data, each participant had three measurements.
# Assume the first two measurements (time = 1, 2) came from data 1 while the last measurement
(time = 3) was from data 2.
# We will create a scenario in which sex is not documented at site 2 and the scaling of pain
scores are different across sites (site 1 uses 0-100 for pain scores while site 2 uses 0-5) - these must
be added and harmonized for complete data for later analysis.
#scenario set up for the knee data
Data_1 <- knee[which(knee$time!=3),]
Data_1$pain <- Data_1$pain * 20
Data_2 <- knee[which(knee$time==3),]
Data_2 <- Data_2[,setdiff(colnames(knee),"sex")]

# harmonization using the example from the knee data
## harmonize pain scales between data 1 and data 2
Data_1$pain <- Data_1$pain / 100 * 5
## supply sex for data 2
Data_2$sex <- sapply(Data_2$id, function(i) return(Data_1$sex[which(Data_1$id==i)[1]]))
## combine data 1 and data 2
Data_All <- rbind(Data_1,Data_2)
## re-order the merged data
Data_All <- Data_All[order(Data_All$id),colnames(knee)]

# check the summary statistics
summary(Data_All)
```

## Appendix 3

The codes below present a scatter plot between the participants' age and by subject id (for data checks) as well as a box plot of participants' age by pain levels.

```
# draw the histogram for age
ggplot(knee, aes(x = age)) +
  geom_histogram(bins = 20, fill = "cornflowerblue", color = "white") +
  labs(title = "Participants by age", x = "Age")

# draw the density for age
ggplot(knee, aes(x = age)) +
  geom_histogram(aes(y = ..density..), bins = 20, fill = "cornflowerblue", color = "white") +
  labs(title = "Participants by age", x = "Age")+
  geom_density(alpha = .2, fill = "antiquewhite3")

# simple scatterplot for age by subject id
ggplot(knee,aes(x = id, y = age)) +
  geom_point() +
  theme(axis.text.x = element_blank()) +
  labs(title = "Scatter plot: age by subject id")

######  draw the scatter plots between continuous variables and categorical variables
# first, must convert sex to a factor variable so it can be used for grouping
knee$sex <- as.factor(knee$sex)
levels(knee$sex) <- c("female", "male")

# draws matrix of graphs for age, pain values, baseline pain value and sex
ggpairs(knee[,c("age","pain","pain.start","sex")], aes(color = as.factor(knee$sex)))+ theme_bw()

###### boxplot for age by sex
ggplot(knee, aes(x = as.factor(sex), y = age)) +
  geom_boxplot() +
  labs(title = "Participants age by sex") +
  xlab("Male")
```

## Appendix 4

The code below provides an example of a bar chart using the patients' VAS pain values at the first time point for the study.

```
# plot the bar chart of pain values
ggplot(knee, aes(x = pain)) +
  geom_bar(fill = "cornflowerblue", color="black") +
  labs(x = "Pain", y = "Frequency", title = "Magnitude of pressure pain")

# plot the bar chart pain values by sex
knee$sex <- as.factor(knee$sex)
ggplot(knee, aes(x = pain, fill = sex)) +
    geom_bar(position="dodge",color="black") +
    labs(x = "Pain", y = "Frequency", title = "Magnitude of pressure pain")
```

## Appendix 5

The code below provides an example of a bar chart using the patients' VAS pain values at the first time point for the study.

```
#data from the package ds_labs
# load in the data of self-reported adult male height in feet
data(outlier_example)
# check the summary statistics
summary(outlier_example)
# a value of 180 was mistakenly reported in centimeters rather than feet
# the outliers can be detected from plots as well
hist(outlier_example, breaks = 100)
```

## Appendix 6

The code below provides an example for testing the normality.

```
#testing the normality for the pressure pain in the knee
shapiro.test(knee$pain)
ks.test(knee$pain, "pnorm")
```

## Appendix 7

```
## test whether the variance of pain values for therapy group 0 is equal to the variance of pain
values for therapy group 1
var.test(knee$pain[knee$th=="0"], knee$pain[knee$th=="1"])

##Barlett test for homogeneity of variance across pain.start values
bartlett.test(pain ~ pain.start, data = knee)
```

## Appendix 8

```
# paired t-test
## compare the difference of pain scores between first and second time points
t.test(knee$pain[which(knee$time==1)], knee$pain[which(knee$time==2)], paired = TRUE)
# ANOVA
## compare the difference of pain scores between three time points
summary(aov(pain~time, data = knee))
# linear mixed model incorporating the subject effect
knee_LMM <- lmer(pain ~ time + (1|id), data = knee)
summary(knee_LMM)
```

## References

1. Kuehl R. Design of Experiments: statistical principles of research design and analysis. 2nd ed. London: Duxbury Press.
2. ASA Physical Status Classification System [Internet]. https://www.asahq.org/standards-and-guidelines/asa-physical-status-classification-system. Accessed 14 Dec 2020.
3. Hawker GA, Mian S, Kendzerska T, French M. Measures of adult pain: visual analog scale for pain (VAS pain), numeric rating scale for pain (NRS pain), McGill pain questionnaire (MPQ), short-form McGill pain questionnaire (SF-MPQ), chronic pain grade scale (CPGS), short Form-36 bodily pain scale (SF-36 BPS), and measure of intermittent and constant osteoarthritis pain (ICOAP). Arthritis Care Res. 2011;63(S11):S240–52.
4. Data Visualization with R [Internet]. https://rkabacoff.github.io/datavis/. Accessed 14 Dec 2020.
5. Tufte E. The visual display of quantitative information. 2nd ed. Cheshire, CT: Graphics Press; 2001. p. 197.
6. Tufte E. Beautiful evidence. 1st ed. Cheshire, CT: Graphics Press; 2006. p. 213.
7. Tufte E. Envisioning information. 1st ed. Cheshire, CT: Graphics Press; 1990. p. 128.

8. Comparisons of superiority, non-inferiority, and equivalence trials [Internet]. https://www.ncbi.nlm.nih.gov/pmc/articles/PMC5925592/. Accessed 14 Dec 2020.
9. Schumi J, Wittes JT. Through the looking glass: understanding non-inferiority. Trials. 2011;12(1):106–12.
10. Vavken P. Rationale for and methods of superiority, noninferiority, or equivalence designs in orthopaedic, controlled trials. Clin Orthop Relat Res. 2011;469(9):2645–53.
11. Mascha EJ, Sessler DI. Equivalence and noninferiority testing in regression models and repeated-measures designs. Anesth Analg. 2011;112(3):678–87.
12. Sheskin D. Handbook of parametric and nonparametric statistical procedures. 3rd ed. Boca Raton, FL: CRC.
13. Box GEP, Cox DR. An analysis of transformations. J R Stat Soc Ser B (Methodological). 1964;26:211. https://rss.onlinelibrary.wiley.com/doi/abs/10.1111/j.2517-6161.1964.tb00553.x. Accessed 14 Dec 2020.
14. Chen G, Lockhart RA, Stephens MA. Box-Cox transformations in linear models: large sample theory and tests of normality. Can J Stat. 2002;30(2):177–209.
15. Teugels JL, Vanroelen G. Box–Cox transformations and heavy-tailed distributions. J Appl Probab. 2004;41:213–27.
16. Hung M, Saltzman CL, Kendall R, Bounsanga J, Voss MW, Lawrence B, et al. What are the MCIDs for PROMIS, NDI, and ODI instruments among patients with spinal conditions? Clin Orthop Relat Res. 2018;476(10):2027–36.
17. Bhardwaj SS, et al. Statistical significance and clinical relevance: the importance of power in clinical trials in dermatology. Arch Dermatol. 2004;140:1520. https://jamanetwork.com/journals/jamadermatology/fullarticle/480877. Accessed 14 Dec 2020.
18. Ranganathan P, Pramesh CS, Buyse M. Common pitfalls in statistical analysis: clinical versus statistical significance. Perspect Clin Res. 2015;6(3):169–70.
19. The use of confidence intervals in reporting orthopaedic research findings—PubMed [Internet]. https://pubmed.ncbi.nlm.nih.gov/19333667/. Accessed 14 Dec 2020.
20. Statistical Significance Versus Clinical Importance of Obser...: Anesthesia & Analgesia [Internet]. https://journals.lww.com/anesthesia-analgesia/fulltext/2018/03000/statistical_significance_versus_clinical.48.aspx. Accessed 14 Dec 2020.
21. Braitman LE. Confidence intervals assess both clinical significance and statistical significance. Ann Intern Med. 1991;114:515. Accessed 14 Dec 2020.
22. Kieser M et al. Assessment of statistical significance and clinical relevance. Stat Med. 2013. Accessed 14 Dec 2020. https://doi.org/10.1002/sim.5634.
23. Altman DG, Bland JM. Statistics notes: absence of evidence is not evidence of absence. BMJ. 1995;311(7003):485.
24. Losina E, Wright J, Katz JN. Clinical trials in orthopaedics research. Part III. Overcoming operational challenges in the design and conduct of randomized clinical trials in orthopaedic surgery. J Bone Joint Surg Am. 2012;94(6):e35.
25. Wiens BL, Zhao W. The role of intention to treat in analysis of noninferiority studies. Clin Trials. 2007;4:286. https://doi.org/10.1177/1740774507079443.
26. Understanding Equivalence and Noninferiority Testing [Internet]. https://www.ncbi.nlm.nih.gov/pmc/articles/PMC3019319/#CR9. Accessed 14 Dec 2020.
27. Nancy Garrick DD. Data and safety monitoring (DSM) guidelines for NIAMS-funded clinical research [internet]. National Institute of Arthritis and Musculoskeletal and Skin Diseases. NIAMS; 2017. https://www.niams.nih.gov/grants-funding/data-safety-monitoring/dsm-guidelines. Accessed 1 Nov 2022.
28. Data and Safety Monitoring Board (DSMB) Guidelines [Internet]. https://www.nidcr.nih.gov/research/human-subjects-research/toolkit-and-education-materials/interventional-studies/data-and-safety-monitoring-board-guidelines. Accessed 1 Nov 2022.
29. Togo K, Iwasaki M. Optimal timing for interim analyses in clinical trials. J Biopharm Stat. 2013;23(5):1067–80.
30. Kumar A, Chakraborty B. Interim analysis: a rational approach of decision making in clinical trial. J Adv Pharm Technol Res. 2016;7(4):118.
31. Todd S, Whitehead A, Stallard N, Whitehead J. Interim analyses and sequential designs in phase III studies: interim analyses and sequential designs in phase III studies. Br J Clin Pharmacol. 2001;51(5):394–9.
32. Chen SY, Feng Z, Yi X. A general introduction to adjustment for multiple comparisons. J Thorac Dis. 2017;9(6):1725–9.
33. Benjamini Y, Hochberg Y. Controlling the false discovery rate: a practical and powerful approach to multiple testing. J R Stat Soc Ser B (Methodological). 1995;57(1):289–300.
34. Anglen J, Burd T, Lowry K, Madsen R. Prevention of heterotopic bone formation and type-II errors: letter to the editor response. J Bone Joint Surg. 2002;84-A(7):1272–3.
35. Goodman SN. The use of predicted confidence intervals when planning experiments and the misuse of power when interpreting results. Ann Intern Med. 1994;121(3):200.
36. Thoma A, Farrokhyar F, Bhandari M, Tandan V. Users' guide to the surgical literature. p. 9.
37. Non-Inferiority Clinical Trials to Establish Effectiveness Guidance for Industry. p. 56.

# CONSORT Reporting Standards

# 18

Madison Thompson and Stephen Lyman

## 18.1 Introduction

First published in 1996, the Consolidated Standards of Reporting Trials statement (CONSORT) consists of a checklist of items that should be included when reporting randomized control trials (RCTs) as well as a flow diagram for following participants through said trials. CONSORT was created to standardize and improve the quality of reporting in RCTs and has since been revised twice to reflect changes in the ever-evolving best practices for RCTs [1, 2]. The standards were designed with the most common type of RCT, parallel group design trials, in mind, though the statement includes extensions that further specify requirements for other study designs (e.g., crossover, cluster), types of data (e.g., harm, patient reported outcome measures), and interventions (e.g., non-pharmacological, herbal) [3, 4].

M. Thompson
Georgetown University School of Medicine, Washington, DC, USA
e-mail: mct91@georgetown.edu

S. Lyman (✉)
Hospital for Special Surgery, New York, NY, USA

Medical Education, Kyushu University School of Medicine, Fukuoka, Japan
e-mail: LymanS@hss.edu


S. Lyman et al. (eds.), *Introduction to Surgical Trials*,
https://doi.org/10.1007/978-3-031-77563-5_18

## 18.2 Development

*The Book of Daniel* in the Bible is believed to document the first clinical trial, occurring sometime around 500 BC [5]. Despite their existence for centuries, however, clinical trials remain plagued with the issues of inconsistent, and worse inaccurate, reporting. Review papers in the 1980s revealed substantial disparities between the information gathered in an RCT versus what was actually published [6].

One such example is the information, or lack thereof, provided on patient randomization. In an RCT, randomization is of paramount importance, yet researchers found that barely 50% of RCTs adequately described the method of randomization employed. While some journals simply reported that randomization occurred rather than describing the specific method (e.g., random number generator), 34% did not mention randomization methodology at all [7]. A review conducted by Controlled Clinical Trials went so far as to assert that "randomization method for most clinical trials is so poor that the reader cannot tell if randomization has been applied properly" [8].

Work on the original CONSORT commenced in 1993 when two independent groups, the Standards of Reporting Trials (SORT) group and Asilomar Working Group on Recommendations for Reporting of Clinical Trials in the Biomedical Literature both convened to discuss essential items that should be included in publications on clinical trials [6].The groups concluded a single, coherent list would ensure the greatest adherence, and in 1996 published the first CONSORT statement of 21 items [1]. This has since evolved into a 25-item checklist and flow sheet with various extensions [4].

## 18.3 Adoption

CONSORT has been endorsed by 585 medical journals, including the *Journal of the American Medical Association*, *New England Journal of Medicine*, *Lancet*, and *British Medical Journal*, and cited nearly 8000 times [9].

Publications abiding by CONSORT standards were found to have significantly better—in some case upwards of 80% more—reporting of information such as allocation concealment, sequence generation method, scientific rationale for the trial, and sample size estimation than papers published in non-endorsing journals [10–12]. Systematic reviews have also found that Jadad reporting quality scores and reporting on specific items such as participant flow and sequence generation significantly improved after journals adopted CONSORT [12, 13].

## 18.4 Consort Checklist and Diagram

The primary CONSORT 25-item checklist (Table 18.1) and participant flow diagram (Fig. 18.1) provide authors with a standardized approach to reporting clinical trials. These standards facilitate adequate appraisal and interpretation of such trials by editors, researchers, and readers alike. The main checklist is geared toward the most common RCT design, two-group parallel design trials, which is utilized in over half of studies [14].

CONSORT designed the checklist to encourage researchers to denote specific page/line numbers in their manuscript where the corresponding information could be found. This was done to ensure accountability, avoid confusion, and reinforce accurate reporting [4].

**Table 18.1** CONSORT 2010 checklist [4]

| Section/Topic | Item no | Checklist item | Reported on page no |
|---|---|---|---|
| **Title and abstract** | | | |
| | 1a | Identification as a randomized trial in the title | |
| | 1b | Structured summary of trial design, methods, results, and conclusions | |
| **Introduction** | | | |
| Background and objectives | 2a | Scientific background and explanation of rationale | |
| | 2b | Specific objectives or hypotheses | |
| **Methods** | | | |
| Trial design | 3a | Description of trial design (such as parallel, factorial) including allocation ratio | |
| | 3b | Important changes to methods after trial commencement (such as eligibility criteria), with reasons | |
| Participants | 4a | Eligibility criteria for participants | |
| | 4b | Settings and locations where the data were collected | |
| Interventions | 5 | The interventions for each group with sufficient details to allow replication, including how and when they were actually administered | |

(continued)

**Table 18.1** (continued)

| Section/Topic | Item no | Checklist item | Reported on page no |
|---|---|---|---|
| Outcomes | 6a | Completely defined pre-specified primary and secondary outcome measures, including how and when they were assessed | |
| | 6b | Any changes to trial outcomes after the trial commenced, with reasons | |
| Sample size | 7a | How sample size was determined | |
| | 7b | When applicable, explanation of any interim analyses and stopping guidelines | |
| Randomization: | | | |
| Sequence generation | 8a | Method used to generate the random allocation sequence | |
| | 8b | Type of randomization; details of any restriction (such as blocking and block size) | |
| Allocation concealment mechanism | 9 | Mechanism used to implement the random allocation sequence (such as sequentially numbered containers), describing any steps taken to conceal the sequence until interventions were assigned | |
| Implementation | 10 | Who generated the random allocation sequence, who enrolled participants, and who assigned participants to interventions | |
| Blinding | 11a | If done, who was blinded after assignment to interventions (for example, participants, care providers, those assessing outcomes) and how | |
| | 11b | If relevant, description of the similarity of interventions | |
| Statistical methods | 12a | Statistical methods used to compare groups for primary and secondary outcomes | |
| | 12b | Methods for additional analyses, such as subgroup analyses and adjusted analyses | |
| **Results** | | | |
| Participant flow (a diagram is strongly recommended) | 13a | For each group, the numbers of participants who were randomly assigned, received intended treatment, and were analyzed for the primary outcome | |
| | 13b | For each group, losses and exclusions after randomization, together with reasons | |
| Recruitment | 14a | Dates defining the periods of recruitment and follow-up | |
| | 14b | Why the trial ended or was stopped | |
| Baseline data | 15 | A table showing baseline demographic and clinical characteristics for each group | |
| Numbers analyzed | 16 | For each group, number of participants (denominator) included in each analysis and whether the analysis was by original assigned groups | |
| Outcomes and estimation | 17a | For each primary and secondary outcome, results for each group, and the estimated effect size and its precision (such as 95% confidence interval) | |
| | 17b | For binary outcomes, presentation of both absolute and relative effect sizes is recommended | |

(continued)

**Table 18.1** (continued)

| Section/Topic | Item no | Checklist item | Reported on page no |
|---|---|---|---|
| Ancillary analyses | 18 | Results of any other analyses performed, including subgroup analyses and adjusted analyses, distinguishing pre-specified from exploratory | |
| Harms | 19 | All important harms or unintended effects in each group | |
| **Discussion** | | | |
| Limitations | 20 | Trial limitations, addressing sources of potential bias, imprecision, and, if relevant, multiplicity of analyses | |
| Generalizability | 21 | Generalizability (external validity, applicability) of the trial findings | |
| Interpretation | 22 | Interpretation consistent with results, balancing benefits and harms, and considering other relevant evidence | |
| **Other information** | | | |
| Registration | 23 | Registration number and name of trial registry | |
| Protocol | 24 | Where the full trial protocol can be accessed, if available | |
| Funding | 25 | Sources of funding and other support (such as supply of drugs), role of funders | |

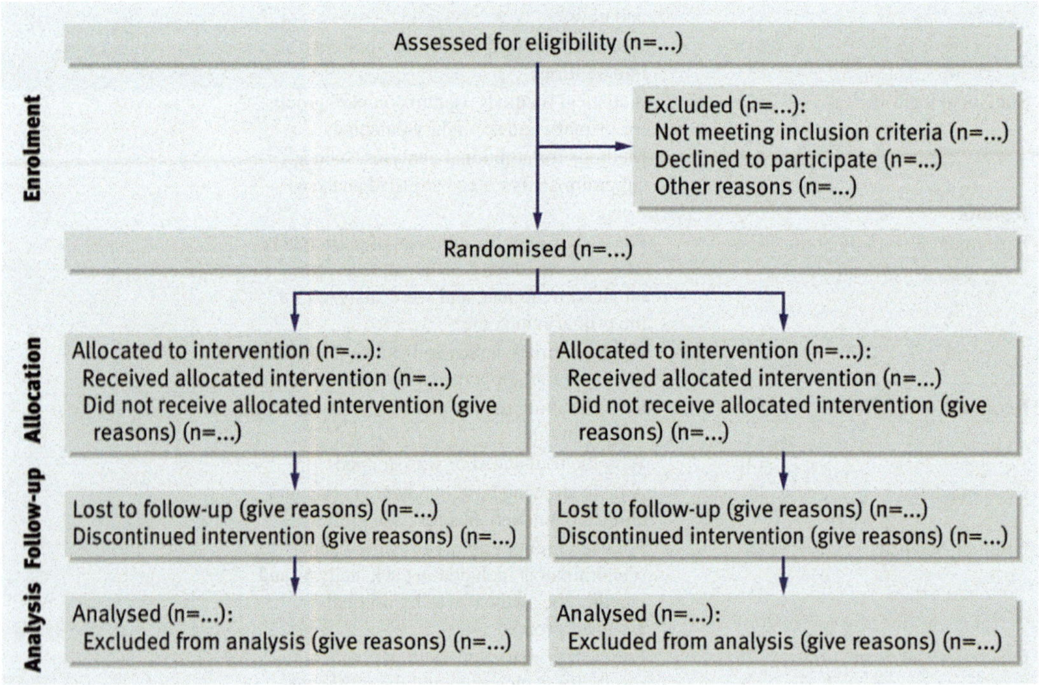


**Fig. 18.1** CONSORT participant flow diagram for parallel trials [4]. (Reproduced under the terms of the Creative Commons Attribution License (http://creativecommons.org/licenses/by/2.0), which permits unrestricted use, distribution, and reproduction in any medium, provided the original work is properly cited)

### 18.4.1 Title

Explicit identification as a randomized trial within a journal title facilitates more efficient indexing, search engine optimization, and identification by readers. A manual search of *Cancer* found that barely 50% of articles considered to be controlled or randomized appeared in the electronic MEDLINE RCT results. The "lost" publications were not indexed properly, often due to the title not explicitly identifying the study as an RCT [6]. Begg and colleagues assert that if continually "lost" in a systemic fashion, there is a vastly increased risk for bias when reviewing literature, as these articles may not be included [15].

### 18.4.2 Abstract

CONSORT provides an abstract-specific checklist (Table 18.2) that expands upon item 1b of the primary checklist (Table 18.1) and enumerates the items that should be included in the abstract in order to provide a succinct yet comprehensive description of the trial. Studies have found that there are often significant discrepancies between information reported in the abstract versus the full journal text [3], providing the impetus for the creation of standardized and consistent reporting standards for both bodies of text.

The average journal article costs upwards of $30 for an unaffiliated reader [16], not to mention takes far longer to read and dissect than brief abstracts that are available free of charge. Readers often use abstracts as a screening tool [3], weighing whether purchasing the full article is worth their time and money. Following the CONSORT guidelines for abstracts provides a transparent and accurate preview of the journal article, improving both cost- and time-efficiency on behalf of future readers and researchers. Again, the checklist provides space for authors to indicate line numbers for accountability.

**Table 18.2** CONSORT extension for abstracts [22]

| Item | Description | Reported on line number |
|---|---|---|
| Authors | Contact details for the corresponding author | |
| Trial design | Description of the trial design (e.g., parallel, cluster, non-inferiority) | |
| Methods: | | |
| Participants | Eligibility criteria for participants and the settings where the data were collected | |
| Interventions | Interventions intended for each group | |
| Objective | Specific objective or hypothesis | |
| Outcome | Clearly defined primary outcome for this report | |
| Randomization | How participants were allocated to interventions | |
| Blinding (masking) | Whether or not participants, care givers, and those assessing the outcomes were blinded to group assignment | |
| Results: | | |
| Numbers randomized | Number of participants randomized to each group | |
| Recruitment | Trial status | |
| Numbers analyzed | Number of participants analyzed in each group | |
| Outcome | For the primary outcome, a result for each group and the estimated effect size and its precision | |
| Harms | Important adverse events or side effects | |
| Conclusions | General interpretation of the results | |
| Trial registration | Registration number and name of trial register | |
| Funding | Source of funding | |

### 18.4.3 Introduction

An introduction should certainly include the reasoning behind why a study was conducted in the first place. CONSORT even cites the Declaration of Helsinki, asserting that it is "unethical to expose humans unnecessarily to the risks of research" and argues that justification of a new trial is in fact critical [3]. Objectives and hypotheses help guide not only researchers through the study but also readers through the manuscript. Quantifiable and qualifiable goals are critical in analyzing the success of any RCT, and clear description of these allows the reader to easily interpret results.

### 18.4.4 Trial Design

Over 50% of RCTs employ a parallel group design [14], and thus the primary CONSORT checklist is written with this type of study in mind. However, CONSORT also includes extensions that cater to the unique requirements and additional features of less common design types such as multi-arm parallel, randomized crossover, cluster, non-inferiority and equivalence, pragmatic, N-of-1, pilot and feasibility, within person, adaptive design trials on their website [17].

It is equally as important that changes in research design and protocol be adequately reported. Time and again reviews have shown that changes in protocols are severely underreported. One such review found that as many as half of the journal articles pertaining to RCTs had unaddressed discrepancies in outcomes [18].

### 18.4.5 Randomization

As discussed earlier, reporting on randomization methods is severely lacking [7, 8]. Perhaps more concerning, though, is that investigators have found less than half the studies that do report on randomization actually use adequate methods [14, 19]. This only raises further concern for the trials that neglect to mention it altogether.

Transparency regarding randomization is paramount for trial replication and validation. RCTs often allocate subjects in a 1:1 pattern, wherein an equal amount of participants receive the placebo and experimental treatments. Justification as for why authors chose a different ratio, perhaps 2:1, can provide further clarity for readers and reviewers as well as better facilitate repeat studies.

Another factor of randomization that has a large bearing on RCT reliability is allocation concealment. One meta-analysis found that trials with unclear or inadequate allocation concealment yielded over 30% greater treatment effect estimates than trials reporting adequate methods [20]. Not even 20% of RCTs on PubMed reported any allocation concealment to begin with [14].

### 18.4.6 Harms

Adverse events are also severely underreported and insufficiently described in RCTs. Analyses have found that barely 40% of surgical trials adequately report adverse events, and information on patient withdrawal due to such events is even less frequent [21, 22]. Omitting such information can severely skew readers' interpretations of findings. A critical tenet of medicine is to "Do no harm," yet how can informed decisions be made without knowing what harms are possible?

## 18.5 Conclusion

> The whole of medicine depends on the transparent reporting of clinical trials [4].

While many of the concepts enumerated in the CONSORT checklist may sound like common practice, a large number of publications fail to meet these standards, running the risk of misinterpretation. In addition to standardizing reporting on concepts such as randomization and participant flow, CONSORT has facilitated massive improvements in study accessibility and replicability. Comprehensive and accurate abstracts demonstrate respect for potential readers' time and money, and standards to ensure objective and transparent reporting overall help limit prejudice. Journals that abide by CONSORT guidelines demonstrate significantly higher quality reporting [10–12], making it no surprise so many have chosen to do so [9].

## References


1. Begg C, Cho M, Eastwood S, et al. Improving the quality of reporting of randomized controlled trials. The consort statement. JAMA J Am Med Assoc. 1996;276:637–9. https://doi.org/10.1001/jama.276.8.637.
2. Moher D, Schulz K, Altman D. The consort statement: revised recommendations for improving the quality of reports of parallel group randomized trials. BMC Med Res Methodol. 2001;1:2. https://doi.org/10.1186/1471-2288-1-2.
3. Moher D, Hopewell S, Schulz K, et al. Consort 2010 explanation and elaboration: updated guidelines for reporting parallel group randomised trials. BMJ. 2010;340:c869. https://doi.org/10.1136/bmj.c869.
4. Schulz KF, Altman DG, Moher D, et al. CONSORT 2010 statement: updated guidelines for reporting parallel group randomised trials. Trials. 2010;11:32. https://doi.org/10.1186/1745-6215-11-32.
5. Collier R. Legumes, lemons and streptomycin: a short history of the clinical trial. CMAJ. 2009;180(1):23–4. https://doi.org/10.1503/cmaj.081879.
6. Williams C. What are the goals of the consort initiative and what will it achieve? Ann Oncol. 1997;8:511–2. https://doi.org/10.1023/a:1008292620190.
7. DerSimonian R, Charette L, McPeek B, Mosteller F. Reporting on methods in clinical trials. N Engl J Med. 1982;306(22):1332–7. https://doi.org/10.1056/NEJM198206033062204.
8. Williams D, Davis C. Reporting of assignment methods in clinical trials. Control Clin Trials. 1994;15(4):294–8. https://doi.org/10.1016/0197-2456(94)90045-0.
9. CONSORT. Endorsers. 2022. https://www.consort-statement.org/about-consort/endorsers1. Accessed 3 Feb 2022.
10. Turner L, Shamseer L, Altman DG, Weeks L, Peters J, Kober T, Dias S, Schulz KF, Plint AC, Moher D. Consolidated standards of reporting trials (CONSORT) and the completeness of reporting of randomised controlled trials (RCTs) published in medical journals. Cochrane Database Syst Rev. 2012;11(11):MR000030. https://doi.org/10.1002/14651858.MR000030.pub2.
11. Turner L, Shamseer L, Altman DG, Schulz KF, Moher D. Does use of the CONSORT statement impact the completeness of reporting of randomised controlled trials published in medical journals? A Cochrane review. Syst Rev. 2012;1:60. https://doi.org/10.1186/2046-4053-1-60.
12. Plint A, Moher D, Morrison A, Schulz K, Altman DG, Hill C, Gaboury I. Does the CONSORT checklist improve the quality of reports of randomised controlled trials? A systematic review. Med J Aust. 2006;185(5):263–7. https://doi.org/10.5694/j.1326-5377.2006.tb00557.x.
13. Vassar M, Jellison S, Wendelbo H, Wayant C, Gray H, Bibens M. Using the CONSORT statement to evaluate the completeness of reporting of addiction randomised trials: a cross-sectional review. BMJ Open. 2019;9(9):e032024. https://doi.org/10.1136/bmjopen-2019-032024.
14. Chan A, Altman D. Epidemiology and reporting of randomised trials published in PubMed journals. Lancet. 2005;365(9465):1159–62. https://doi.org/10.1016/S0140-6736(05)71879-1.
15. Begg C, Berlin J. Publication bias: a problem in interpreting medical data. J R Stat Soc Ser A. 1988;151(3):419–63. https://doi.org/10.2307/2982993.
16. Duke University. Paywalls and Information Costs. 2022. https://sites.duke.edu/library101_instructors/2018/09/05/paywalls-and-information-costs/. Accessed 21 Feb 2022.
17. CONSORT. Endorsers. 2022. http://www.consort-statement.org/extensions. Accessed 16 Feb 2022.
18. Dwan K, Altman D, Arnaiz J, Bloom J, Chan A, Cronin E, Decullier E, Easterbrook P, Von Elm E, Gamble C, Ghersi D, Ioannidis J, Simes J, Williamson P. Systematic review of the empirical evidence of study publication bias and outcome reporting bias. PLoS One. 2008;3(8):e3081. https://doi.org/10.1371/journal.pone.0003081.
19. Hopewell S, Dutton S, Yu L, Chan A, Altman D. The quality of reports of randomised trials in 2000 and 2006: comparative study of articles indexed in pubmed. BMJ. 2010;340:c723. https://doi.org/10.1136/bmj.c723.
20. Wood L, Egger M, Gluud L, Schulz K, Jüni P, Altman D, Gluud C, Martin R, Wood A, Sterne J. Empirical evidence of bias in treatment effect estimates in controlled trials with different interventions and outcomes: meta-epidemiological study. BMJ. 2008;336(7644):601–5. https://doi.org/10.1136/bmj.39465.451748.ad.
21. Rosenthal R, Hoffmann H, Dwan K, Clavien P-A, Bucher HC. Reporting of adverse events in surgical trials: critical appraisal of current practice. World J Surg. 2014;39(1):80–7. https://doi.org/10.1007/s00268-014-2776-8.
22. Hopewell S, Clarke M, Moher D, Wager E, Middleton P, Altman D, Schulz K. CONSORT for reporting randomized controlled trials in journal and conference abstracts: explanation and elaboration. PLoS Med. 2008;5(1):e20. https://doi.org/10.1371/journal.pmed.0050020.

# Part IV

# Regulatory Standards

# The Regulatory Pathway to Market Class III Surgical Medical Devices in the United States

19

Sandra Navarrete, Daniel R. Lee, and Jason L. Koh

## 19.1 Introduction

The United States (US) Food and Drug Administration (FDA) regulates the safety and effectiveness of drugs, biologics, and devices under its authorities enacted under the Federal Food, Drug and Cosmetic Act (FD&C Act) and the Public Health Service Act (PHS Act). Per the FD&C Act Section 201(h), devices or medical products can be an instrument, implement, machine, implant or an apparatus but does not achieve its primary intended purposes through chemical action within or on the body and is not dependent upon being metabolized for the achievement of its primary intended purposes (U.S. Food and Drug Administration, 2022) [1]. Medical devices and radiologic products are overseen by the Center for Devices and Radiological Health (CDRH). A medical device can be marketed only if they have been approved or cleared by the FDA.

Regulatory controls are based on the risk of the device to ensure reasonable safety and effectiveness of a device. Devices, in general, fall into three categories which are based on their intended use: therapeutic, esthetic, and diagnostic (Table 19.1).

There are several pathways to market a device which are based on the risk posed to the consumer. Class I devices are considered low risk and are exempt from any pre-market notifications but need to employ general controls associated with registration and listing and compliance with any Current Good Manufacturing Practices (CGMPs) as required by the FDA Quality System Regulations (QSRs). Class II devices are considered moderate risk and are subject to the aforementioned general controls as well as additional controls that can be device-specific. Class III devices are high-risk and are subject to pre-market approval (PMA) requirements to demonstrate that the product is safe and effective for its intended use.

Per the FDA, medical device and biologics approval pathways include Pre-market Notification (510k), De Novo Classification Request, Exempt, Pre-market Approval (PMA), Product Development Protocol (PDP), Humanitarian Use Exemption (HDE), and Biologics License Application (BLA) (U.S. Food and Drug Administration, 2022) [2].

S. Navarrete
Independent Consultant, Austin, TX, USA

Biomedical Consultant @ Independent, Austin, TX, USA

D. R. Lee
CellRight Technologies, LLC, Universal City, TX, USA
e-mail: dlee@cellrighttechnologies.com

J. L. Koh (✉)
Mark R. Neaman Family Chair of Orthopaedic Surgery, Orthopaedic & Spine Institute, Endeavor Health, Evanston, IL, USA

University of Chicago Pritzker School of Medicine, Chicago, IL, USA

Northwestern University McCormick School of Engineering, Evanston, IL, USA


S. Lyman et al. (eds.), *Introduction to Surgical Trials*,
https://doi.org/10.1007/978-3-031-77563-5_19

**Table 19.1** Types of medical devices

| Categories | Description |
|---|---|
| Therapeutic devices | Intended to treat a specific condition or disease |
| Esthetic devices | Intended to provide a desire change in visual appearance through a physical modification of the structure of the subject's body |
| Diagnostic devices | Intended to be used alone or with other information to help assess a health condition |
| Device with more than one use | Intended use in more than one category such as one that diagnoses but can also be therapeutic |

The purpose of this chapter is to outline the regulatory pathway for Class III surgical medical devices in the United States and present an overview of the types of and considerations required for marketing such devices. Demonstrating effectiveness in well-controlled investigation(s) resulting in clinical trial data are cost and time intensive considerations in order to receive marketing approval.

Ascertaining how to get a medical device approved for market use can be daunting, however when formulating a strategic approach by categorizing the medical device by *type* and *class* will create a path for success. The FDA defines a medical device as an instrument, apparatus, implement, machine contrivance, implant, in vitro reagent, or other similar or related article, including a component part, or accessory (U.S. Food and Drug Administration, 2022) [1].

(A) recognized in the official National Formulary, or the United States Pharmacopeia, or any supplement to them,
(B) intended for use in the diagnosis of disease or other conditions, or in the cure, mitigation, treatment, or prevention of disease, in man or other animals, or,
(C) intended to affect the structure or any function of the body of man or other animals, and which does not achieve its primary intended purpose through chemical action within or on the body of man or other animals and which does not achieve its primary intended purpose through chemical action or on the body of man or other animals and which is not dependent upon being metabolized for the achievement of its primary intended purposes. The term "device" does not include software functions excluded pursuant to section 520(0).

## 19.2 Medical Device Classification

To understand the medical device regulatory pathway, one must understand the risk-based classification as defined by the FDA. Device class is the level of control necessary to provide assurance that the device is safe and effective. Class I devices have the least regulatory control and Class III devices have the most stringent control (Table 19.2). General controls are the baseline requirements of the Food, Drug and Cosmetic Act that apply to all device classes.

Special controls are specific to Class II devices and are those in which general controls are insufficient to provide assurance of safety and effectiveness of a device and for which there is insufficient information to establish special controls to provide such assurance (U.S. Food and Drug Administration, 2018) [3].

If a Class I or Class II device is non-exempt from pre-market submission, they will require a 510(k) (U.S. Food and Drug Administration 2020) [4]. A pre-market 510(k) is a submission made to the FDA to show that a device is substantially equivalent (i.e., safe and effective) to a legally marketed medical device (Table 19.3). These pre-market special controls may include pre-market data requirements and performance standards to demonstrate equivalence.

Class III devices require the most stringent type of regulatory application called the pre-market application (PMA). A 510(k) is the appropriate route for a Class III device only if the device was on the market prior to the medical device amendments in 1976 or substantially equivalent to such a device and a PMA has not been requested (U.S. Food and Drug Administration 2020) [4].

An applicant must receive FDA approval of a PMA application prior to marketing a device. The FDA will scientifically review the PMA to ensure it contains evidence that it is safe and effective for its intended use. PMA regulations can be found in Title 21 Code of Federal

**Table 19.2** Device classification

| Device Class | Regulatory controls | Submission type or exemption | Special controls | Risk | Medical device example |
|---|---|---|---|---|---|
| Class I | General controls | 510(k)<br>510(k) exempt | – | Lowest risk | Surgical masks<br>Latex gloves |
| Class II | General controls and special controls | 510(k)<br>510 (k) exempt | • Performance standards<br>• Post-market surveillance<br>• Patient registries<br>• Special labeling requirements<br>• Pre-market data requirements<br>• Guidelines | Moderate risk | Contact lenses<br>Blood transfusion devices |
| Class III | General controls and PMA | PMA | – | Greatest risk | Renal stents<br>Cochlear implants |

**Table 19.3** Substantial equivalence

| Substantial equivalence defined by the FDA |
|---|
| • has the same intended use as the predicate; **and**<br>• has the same technological characteristics as the predicate;**or**<br>• has the same intended use as the predicate; **and**<br>• has different technological characteristics and does not raise different questions of safety and effectiveness; **and**<br>• the information submitted to FDA demonstrates that the device is as safe and effective as the legally marketed device |

(U.S. Food and Drug Administration, 2022) [5]

**Table 19.4** Pre-Market and Post-Market Considerations

| Pre-market | | | Post-market |
|---|---|---|---|
| Preclinical study | Feasibility (Pilot) trial | Pivotal trial | Post-market trial |
| • Device prototype<br>• Animal studies<br>• Controlled laboratory settings | • Single center<br>• Limited human subjects<br>• Direct objectives<br>• Gathering data for design and minimize risk to patients | • Safety and effectiveness<br>• Controlled<br>• Test hypotheses<br>• 510 k<br>• PMA | • Design depends on the objective<br>• Comparative studies and/or support claims |

Regulations (CFR), Part 814 (U.S. Food and Drug Administration, 2019) [6]. Class III surgical medical devices will require a PMA to be marketed in the US for human use.

## 19.3 Pre-Market and Post-Market Medical Devices

Conducting clinical research requires an understanding of the FDA regulatory framework. A medical device is classified as either a pre-market device or a post-market device (Table 19.4). Pre-market medical devices will be studied under the auspices of preclinical, pilot and pivotal clinical trials. Post-market devices will undergo post-market surveillance trials. In general, new and innovative surgical medical devices will undergo each of the types of clinical trials' presented.

## 19.4 Regulatory Framework

Clinical studies of medical devices must meet certain regulatory requirements. These standards are found in FDA regulations under 21 CFR Parts 50 (informed consent), 54, 56 (institutional review boards - IRBs) and 812 (investigational device exemption (IDE) and relate to good clinical practice (GCP) requirements. If a study is conducted outside the U.S., it will comply with most of these regulations and have applications for any studies which are conducted outside the United States. Compliance to U.S. regulations for studies conducted outside the U.S. are especially important if the data is used to support approval of a medical device in the United States. Clinical study legal requirements include: reasonable assurance of safety and effectiveness, valid scientific evidence, benefit–risk assessment, clinical study level of evidence and regulation, least burdensome concept and principles of study design, and approval of an investigational device exemption.

## 19.5 Investigational Device Exemption (IDE)

An Investigational Device Exemption (IDE) permits the collection of safety and efficacy data via clinical trial to support the PMA or prior notification 510(k) in some cases. All clinical evaluations of investigational devices, unless exempt, must have an approved IDE before the start of a clinical trial (Table 19.5). Per the FDA, the approved IDE permits a device to be shipped lawfully for the purpose of clinical investigation since the device under IDE is not approved for commercial distribution. Furthermore, the sponsor of the study does not need to submit a PMA or 510(k) while the device is under investigation. Sponsors are also exempt for the Quality System (QS) regulations except for the requirements for design controls (U.S. Food and Drug Administration, 2022) [7].

An IDE application of a significant risk device should submit an IDE application to the FDA. Table 19.6 outlines Significant Risk and Non-Significant risk devices. The sponsor of the application should show that the risks of human subjects are outweighed by the anticipated benefits and that the device will be effective. An IDE clinical trial cannot begin until the FDA and Institutional Review Board (IRB) has given approval.

Per the FDA, an IDE application can be submitted to the FDA via eCopy and must include the sections provided in CFR 812.20 (U.S. Food and Drug Administration, 2020) [9] (Table 19.7).

An IDE applicant may request to meet with the FDA as part of the pre-submission process to obtain feedback on clinical matters (U.S. Food and Drug Administration, 2021) [10]. The Q submission process is one in which interactions between the FDA and sponsor of the investigational medical device are recorded before their submission. These meetings will be given a "Q" designation and referred to as a Q submission. The FDA may withhold approval if a request for more information is made. Once an IDE is approved, a clinical investigation can begin. Investigational devices must be labeled for "investigational use" while utilized in a clinical trial.

**Table 19.5** Requirements of clinical evaluation of devices not cleared for marketing

| Requirements of clinical evaluation of devices not cleared for marketing |
|---|
| • an investigational plan approved by an institutional review board (IRB). If the study involves a significant risk device, the IDE must also be approved by FDA;<br>• informed consent from all patients;<br>• labeling stating that the device is for investigational use only;<br>• monitoring of the study and;<br>• required records and reports. |

(U.S. Food and Drug Administration, 2022) [7]

**Table 19.6** Significant risk and non-significant risk

| Significant risk (SR) | Non-significant risk (NSR) |
|---|---|
| Under 21 CFR 812.3(m), an SR device means an investigational device that:<br>• Is intended as an implant and presents a potential for serious risk to the health, safety, or welfare of a subject<br>• Is purported or represented to be for use supporting or sustaining human life and presents a potential for serious risk to the health, safety, or welfare of a subject;<br>• Is for a use of substantial importance in diagnosing, curing, mitigating, or treating disease, or otherwise preventing impairment of human health and presents a potential for serious risk to the health, safety, or welfare of a subject; or<br>• Otherwise presents a potential for serious risk to the health, safety, or welfare of a subject | An NSR device study is one that does not meet the definition for an SR device study |
| SR device studies must follow all the IDE regulations at 21 CFR 812.<br>• SR device studies must have an IDE application approved by FDA before they may proceed | • NSR device studies must follow the abbreviated requirements at 21 CFR 812.2(b)<br>• These abbreviated requirements address labeling, IRB approval, informed consent, monitoring, records, reports, and prohibition against promotion. However, there is no need to make progress reports or final reports to FDA<br>• NSR device studies do not have to have an IDE application approved by FDA<br>• Sponsors and IRBs do not have to report the IRB approval of an NSR device study to FDA. This means that an IRB may approve an NSR device study and an investigator may conduct the study without FDA knowing about it<br>• An IRB's NSR determination is important because the IRB serves as the FDA's surrogate for review, approval, and continuing review of the NSR device studies. An NSR device study may start at the institution as soon as the IRB reviews and approves the study and without prior approval by FDA |
| • The sponsor must submit an IDE application to FDA and obtain the agency's approval of the study. [(See 21 CFR 812.20(a) (1) and (2)]<br>• The sponsor must advise its clinical investigators about the SR status and obtain their agreement to comply with the applicable regulations governing such studies (i.e., 21 CFR Parts, 50, 56, 812) (See 21 CFR 812.43(c) [4](i)]. Sponsors should provide the IDE number and/or a copy of the IDE approval letter to the IRB when requested.<br>• Sponsors may send their SR device study to an IRB for review before the IDE application is approved by FDA. However, FDA cautions that an SR device study may not begin until FDA approves the IDE. | If the sponsor identifies a study as NSR, the sponsor must provide the reviewing IRB an explanation of its determination [21 CFR 812.2(b) (1)(ii)] and should provide any other information that may help the IRB in evaluating the risk of the study. For example, a Contains Nonbinding Recommendations 5 description of the device, reports of prior investigations with the device, the proposed investigational plan, subject selection criteria, and other information the IRB may need.<br>• If FDA has determined that the study is NSR, the sponsor should so inform the IRB. By providing such risk determination information to the IRB, the IRB's workload should be reduced and the review process should be facilitated |
| Require IDE application to the FDA | Do not pose significant risk to patients and do not require an IDE application to the FDA. They are subject to abbreviated IDE regulations and must be approved by an IRB |

(U.S. Food and Drug Administration, 2006) [8]

**Table 19.7** IDE required elements

| | Required elements | Specific contents |
|---|---|---|
| 1 | Name and address of sponsor | – |
| 2 | Report of prior investigations (§ 812.27). A report of prior investigations must include reports of all prior clinical, animal, and laboratory testing of the device. It should be comprehensive and adequate to justify the proposed investigation | • A bibliography of all publications, whether adverse or supportive, that are relevant to an evaluation of the safety and effectiveness of the device<br>• Copies of all published and unpublished adverse information<br>• Copies of other significant publications if requested by an IRB or FDA<br>• A summary of all other unpublished information (whether adverse or supportive) that is relevant to an evaluation of the safety and effectiveness of the device<br>• If nonclinical laboratory data are provided, a statement that such studies have been conducted in compliance with the Good Laboratory Practice (GLP) regulations in 21 CFR Part 58. If the study was not conducted in compliance with the GLP regulations, include a brief statement of the reason for noncompliance |
| 3 | Investigational plan (§812.25) | The investigational plan shall include the following items in the following order:<br>• Purpose (the name and intended use of the device and the objectives and duration of the investigation)<br>• Protocol (a written protocol describing the methodology to be used and an analysis of the protocol demonstrating its scientific soundness)<br>• Risk analysis (a description and analysis of all increased risks to the research subjects and how these risks will be minimized; a justification for the investigation; and a description of the patient population including the number, age, sex, and condition)<br>• Description of this device (a description of each important component, ingredient, property, and principle of operation of the device and any anticipated changes in the device during the investigation)<br>• Monitoring procedures (the sponsor's written procedures for monitoring the investigation and the name and address of each monitor.<br>• Additional records and reports (a description of any records or reports of the investigation other than those required in Subpart G of the IDE regulations) |
| 4 | A description of the methods, facilities, and controls used for the manufacture, processing, packing, storage, and installation of the device | – |
| 5 | An example of the agreement to be signed by the investigators and a list of the names and addresses of all investigators. Information that must be included in the written agreement are found in § 812.43 | – |
| 6 | Certification that all investigators have signed the agreement, that the list of investigators includes all investigators participating in the study, and that new investigators will sign the agreement before being added to the study | |
| 7 | A list of the names, addresses, and chairpersons of all IRBs that have or will be asked to review the investigation and a certification of IRB action concerning the investigation (when available) | – |

(continued)

**Table 19.7** (continued)

| | Required elements | Specific contents |
|---|---|---|
| 8 | The name and address of any institution (other than those above) where a part of the investigation may be conducted | – |
| 9 | The amount, if any, charged for the device and an explanation of why sale does not constitute commercialization | – |
| 10 | Please note that an environmental assessment as required under 21 CFR 25.40 or a claim for categorical exclusion under 21 CFR 25.30 or 25.34 is no longer required. [§25.34(g)] | – |
| 11 | Copies of all labeling for the device | – |
| 12 | Copies of all informed consent forms and all related information materials to be provided to subjects as required by 21 CFR 50, Protection of Human Subjects | – |
| 13 | Any other relevant information that FDA requests for review of the IDE application. Information previously submitted to FDA in accordance with Part 812 may be incorporated by reference | – |

## 19.6 IDE Clinical Trial Design Considerations

Clinical trials are intended to add to medical knowledge but those used in regulatory approvals are designed to demonstrate safety and effectiveness of the device and if the device should be approved for use in the general population. There are several clinical trial design considerations an IDE applicant must review. As previously discussed, device clinical trials can fall into three categories and are differentiated by size as well as objectives: pilot studies, pivotal studies for safety and effectiveness and post market studies. The U.S. Department of Health and Human Services (HHS), Food and Drug Administration (FDA), Center for Devices and Radiological Health (CDRH) and the Center for Biologics Evaluation and Research (CBER) have numerous resources to guide investigators through clinical trials.

### 19.6.1 Feasibility (Pilot) Study Considerations

With respect to devices, there is little formal guidance on the need for feasibility or pilot studies. Class III devices are subject to one well-controlled and executed study to demonstrate the safety and effectiveness of devices. Given the cost and time required to conduct a pivotal trial, a feasibility study may be warranted to reduce variability and fine tune pivotal studies. Some information on the need for preliminary research is described in an FDA clinical trial guidance document [11]. Feasibility studies are often used to explore whether a device has the anticipated value, the potential to become a marketable device and to collect some human experience data. Usually these single center studies involving a limited number of subjects are used to gather more information on the product and on trial management, logistics and planning prior to a pivotal study. Such data can be of use in optimizing the design of the study or making modifications to the device. Common considerations for feasibility studies include [12]:

- Preliminary safety assessments - used to identify any safety considerations or adverse events not previously noted in the previous limited clinical experiences or identified in nonclinical testing and evaluation.
- Preliminary Performance Evaluations - are used to assess device performance, as well as aspects related to the patient and the user.

Device performance in a pilot trial helps to identify the best clinical benefit and outcomes to measure in the pivotal trial which also provides data which can be used in sample size determination. Pilot studies also help assess the ease of use of the product and identify any additional requirements needed during use in the pivotal trial. Pilot studies also are used to assess the performance of the device and how well it meets its specifications.

- Validation of Outcome Measures - the selection of the right outcome measure and the claims desired for a device are critical in establishing the effectiveness of a device and pivotal trial success criteria. The outcome measures will also influence the sample size and the selection of a control group.
- Validation of Methods for Measuring Outcomes - being able to reliably measure outcomes is also assessed in a pilot study. Outcomes that can be measured via instruments or validated assays are a straightforward matter, but subjective endpoints such as pain and quality of life may be more challenging. In some cases the pilot study is used to validate a new or modified methodology to assess outcomes.

Feasibility studies, though not required by the FDA, can be beneficial in clarifying the most appropriate indications for use, identifying and validating primary end points, choosing a control group, providing data for sample size calculations, and defining success criteria.

### 19.6.2 Pivotal Study Considerations

Pivotal device studies are used to develop the data necessary to evaluate safety and effectiveness of a device for its identified use. The definitive evidence developed will be used for the determination of safety and effectiveness of the device in the pre-market approval application (PMA) and assesses the overall benefit-risk. Much of the information contained in this section is collected from an FDA document, "Guidance for Industry, Clinical Investigators and Food and Drug Administration Staff" [13]. The guidance describes the principles of designing pivotal clinical trial designs and can assist in designing adequate studies to provide reasonable assurance of safety and effectiveness for a pre-market submission.

Several types of studies can be used in a pivotal study to determine if a device demonstrates safety and effectiveness. This section will focus on clinical outcome studies and will review general considerations as well as those considerations relevant to this type of study.

### 19.6.3 Bias and Variance

A general consideration of studies is to collect meaningful data so one needs to remove the possibility of any bias which is a systematic, nonrandom error in the estimate of a treatment and can lead to an incorrect determination of safety and effectiveness. A study can be used to eliminate, reduce or estimate bias since bias can risk the validation of study results. Variance needs to be minimized and requires evaluating clinical and statistical significance in addition to increasing sample size.

### 19.6.4 Study Objectives

The study objectives should be the supporting data which aligns with the intended use of the device and the claims which will be used after market approval. Hypothesis testing in a study should also align with any desired claims for the device.

### 19.6.5 Subject Selection

The subjects enrolled into a pivotal study should reflect the target population for the device. Frequently there are specific enrollment criteria, eligibility criteria that describe the key characteristics of the intended target population. In many studies, subject selection is described as inclusion/exclusion criteria. One should also be prepared to defend how the target population for the study was selected and for adequate representation from all populations.

## 19.6.6 Stratification for Subject Selection

Many studies are conducted at multiple sites, so it is important that all sites select subjects that represent the target population. This may go beyond just following inclusion/exclusion criteria but can include subgroup subjects from all sites where differences may be expected. An example of this may be males and females are listed in the inclusion criteria, but the study should have balanced numbers of men and women.

## 19.6.7 Site Selection

Pivotal studies frequently are performed at multiple sites. Each site should be selected based on their appropriateness for the intended use of the device. Multicenter sites have the advantages of easier and faster recruitment and assure a more representative group of subjects. The challenge is achieving consistent results from all study sites, especially with differences in surgical skills, surgical technique and learning curves.

## 19.6.8 Comparative Study Designs

Comparative studies compare two or more treatments. Parallel group studies assign subjects to one of the devices being compared then comparisons are made between the groups. A paired design occurs if there is an opportunity to test each treatment at the same time in each subject. This lessens any variability since it eliminates variability between subjects. In the cross-over design, each subject may receive each treatment at different times and if the effects of one treatment do not affect the following treatment. Also, the sequence of the treatments should be specified.

## 19.6.9 Clinical Outcome Studies

In a clinical outcome study, one must consider a number of important factors. Table 19.8 provides various key considerations.

For additional detailed discussion on controls, one is referred to the FDA guidance document for more detailed discussions on controls.

## 19.6.10 Placebo Effect

A concern in many studies is that the treatment may have no effect but there may still be a demonstration of effectiveness. To address this a placebo control, a totally ineffective treatment that is usually blinded, is used to identify this in studies gut is used infrequently with surgical devices. The bias introduced by a placebo could address whether subjects have an expectation of benefit or that they are participating in a study.

## 19.6.11 Non-Comparative Study Designs

Single Group Studies with Objective Performance Criteria (OPC).

Objective Performance Criteria use a well-described and publicly available control from historical data or other clinical studies or registries to set the criteria.

Single Group Studies with Performance Goals (PG).

Performance goals may be set as a numerical value. PG may be based on the upper or lower limits of the confidence interval of a safety or effectiveness endpoint. This level of evidence is weaker than an OPC.

## 19.6.12 Observational Studies or Registries

Bias issues affect the reliability of using observational studies or registries since the assignment of therapy may have been based on a correct or incorrect prognosis. A meta-analysis may be use-

**Table 19.8** Clinical outcome considerations

| | |
|---|---|
| Endpoints | • Key study variables that will demonstrate device performance and are known as primary and secondary endpoints<br>• Should be clinically meaningful and objective<br>• Protocol describes how it is measured and how and who will analyze<br>• Study duration needs to be considered by study sponsors<br>• Composite, multiple or surrogate endpoints can be considered |
| Randomization | • Method of selecting subjects that provides assurance that subjects are suitable for the study and are comparable at baseline<br>• Assigns subjects to test groups to minimize bias<br>• Assure comparability and balance between groups |
| Blinding | • Limiting the knowledge of intervention assignment<br>• To prevent knowledge of the intervention which can influence the study outcome in the subject, evaluators, others<br>• Blinding of subjects to the intervention throughout the study duration is desirable<br>• If blinding is not possible with the subject or investigator, third party evaluators may be employed who are blinded to the intervention |
| Controls | • Comparison of the treatment with a control to provide a quantitative evaluations<br>• Types of controls:<br>  • Concurrent<br>    • no treatment (no intervention)<br>      Placebo (intervention with no effect)<br>      Active treatment (intervention that delivers a known effect)<br>      Subject as own concurrent<br>    • Subject as own (baseline compared to endpoint)<br>    • Historical (different group treated in the past where data available from same outcomes) |

ful if a solid methodology is used to select studies for inclusion in the analyses. A basic literature summary is a historical review but lacks any additional analyses and is not useful to demonstrate the effectiveness of a treatment.

### 19.6.13 Sustaining the Quality of Clinical Studies

Setting up a study to obtain quality data throughout the study enables one to collect scientifically valid information on safety and effectiveness. This includes:

- Handling Clinical Data—Studies should have a data management plan and provide adequate training so that the level of evidence, minimizing bias and collecting reliable, useful data is achieved.
- Study Conduct—Studies are also assessed to ensure that activities were conducted under GCPs. Planning and managing study under accepted guidelines help to insure collection of quality data and support the approval of the device. Study progress reports are routinely reviewed to note adherence to accepted practices. These reviews will assess if there are any deviations from randomization procedures, blind is maintained, protocols are followed, subjects followed according to protocol, data monitoring is conducted and optimum clinical care is employed.

### 19.6.14 Study Analysis

Study protocols need to have a detailed statistical analysis plan (SAP) which needs to be defined at the protocol stage and adhered to at the completion to support the validity of data generated by the study. The SAP should have as much detail as possible and includes the statistical analysis for the primary endpoint and the determined sample size but also should have options if assumptions are not valid or there is missing data. If any changes are encountered due to an interim analysis or adverse safety event, then a new SAP should be submitted before any outcome data becomes available.

### 19.6.15 Investigational Plan or Protocol

This written document provides the detailed plan for the design, conduct, assumptions and analysis of the clinical study. The key components include:

- scientific rationale,
- definition of the subject populations including inclusion/exclusion criteria,
- proposed intended use of the device,
- listing of study endpoints,
- statement of the procedures to be employed with the subjects,
- statistical analysis plan.

The protocol should clearly document the rationale regarding decisions made about the study, the clinical design, and the selection of the endpoints.

### 19.6.16 Guidance Documents

For many devices, the FDA has developed clinical trial guidance documents to aid investigators in their planning and requirements for marketing approval of numerous type devices. It is in the best interests of investigators to thoroughly review the available guidance since they will be used in the review of any market approvals. If there is not a specific document for a device, review of a closely related product may be helpful in identifying aspects which should be included in protocols. The FDA has additional resources related to *Good Clinical Practice and Clinical Trials* [14] and investigators should be referenced as protocols and plans are developed.

Clinical studies require much time, are costly and are burdensome so one should be aware of the many factors that could lead to success or failure. To aid in increasing the chances for success, one should become aware of the many factors that can improve the likelihood of success via a review of the literature from successful clinical trials [15].

## 19.7 Conclusion

Medical devices will follow a series of pre-market to post-market clinical trials. Each of these types of trials serves a specific purpose relative to the medical device that is under investigation. In general, all surgical medical devices will undergo pre-market and post-market rigor. A medical device will be classified as a Class I, Class II or Class III device in the United States. Class III devices undergo the most regulatory rigor. These devices are used to sustain human well-being, extend human life, and reduce the risk of injury.

A pre-market novel, significant risk Class III (surgical) medical device would follow the path of a PMA and undergo an IDE in support of the PMA. Clinical trials performed under IDE are conducted to confirm medical devices are safe and effective and perform according to the proposed labeling. Pivotal studies can be used for market approval of therapeutic devices. All of these devices may have different levels of complexity, require user skill and training, involve a learning curve, and are numerous type devices. Time, cost considerations, and regulatory oversight must be planned within the clinical trial and add to the overall go-to-to market timeline.

## References

1. How to determine if your product is a medical device [Internet]. U.S. Food and Drug Administration. FDA. https://www.fda.gov/medical-devices/classify-your-medical-device/how-determine-if-your-product-medical-device. Accessed 22 Feb 2023.
2. How to study and market your device [Internet]. U.S. Food and Drug Administration. FDA. https://www.fda.gov/medical-devices/device-advice-comprehensive-regulatory-assistance/how-study-and-market-your-device. Accessed 22 Feb 2023.
3. Regulatory controls [Internet]. U.S. Food and Drug Administration. FDA. https://www.fda.gov/medical-devices/overview-device-regulation/regulatory-controls. Accessed 22 Feb 2023.

4. Classify your medical device [Internet]. U.S. Food and Drug Administration. FDA. https://www.fda.gov/medical-devices/overview-device-regulation/classify-your-medical-device. Accessed 22 Feb 2023.
5. Center for Devices, Radiological Health. Premarket notification 510(k) [Internet]. U.S. Food and Drug Administration. FDA. https://www.fda.gov/medical-devices/premarket-submissions-selecting-and-preparing-correct-submission/premarket-notification-510k. Accessed 22 Feb 2023.
6. Premarket approval (PMA) [Internet]. U.S. Food and Drug Administration. FDA. https://www.fda.gov/medical-devices/premarket-submissions-selecting-and-preparing-correct-submission/premarket-approval-pma. Accessed 22 Feb 2023.
7. Investigational Device Exemption (IDE) [Internet]. U.S. Food and Drug Administration. FDA. https://www.fda.gov/medical-devices/premarket-submissions-selecting-and-preparing-correct-submission/investigational-device-exemption-ide. Accessed 22 Aug 2024.
8. Significant Risk. Information sheet guidance for IRBs, clinical investigators, and sponsors [Internet]. Fda.gov. https://www.fda.gov/media/75459/download. Accessed 22 Feb 2023.
9. IDE application [Internet]. U.S. Food and Drug Administration. FDA. https://www.fda.gov/medical-devices/investigational-device-exemption-ide/ide-application. Accessed 22 Feb 2023.
10. Center for Devices, Radiological Health. Requests for feedback and meetings for medical device submissions: The Q-submission program [Internet]. U.S. Food and Drug Administration. FDA. https://www.fda.gov/regulatory-information/search-fda-guidance-documents/requests-feedback-and-meetings-medical-device-submissions-q-submission-program. Accessed 22 Feb 2023.
11. Center for Devices, Radiological Health. Investigational device exemptions (IDEs) for early feasibility medical device clinical studies, including certain first in human (FIH) studies [Internet]. U.S. Food and Drug Administration. FDA. https://www.fda.gov/regulatory-information/search-fda-guidance-documents/investigational-device-exemptions-ides-early-feasibility-medical-device-clinical-studies-including. Accessed 22 Feb 2023.
12. Jun. Chartting a course in medical device clinical trials [Internet]. mddionlinecom. 1997. https://www.mddionline.com/rd/chartting-course-medical-device-clinical-trials. Accessed 22 Feb 2023.
13. Design considerations for pivotal clinical investigations for medical devices guidance for industry, clinical investigators, institutional review boards and food and drug administration staff [Internet]. Fda.gov. 2011. https://www.fda.gov/media/87363/download. Accessed 22 Feb 2023.
14. Office of the Commissioner. Regulations: Good clinical practice and clinical trials [Internet]. U.S. Food and Drug Administration. FDA. https://www.fda.gov/science-research/clinical-trials-and-human-subject-protection/regulations-good-clinical-practice-and-clinical-trials. Accessed 22 Feb 2023.
15. Fogel DB. Factors associated with clinical trials that fail and opportunities for improving the likelihood of success: a review. Contemp Clin Trials Commun. 2018;11:156–64. https://doi.org/10.1016/j.conctc.2018.08.001.

# 20 Regulatory Standards for Surgical Trials in Asia: The Japanese Experience

Yuichi Hoshino

## 20.1 Introduction

Clinical surgical trials are required to prove the efficacy of surgical innovations. Historically, novel surgical techniques have evolved through the creativity of inventive surgeons with the help of an unconstrained regulatory apparatus. However, our understanding of modern research ethics and an increasingly robust regulatory system have made this avenue of innovation largely obsolete. Too many catastrophes of technological innovation have been observed to ignore the potential pitfalls of unrestrained surgical experimentation.

Japan is no exception. There have been several cases of research misconduct in Japan. As a result, strict regulations on clinical research have been established. However, surgical trials can be exempt from strict regulations so long as the study is observational (i.e., non-randomized) or exclusively involves an established surgical technique without use of novel surgical products. Even in such exemptions, there are still some regulations when introducing a new technique in our clinical practice.

Y. Hoshino (✉)
Department of Orthopaedic Surgery, Graduate School of Medicine, Kobe University, Kobe, Japan
e-mail: you.1.hoshino@gmail.com

## 20.2 Clinical Medical Research Regulation in Japan

All clinical trials in Japan have to follow the Clinical Trial Act, which was passed into law in 2017 with enforcement beginning in 2018. The Clinical Trial Act originated out of reflection on multiple episodes of scientific misconduct by Japanese medical researchers which were revealed in early 2010s, such as the Valsartan Scandal [1]. The main fraud of the scandal was a data manipulation in favor of an antihypertensive drug in a published paper. Moreover, several types of misconducts were revealed simultaneously. One of the researchers was an employer from the pharmaceutical company which provided the antihypertensive drug. Research teams have received more than 1.1 billion yen as unrestricted grants from the company. Also, a publisher of the paper was involved in the promotion of the antihypertensive drug.

The main purpose of this act is to maintain public confidence in Japan toward clinical research, and to facilitate implementation of ethical clinical research by requiring researchers to carefully monitor adverse events, adhere to best clinical and research practices, and to appropriately manage conflict of interest. The act also obligates companies to disclose the conditions under which they provide funding to researchers studying their products. The Act was established mainly for controlling trials of pharmaceutical agents, but medical devices are included in the


S. Lyman et al. (eds.), *Introduction to Surgical Trials*,
https://doi.org/10.1007/978-3-031-77563-5_20

scope of this act. Therefore, surgical trials are also subject to the Act if experimental medical devices are the focus of the trial.

In preparation for clinical trials, it is necessary to pass several review steps, to obtain permission from an administrator from each relevant medical organization, and to submit the study protocol to the Japanese Ministry of Health, Labor and Welfare. After the execution plan is published in the ministry database and registered in the Japan Registry of Clinical Trials (jRCT), the clinical trial is permitted to launch. Every trial undergoes safety monitoring and is required to submit an annual report. All trial-related medical complications must be reported immediately. Furthermore, any trial modifications must be reported to the ministry for review before implementation. Completion of the trial should be publicly reported while disclosing all relevant results in the ministry database.

As mentioned earlier, clinical trials in Japan are strictly controlled by the Clinical Trial Act. However, there are two exceptions for surgical trials from the Act.

1. Observational Studies: Strictly speaking, clinical care in observational studies is not modified for research purposes but is determined based on the surgeon's consideration of the best care for each individual patient. In such cases, observational studies are not required to adhere to the Act. Without any randomization or study arm allocation outside the patients' best interests, clinical information and study-related samples may be collected for research.
2. Surgical Trials Using Only Established Medical Devices: Comparison of surgical techniques using alternative approved medical devices could be categorized within this exemption.

The decision on whether a study is exempt based on either of these criteria is made locally by the internal review board of the initiating medical organization.

## 20.3 Clinical Research on Surgical Technique

There has been a long debate about whether surgical trials focused on surgical techniques should be exempt from legal regulations. Currently, as mentioned earlier, a comparative study between different surgical techniques can be exempted with approval only from an internal review board. The rationale for the exemption is that such studies have low participant and social risk since the medical devices being used are already available in routine clinical practice outside trial participation. Newly introduced surgical techniques are typically innovated in an attempt to improve clinical care for the benefit of patients without external financial interest from a device or pharmaceutical manufacturer. Accordingly, the expectation of regulation on surgical trials specifically focused on surgical technique evaluation is limited in Japan.

On the other hand, even when clinical research regulations are imposed on surgical trials to closely monitor the evaluation of surgical innovations, it is still practically difficult to exert stringent restriction in Japanese clinical practice. Once a novel surgical technique is proposed by a surgeon as the preferred remedy for a given indication and a patient has consented to surgery, the technique is no longer experimental, but enters clinical practice. In reality, new surgical innovations have been rarely introduced as a subject of research under the Clinical Trial Act [2, 3]. Therefore, surgical trials are not commonly controlled by the Act's regulations.

One of the infamous clinical surgical trial failures of a newly introduced surgery is the first heart transplant from a brain-dead donor in Japan, remembered today as the 'Wada Incident'. In 1968, Professor Jurō Wada of Sapporo Medical College attempted a heart transplant, but the recipient died less than 3 months postoperatively. Several questions were raised after the failure concerning both the choice of the recipient and the brain death diagnosis of the donor.

Consequently, Dr. Wada was charged with a double murder. Ethical guidelines and regulations supporting the transplant surgery was not fully established. Currently, the Organ Transplant Law has allowed organ procurement from brain-dead donors who had left written consent since 1997. However, the number of transplant surgeries in Japan is still relatively low among developed countries.

Fortunately, even when a surgical trial is exempted from the Clinical Trial Act, there is a guideline for clinical trials in Japan, namely the "ethical guidelines for medical and health research involving human subjects" [4], which began enforcement in 2015. The guideline mainly focuses on ethical issue about clinical research and requires each institution to set up an internal regulatory administration. Those clinical trials which are exempted from the Clinical Trial Act should follow these guidelines which are relatively manageable without obligatory national registration and required annual reporting.

Additionally, the clinical introduction of a new surgical technique is regulated by a local internal order. According to an amendment to the Enforcement of Medical Care Act, which was introduced in 2016, a new surgical technique requires approval from the department head or, for a difficult case, the medical safety administration of the hospital prior to the surgery. This requirement is especially true when the surgery is the first case for the hospital and has the potential to cause severe or even fetal consequences. This order does not directly control surgical trials but has some regulatory effect at the time novel surgery may be introduced, which may include patients involved in an observational surgical trial.

## 20.4 Conclusion

Japanese regulations on clinical trial are well organized in general, but surgical trials can be exempted when focusing solely on surgical techniques. However, such pure surgical technique comparisons still need to go through following ethical guidelines and established clinical regulatory standards in Japan.

## References

1. Sawano T, et al. Payments from pharmaceutical companies to authors involved in the valsartan scandal in Japan. JAMA Netw Open. 2019;2(5):e193817.
2. Loz M. Surgical innovation as sui generis surgical research. Theor Med Bioeth. 2013;34(6):447–59.
3. Reitsma AM, Moreno JD. Ethical regulations for innovative surgery: the last frontier? J Am Coll Surg. 2002;194(6):792–802.
4. Website. https://www.mhlw.go.jp/file/06-Seisakujouhou.../0000080278.pdf.

# Part V

# Alternatives to the Classic RCT

# 21 Pragmatic Trials

Udit Dave and Daphne I. Ling

## 21.1 Randomized Controlled Trials

Randomized controlled trials (RCT) are conducted with individuals randomly assigned to a treatment. Prior to the initiation of a RCT, it is important to determine whether the trial will advance the field, to ensure reliable parameter estimates exist, and to have sufficient preliminary evidence to validate the need to conduct a trial [1]. RCT should be conducted when there is clinical equipoise, which is the uncertainty that a given intervention works better than another [2]. RCT are known for having high internal validity [3].

In the field of orthopedics, RCT have particular limitations. A major weakness associated with this study design is challenges with recruitment. It is difficult to obtain consent from patients to participate in a randomized study because they are hesitant to not know which procedure they will undergo. For surgical interventions, blinding is also not possible [4]. Many patients do not attend their follow-up appointments after undergoing a surgical procedure, particularly if they do not experience any post-surgical complications [2]. In addition, RCT are conducted under highly-controlled conditions, which means that their results may have minimal external validity [5]. RCT can yield an evaluation of the efficacy of the intervention, which refers to its performance under ideal circumstances. However, it is important for surgical interventions to be evaluated for its effectiveness, which refers to its performance in real-world settings in which factors are not highly controlled [6].

## 21.2 Cluster-Randomized Controlled Trials

Cluster RCT are conducted by randomly assigning entire groups to a treatment rather than designating the treatment for each individual [7]. Each cluster is the unit of analysis and its members share either geographic, physical, or social connections [8]. It is important for the treatment and control groups to be comprised of the same number of clusters, but it is common for each cluster to have an imbalanced number of individuals between groups [9]. Although cluster RCT are effective at reducing the effects of contamination or cross-over between individuals, a major weakness of this study design is the limited opportunity for the even distribution of confounding variables [10].

U. Dave
Georgetown University, Washington, DC, USA
e-mail: Urd3@georgetown.edu

D. I. Ling (✉)
Hospital for Special Surgery, New York, NY, USA
e-mail: lingd@hss.edu


S. Lyman et al. (eds.), *Introduction to Surgical Trials*,
https://doi.org/10.1007/978-3-031-77563-5_21

## 21.3 Pragmatic Trials

Clinical trials are generally classified as either exploratory, explanatory, or pragmatic [11]. Exploratory trials involve a preliminary evaluation of new interventions. Explanatory trials evaluate known interventions under favorable conditions. Pragmatic trials are used to evaluate interventions in real-world settings. Pragmatic trials were developed as one solution to the limitation of other trial designs that evaluate efficacy instead of effectiveness [12]. That is, the findings from published studies do not always translate into clinical practice. A pragmatic trial asks the question: "Does this intervention work in real life?" [13]. This approach can incorporate a broader definition of the surgical intervention being studied, which better accounts for the inherent variability associated with surgery [11]. The increased external validity of a pragmatic trial is a distinct advantage over trials with exploratory or explanatory designs [13]. In order to properly evaluate the effects of a treatment in routine practice, pragmatic trials need to be conducted with a diverse patient population. Historically, individuals who are young, old, or sick tend to be underrepresented in clinical trials [14]. This limitation forces clinicians to rely on available data to extrapolate potential outcomes for such patients, which in turn affects the appropriateness of the treatment they receive. Furthermore, pragmatic trials have the potential to yield information about long-term surgical outcomes, which enables a realistic evaluation of post-intervention quality of life [11].

Despite the differences between explanatory and pragmatic trials, it is important to recognize that explanatory and pragmatic trials are not dichotomous since trials will often contain characteristics of both study designs [13]. Attributes of explanatory and pragmatic trials are compared in Table 21.1.

Recognizing that most clinical trials are not strictly of an explanatory or pragmatic nature, the Pragmatic-Explanatory Continuum Indicator Summary (PRECIS) tool was developed to mea-

**Table 21.1** A comparison of study characteristics between pragmatic and explanatory trials

| Characteristic | Explanatory | Pragmatic |
|---|---|---|
| Study objective | Determine intervention efficacy in ideal setting | Determine intervention effectiveness in real-world setting |
| Study population | Highly specific, homogeneous patient population | Diverse, representative, heterogeneous patient population |
| Sample size | Small | Large |
| Blinding | Clinicians, participants, and analysts are blinded if possible | Analysts are blinded |
| Surgeon population | Surgeons are experts in the intervention being evaluated and expertise is standardized to focus on experimental intervention | Surgeons have varying levels of familiarity with the intervention being evaluated to account for a wide range of surgeon training and performance |
| Study setting | Contextual factors standardized to focus on experimental intervention | Contextual factors optimized to evaluate their impact on the intervention |
| Intervention type | Highly specific, controlled definition of intervention | Less strict definition of intervention to account for natural variability in clinical practice |
| Comparison type | Low flexibility of comparison intervention, placebo may be used instead of standard of care | High flexibility of comparison intervention, standard of care often used |
| Measurement technique | Primary outcome may serve as a proxy for other downstream outcomes | Primary outcome is measured under normal clinical settings without the need for a special measurement strategy |
| Follow-up procedure | Frequent follow-up appointments to maximize data collection regardless of complications | Less formalized follow-up appointments, outcomes can be evaluated with use of administrative databases |

(continued)

**Table 21.1** (continued)

| Characteristic | Explanatory | Pragmatic |
|---|---|---|
| Patient compliance | Compliance is highly monitored and may be used as a prerequisite for inclusion in the study | Patient compliance may not be monitored or actively controlled |
| Physician compliance | Physician compliance to protocol is closely monitored | Physician compliance may not be monitored or actively controlled |
| Scope of outcomes | Short-term outcomes | Long-term outcomes such as patient-reported quality of life |
| Validity of results | High internal validity, acceptable external validity | High external validity, acceptable internal validity |

Adapted from Cook [11], Patsopoulos [13], Brewin [15], Thorpe [16], Farrokhyar [17]

sure this gradient [16]. The PRECIS tool resembles a bicycle wheel. There is an "E" in the center that is indicative of trials that are more explanatory than pragmatic. The spokes of the wheel represent the ten characteristics of a pragmatic trial: (1) flexibility of the comparison intervention, (2) practitioner expertise (experimental intervention), (3) flexibility of the experimental intervention, (4) eligibility criteria, (5) primary analysis, (6) practitioner adherence, (7) participant compliance, (8) outcomes, (9) follow-up intensity, and (10) practitioner expertise (comparison). These characteristics are plotted, and graphs that present points farther out on the spokes are indicative of trials that are more pragmatic than explanatory [16]. The PRECIS model has been further updated by the PRECIS-2 tool [18]. This newer model has a similar basis as PRECIS for determining the relative pragmatism of a study, but PRECIS-2 has more lax criteria for fulfilling the characteristics required of a pragmatic trial. Additionally, the PRECIS-2 tool only evaluates nine categories: (1) eligibility, (2) recruitment, (3) setting, (4) organization, (5) flexibility: delivery, (6) flexibility: adherence, (7) follow-up, (8) primary outcome, and (9) primary analysis. Each of the nine axes in PRECIS-2 are evaluated from one to five with five being the most pragmatic [18].

## 21.4 Limitations of Pragmatic Trials

Similar to all trial designs, limitations exist that are inherent to pragmatic trials. Despite the high external validity of a pragmatic trial, the extent to which the results are generalizable can be difficult to assess. For example, treatment in drastically different settings that were not evaluated in a pragmatic trial can still limit the external validity of the trial [13]. Furthermore, increasing variability between groups in a pragmatic trial does not necessarily reduce the variability between different trials. Therefore, each pragmatic trial only has a specific external validity that does not automatically overlap with the results of similar trials with different compositions of healthcare delivery systems, physicians, or patients [13]. Additionally, pragmatic trials are not well-suited to determining the effectiveness of complex surgical interventions because of the potentially steep learning curve and the fact that such procedures are unlikely to be successful in clinical settings that may lack the specific attributes that enabled the intervention to be successful in a particular trial [13].

Other limitations exist with regard to the proper execution of a pragmatic trial. Pragmatic trials are often more expensive compared to explanatory trials due to their broader scope. Pragmatic trials require a large amount of resources for patient follow-up in a variety of different settings [13]. Cost and feasibility are major limitations that researchers must consider before deciding to implement a pragmatic trial to evaluate the effectiveness of an intervention. Furthermore, since the level of pragmatism in any given trial is measured on a spectrum, it is not possible to ascertain whether a trial will be fully pragmatic without also having some of the inherent limitations of an explanatory trial [16, 18].

## 21.5 Examples of Surgical Pragmatic Trials

Surgical pragmatic trials often involve patient-reported outcome measures (PROM), which can be used to determine patients' overall levels of pain, quality of life, and general satisfaction following a procedure [19]. PROM allow clinicians to incorporate the perspective of the patient into their care by quantifying self-reported improvement [20, 21]. In the USA, PROM have become a staple in healthcare due to the Medicare Access and CHIP Reauthorization Act (MACRA) and the shift toward a value-based system in which reimbursement to providers is based on clinical outcomes [22]. With this change, it has become imperative for clinicians to take into account the patients' perspective when choosing treatment plans and to provide evidence of the value of an intervention as it relates to a procedure's clinical and cost effectiveness [23].

Surgical pragmatic trials can also demonstrate bias toward a specific intervention. An analysis of the Australasian Laparoscopic Colon Cancer Study was conducted to determine reasons for patient exclusion from the study [24]. Participating surgeons were given surveys over a six-month period to record the number of patients excluded from the study and the reasons for which they were excluded. Results demonstrated that only 45% of patients eligible for participation in the study were selected. The leading reason for exclusion from the trial was patient preference for one surgery over another. Similarly, almost one-third of exclusions were due to surgeons' preferences for a certain surgery. The remaining exclusions were due to time issues, patient anxiety, and issues in the patient-doctor relationship such as disorganization and poor communication [24]. This study illustrates the potentially large impact of patient and provider preferences on enrollment in a pragmatic surgical trial.

Pragmatic trials have been utilized in orthopedic settings as well. A pragmatic design was used in a study to determine the clinical effectiveness of Hylan G-F 20, a viscosupplement given as a set of three injections over the course of one week for knee osteoarthritis [25]. A total of 244 patients were enrolled in a pragmatic trial in which they received either the standard of care alone or the standard of care plus Hylan G-F 20 injections. The standard of care could include drug interventions such as NSAIDs, analgesics, and corticosteroid injections as well as supportive measures including weight loss programs, counseling and education, physical therapy, application of heat and ice, or rest [25]. Follow-up phone calls were made at the first and second month post-treatment and then every 2 months afterwards. This study exemplifies a pragmatic design because rather than measuring the hylan G-F 20 treatment against a placebo injection, which would measure efficacy, this study evaluated the treatment's effectiveness compared to other appropriate care regimens. The hylan G-F 20 injections were found to improve overall knee health and health-related quality of life, as measured on the Western Ontario and McMaster Universities Osteoarthritis Index (WOMAC), Short-Form Health Survey (SF-36), and Health Utilities Index (HUI3), to a greater extent than only providing the standard of care in treating knee osteoarthritis [25].

An example of a pragmatic design in orthopedic surgery was found in a study comparing the effects of treating unstable ankle fractures with either close contact casting or surgery [26]. Ankle fractures are known to cause morbidity in older individuals, and although ankle surgery is the standard of care to treat fractures, such surgeries are accompanied with risks of infection and healing complications. This study aimed to evaluate whether treating an ankle fracture with a close contact cast could produce a similar outcome as surgery but with less resource consumption and fewer complications [26]. A total of 620 individuals over the age of 60 years with unstable ankle fractures were recruited from 24 hospitals and trauma centers in the United Kingdom and were randomly assigned to ankle surgery or close contact casting. This study was pragmatic because patients were selected from both major trauma centers and local hospitals. In addition, the study protocol allowed for the usual access to care beyond the random assignment of casting or surgery, which enabled the effectiveness of casting to be evaluated and the results to be more generalizable. The study findings showed that casting produces similar outcomes compared to surgery in older adults six months after suffering unstable ankle fractures [26].

## 21.6 Stepped-Wedge Trials

Designing a stepped-wedge trial is one solution to the situation in which conducting a standard RCT and withholding the intervention from one group would be unethical. Stepped-wedge trials are a recent methodological development in which time is divided into intervals and participants or clusters are selected at random to receive the intervention at specified intervals [27]. That is, groups are randomized by time rather than by assignment to the treatment intervention. By the end of a stepped-wedge trial, all participants have received the intervention, which makes frequent measurement and detailed follow-up particularly important [27]. There are two main types of stepped-wedge trial designs: cross-sectional and cohort [28]. In a cross-sectional stepped-wedge trial, different individuals from each group are evaluated at each time point. In a cohort stepped-wedge trial, the same individuals are evaluated at each time point. Cohort stepped-wedge trials can be further classified as either open or closed. In an open trial, individuals may be added to or removed from the study once the trial has begun; however, in a closed trial, no individuals may be added once the trial has begun [28].

## 21.7 Considerations for Analysis

Problems with analysis may arise if there is cross-over between the intervention and control groups, meaning a patient has received an intervention different from the one to which they were randomly assigned [11]. In this type of scenario, per-protocol analysis is valuable because it allows for cross-over cases to be excluded or analyzed in the group based on the actual treatment received. This type of scenario may be less common in surgical trials where patients have already undergone the procedure and have received the full treatment [4]. Intention-to-treat analysis does not account for this specific violation of randomization, but it keeps intact the removal of measured and unmeasured confounding from the randomization process. Thus, it may be best practice to report the results from both analytical approaches [11].

In cluster RCT and pragmatic trials, interventions tend to be heterogeneous, which contribute to variance between clusters. Since there are differences in the quality and fidelity of an intervention across clusters, the statistical power of a trial is increased by adding more groups to a study rather than by adding more members to individual groups [27]. The intra-class correlation (ICC) can be used to measure the similarity among members of a cluster. The ICC ranges from 0 to 1, and a higher value indicates that members of a group are more similar: values less than 0.5 indicate poor similarity, values between 0.5 and 0.75 indicate moderate similarity, values between 0.75 and 0.9 indicate good similarity, and values above 0.9 indicate excellent similarity [29].

Stepped-wedge trials are associated with unique analysis issues. Confounding by time through staggered implementation makes time correlated with the intervention itself, which can subsequently have an effect on the outcome. This phenomenon is called a secular trend [30]. To correct for secular trends, analysis must be time-adjusted. Common time-dependent factors include calendar time, seasonality, and external events that can all potentially impact the effect of the intervention [30]. In addition, patient responses to the intervention can also become stronger or weaker over time, meaning that it is important for any analyses to account for time instead of assuming that an intervention has a constant effect on individuals [28].

Regression analysis can be used to adjust for both fixed and time-varying covariates. Fixed covariates are non-repeated measures, whereas time-varying covariates are repeated measures that are often important in stepped-wedge trials. In addition, the presence of correlated measurements within groups of a cluster RCT also requires statistical adjustments to account for both within-cluster and between-cluster variability [31]. This approach will lead to wider confidence intervals and can reduce the precision around effect estimates. Generalized estimating equations (GEE) should be used to account for the correlation among repeated measures or within clusters [32]. The estimates that are given by this type of regression model are robust against misspecification, which occurs when models do not account for all the parameters that should be included [33].

## 21.8 Conclusions

Pragmatic trials are a useful tool that can be used to determine the effectiveness of an intervention in a real-world setting that is not meticulously controlled. They go beyond the explanatory nature of typical RCT to measure the utility of a treatment in routine clinical practice. Pragmatic trials allow for evaluations to be conducted in more diverse patient populations under a broader range of conditions. For surgical procedures, pragmatic trials can determine the overall utility of a treatment intervention that is being implemented by a large number of surgeons in a wide variety of hospital settings. The expanded use of pragmatic trials and newly introduced methods such as stepped-wedge trials, in which all participants receive the intervention according to a staggered treatment schedule, provide researchers with advantageous ways to evaluate the appropriateness of new interventions in clinical settings.

## References


1. Bhide A, Shah PS, Acharya G. A simplified guide to randomized controlled trials. Acta Obstet Gynecol Scand. 2018;97(4):380–7.
2. Lyman S, Nakamura N, Cole BJ, Erggelet C, Gomoll AH, Farr J II. Cartilage-repair innovation at a standstill: methodologic and regulatory pathways to breaking free. J Bone Joint Surg Am. 2016;98(63):1–8.
3. Spieth PM, Kubasch AS, Penzlin AI, Illigens BM, Barlinn K, Siepmann T. Randomized controlled trials—a matter of design. Neuropsychiatr Dis Treat. 2016;12:1341–9.
4. Simunovic N, Devereaux PJ, Bhandari M. Design considerations for randomised trials in orthopaedic fracture surgery. Int J Care Injured. 2008;39(6):696–704.
5. Malavolta EA, Demange MK, Gobbi RG, Imamura M, Fregni F. Randomized controlled clinical trials in orthopedics: difficulties and limitations. Rev Bras Ortop. 2011;46(4):452–9.
6. Glasgow RE, Lichtenstein E, Marcus AC. Why don't we see more translation of health promotion research to practice? Rethinking the efficacy-to-effectiveness transition. Am J Public Health. 2003;93(8):1261–7.
7. Anderson ML, Califf RM, Sugarman J. Ethical and regulatory issues of pragmatic cluster randomized trials in contemporary health systems. Clin Trials. 2015;12(3):276–86.
8. Murray DM. Pragmatic and group-randomized trials in public health and medicine. 2016. https://prevention.nih.gov/education-training/pragmatic-and-group-randomized-trials-public-health-and-medicine.
9. You Z, Williams OD, Aban I, Kabagambe EK, Tiwari HK, Cutter G. Relative efficiency and sample size for cluster randomized trials with variable cluster sizes. Clin Trials. 2011;8(1):27–36.
10. Klar N, Donner A. Current and future challenges in the design and analysis of cluster randomization trials. Stat Med. 2001;20:3729–40.
11. Cook JA. The challenges faced in the design, conduct and analysis of surgical randomised controlled trials. Trials. 2009;10:9.
12. Ford I, Norrie J. Pragmatic trials. N Engl J Med. 2016;375:454–63.
13. Patsopoulos NA. A pragmatic view on pragmatic trials. Dialogues Clin Neurosci. 2011;13:217–24.
14. Basch E, Schrag D. The evolving uses of "Real-World" data. J Am Med Assoc. 2015;321(14):1359–60.
15. Brewin CR, Bradley C. Patient preferences and randomised clinical trials. BMJ. 1989;299:313–5.
16. Thorpe KE, Zwarenstein M, Oxman AD, Treweek S, Furberg CD, Altman DG, et al. A pragmaticeexplanatory continuum indicator summary (PRECIS): a tool to help trial designers. J Clin Epidemiol. 2009;62:464–75.
17. Farrokhyar F, Karanicolas PJ, Thoma A, Simunovic M, Bhandari M, Devereaux PJ, et al. Randomized controlled trials of surgical interventions. Ann Surg. 2010;251(3):409.
18. Loudon K, Treweek S, Sullivan F, Donnan P, Thorpe KE, Zwarenstein M. The PRECIS-2 tool: designing trials that are fit for purpose. BMJ. 2015;350:h2147.
19. Cepeda NA, Polascik BA, Ling DI. A primer on clinically important outcome values; 2019. p. 1–7.
20. Copay AG, Chung AS, Eyberg B, Olmscheid N, Chutkan N, Spangehl MJ. Minimum clinically important difference: current trends in the orthopaedic literature, part I: upper extremity: a systematic review. J Bone Joint Surg Rev. 2018;6(9):e1.

21. Copay AG, Eyberg B, Chung AS, Zurcher KS, Chutkan N, Spangehl MJ. Minimum clinically important difference: current trends in the orthopaedic literature, part II: lower extremity: a systematic review. J Bone Joint Surg Rev. 2018;6(9):e2.
22. Saleh KJ, Shaffer WO. Understanding value-based reimbursement models and trends in orthopaedic health policy: an introduction to the medicare access and CHIP reauthorization act (MACRA) of 2015. J Am Acad Orthop Surg. 2016;24(11):e136–47.
23. Riddle DL, Golladay GJ, Hayes A, Ghomrawi HMK. Poor expectations of knee replacement benefit are associated with modifiable psychological factors and influence the decision to have surgery: a cross-sectional and longitudinal study of a community-based sample. Knee. 2017;24(2):354–61.
24. Abraham NS, Hewett P, Young JM, Solomon MJ. Non-entry of eligible patients into the Australasian laparoscopic colon cancer study. ANZ J Surg. 2006;76(9):825.
25. Raynauld JP, Torrance GW, Band PA, Goldsmith CH, Tugwell P, Walker V, et al. A prospective, randomized, pragmatic, health outcomes trial evaluating the incorporation of hylan G-F 20 into the treatment paradigm for patients with knee osteoarthritis (part 1 of 2): clinical results. Osteoarthr Cartil. 2002;10:506–17.
26. Willett K, Keene DJ, Mistry D, Nam J, Tutton E. Close contact casting vs surgery for initial treatment of unstable ankle fractures in older adults: a randomized clinical trial. JAMA. 2016;316(14):1455–63.
27. Hughes JP, Granston TS, Heagerty PJ. Current issues in the design and analysis of stepped wedge trials. Contemp Clin Trials. 2015;45:55–60.
28. Copas AJ, Lewis JJ, Thompson JA, Davey C. Designing a stepped wedge trial: three main designs, carry-over effects and randomisation approaches. Trials. 2015;16(352):352.
29. Koo TK, Li MY. A guideline of selecting and reporting Intraclass correlation coefficients for reliability research. J Chiropr Med. 2016;15(2):155–63.
30. Hemming K, Taljaard M, Forbes A. Analysis of cluster randomised stepped wedge trials with repeated cross-sectional samples. Trials. 2017;18(1):101.
31. Hussey MA, Hughes JP. Design and analysis of stepped wedge cluster randomized trials. Contemp Clin Trials. 2007;28(2):182–91.
32. Cui J, Qian G. Selection of working correlation structure and best model in GEE analyses of longitudinal data. Commun Stat Simul Comput. 2007;36(5):987–96.
33. Kasza J, Forbes AB. Inference for the treatment effect in multiple-period cluster randomised trials when random effect correlation structure is misspecified. Stat Methods Med Res. 2019;28:3112–22.

# 22 Prospective Cohort Studies

Jose F. Vega, W. Alex Cantrell, and Kurt P. Spindler

## 22.1 Introduction

At its very core, a prospective cohort study is one in which a group of individuals who share certain risk factors both modifiable and non-modifiable are followed for a pre-specified period of time during which the investigators monitor for the development of a specific outcome(s). These risk factors thought to potentially impact the outcome are defined a priori and collected at the beginning of the study and then in real time as the study progresses. At the conclusion of the study, advanced statistical methods such as regression modeling are typically used to help the investigators understand how the risk factors of the study population impact the outcome. In this chapter, we hope to provide the reader with a more in-depth look at prospective cohort studies so that they may better understand the defining features of a prospective cohort study, the types of questions that are best addressed with this study design, the strengths and weaknesses of prospective cohort studies, and what pitfalls to avoid when conducting their own prospective cohort studies.

J. F. Vega
Cleveland Clinic Marymount Hospital,
Chicago, IL, USA

W. A. Cantrell
Investigation Performed at the Cleveland Clinic,
Cleveland, OH, USA

K. P. Spindler (✉)
My Cleveland Clinic, Cleveland, OH, USA
e-mail: spindlk@ccf.org

## 22.2 Defining a Prospective Cohort Study

Modern day prospective cohort studies such as those utilizing the Multicenter Orthopaedic Outcomes Network (MOON) cohort or the Framingham Heart Study cohort require a large team of multidisciplinary researchers, are incredibly expensive (millions of dollars) and follow participants for long periods of time (the Framingham Heart Study enrolled its first participant in 1948).However, the first recorded prospective cohort study was conducted by a single individual, cost nothing, and followed participants for only 10 days—but still took more than 400 years to get published. This was, of course, the study conducted by King Nebuchadnezzar around 600 B.C., in which he aimed to determine how diet impacted vitality (eventually published in *The Bible* as part of the "Book of Daniel").

In this first-ever-recorded prospective cohort study, Nebuchadnezzar, then king of Babylonia (modern day Iraq), sought to require that all members of the royal family consume exclusively meat and wine (in order to stay as vivacious as possible, of course). Unfortunately,


S. Lyman et al. (eds.), *Introduction to Surgical Trials*,
https://doi.org/10.1007/978-3-031-77563-5_22

some of the royal family youths (including Daniel) had strong herbivorous tendencies and refused to give up their leafy-green-loving ways. With his interest piqued, King Nebuchadnezzar agreed to allow his vegetarian relatives to continue their diet of choice for 10 days, at which time the king would compare how physically well the bean eaters compared to the carnivorous faction of the family. The study results - "At the end of the ten days they looked healthier and better nourished than any of the young men who ate the royal food."

Although King Nebuchadnezzar's rudimentary study of meat-eating wine drinkers and legume-loving vegetarians would never hold up to today's rigorous research standards, it has all the makings of a simple prospective cohort study, and sometimes simple studies make for good examples.

The basic tenets of a prospective cohort study include: an a priori clinical question (how does diet impact physical wellness?), a group of individuals that share certain characteristics (members of the Babylonian royal family) but are otherwise different (some ate meat, some preferred vegetables), a *lack of* experimental group (remember, nobody was assigned to adopt the vegetarian diet or vice versa), baseline data, an observation period (ten days), and longitudinal data (visual vitality assessment at the conclusion of the study period).

## 22.3 The Clinical Question

A true prospective cohort study starts with a clinical question such as, "What impacts the rate of post-traumatic osteoarthritis development following anterior cruciate ligament reconstruction (ACLR)?" or "What are risk factors for cardiovascular disease (CVD)?" Questions such as these could be studied via multiple different study designs including case control, retrospective cohort study, or case series, and, while each of those study designs can provide useful information, a well-designed prospective cohort study will yield stronger conclusions.

Questions that lend themselves to investigation via prospective cohort study typically involve identification of risk factors for an outcome that is fairly common. The size of the proposed cohort determines how common the outcome of interest must be before the investigators should consider alternative study designs such as case series, case control, or other retrospective methods. For example, investigators attempting to identify risk factors for anterior cruciate ligament (ACL) injury have produced strong evidence by following student-athletes from a handful of high schools and colleges over a three and a half year period [1]. In contrast, a much larger group of investigators aimed to identify risk factors for infection after revision ACLR. This question, with such a rare outcome of interest, required following thousands of revision ACLR patients (a relatively small group to begin with, which took nearly a decade to assemble) only to capture 9 infections [2]. Remember, as a general rule of thumb, one needs 10 "positive" events for each variable that can be included in a regression analysis. To control for age, sex, and body mass index (BMI) alone, one would need at least 30 infections. Consider that the reported infection rate is less than 1% and some simple math yields a study population of at least 3000!

Additionally, prospective cohort studies lend themselves to "natural experiments." What we mean by this is that randomized controlled trials, which are the gold standard for drawing conclusions about causation because of their ability to minimize unknown biases, are not always ethical or practical to conduct. For example, if one wishes to understand how concomitant chondral injury affects, the risk of developing post-traumatic osteoarthritis (PTOA) in the setting of an ACL injury, one could conduct a randomized trial in which patients with ACL injuries and no chondral damage are randomized to one of two groups. In the first group—the control group—study participants undergo routine ACLR. In the second group—the experimental group—the junior resident is allowed to perform the diagnostic arthroscopy before the attending surgeon performs the reconstruction. If done properly, the randomization process minimizes both known and unknown bias that might exist between the two groups at baseline. One could then obtain serial radiographs and patient-reported outcome measures (PROMs) from these two groups over time to determine how the chondral injury inflicted by the young, budding arthroscopist affects the rate of PTOA. Sadly, this study has yet to enroll any participants for some reason.

Instead, investigators design a prospective cohort study aimed at identifying risk factors for the development of PTOA following ACL injury and assemble a cohort that includes a large number of participants that have concomitant chondral injuries (which are "randomly assigned" by Mother Nature at the time of injury). At the conclusion of their study, the investigators can assess baseline chondral status (normal versus injured) as a risk factor for outcomes [3].

## 22.4 Curating the Cohort

Once a relevant clinical question has been developed, the study cohort can begin to be assembled. As with any other study design, the investigators must create a set of inclusion and exclusion criteria. How specific these criteria should be depends on how large of a cohort the investigators intend to follow. Larger cohorts can accommodate more heterogeneity among the participants because modern statistical methodology allows biostatisticians to "control for" multiple variables. More heterogeneity can help to strengthen conclusions from the proposed study by making the results more generalizable. Regardless of the size of the proposed cohort, all participants will share some characteristic. In the MOON cohort, for example, all participants have undergone primary and revision ACLR by one of a handful of surgeons during a specific time period. Beyond that, the participants differ greatly in terms of age, activity level, concomitant injuries, and more.

One of the biggest factors in settling on the final cohort size is cost. While the initial enrollment of participants into the cohort can be done while keeping expenses low, following participants until the end of the study period comes with significant costs. These costs are both quantifiable (such as salaries for full time employees whose job it is to call participants during the study period, fees for maintaining secure data storage, etc.) and hidden (such as time that investigators spend reaching out to patients to increase follow-up rates). The larger the cohort, the greater the cost. Additionally, the longer the cohort is to be followed, the more expensive the cohort becomes.

Equally as important, *not* investing the necessary amount of resources to maintain a scientifically valid follow-up rate (typically considered ~80% or greater) is wasteful, as the risk that the study results are significantly biased increases as the proportion of participants "lost to follow-up" increases.

## 22.5 Study Design: Obtaining Longitudinal Data

Arguably the greatest strength of a well-designed prospective cohort study is the ability to measure changes in individual participants over time. For example, a subset of the MOON cohort (yes, one can even have cohorts within cohorts, more formally known as nested cohorts) was asked to return to clinic 2 years following their index ACLR for standardized radiographs and physical examination. The follow-up radiographs were then compared to the opposite "normal knee" allowing the investigators to calculate the incidence of radiographic post-traumatic osteoarthritis, and, using regression modeling techniques, identify predictors of early-onset radiographic post-traumatic osteoarthritis [4]. Thanks to this well throughout out study design, the investigators were able to answer two clinical questions—(1) What is the incidence of radiographic post-traumatic knee arthritis following ACLR? And (2) What are risk factors for development of early radiographic post-traumatic osteoarthritis?—with one cohort. That same nested cohort has since returned for another set of radiographs 8 years later (10 years following their primary ACLR), allowing for another round of comparisons to be made [5]. Without valid baseline data (demographics, injury, and treatments), such analyses cannot be completed, and valuable information would remain unknown.

The take-home message is that a well-designed prospective cohort study starts with robust baseline data that is collected in a systematic fashion and with a specific clinical question (or questions) in mind. Additionally, when designing a prospective cohort study and compiling a list of the appropriate baseline variables to collect, a wise investigator thinks broadly, such that the data extracted from the cohort may be used to answer multiple clinical questions concurrently and answer them thoroughly. This is in contrast to registries, which collect baseline and follow up data (typically on much larger populations and at much lower follow up rates) without a specific clinical question and are better suited for retrospective studies (the conclusions of which may lead to a prospective cohort study or randomized trial).

## 22.6 The Achilles Heel of Prospective Cohort Studies: Confounding

The greatest weakness of even the most thoughtfully designed prospective cohort studies is the potential bias introduced by confounding variables. A true confounder has three characteristics: (1) it is a risk factor for the outcome of interest, (2) it is associated with the observed exposure, and (3) it is *not* an intermediate on the causal pathway between the exposure and the outcome.

A classic example of confounding can be seen in some of early studies aimed at identifying a potential relationship between coffee consumption and pancreatic cancer. In these early studies, which were mostly performed as case control studies, the investigators interviewed a group of patients with biopsy-proven pancreatic adenocarcinoma (the cases) and a separate group of hospitalized patients (the controls). Participants were queried on a variety of variables including coffee consumption. In the end, the investigators found that participants with pancreatic cancer were more likely to report being coffee drinkers compared to participants who did not have pancreatic cancer. Furthermore, those participants with pancreatic cancer reported significantly higher amounts of regular coffee consumption compared to those without pancreatic cancer, suggesting that there may be a dose response. What these early investigators failed to account for was the strong positive association between coffee drinking and smoking. As it turns out, coffee drinkers, especially those reporting high levels of consumption (more than five cups per day), were much more likely to be smokers, and smoking happens to be one of the strongest risk factors for pancreatic cancer. Smoking was the confounding variable that the investigators failed to account for in their initial analyses. After stratifying the rates of pancreatic cancer by smoking status, the association between coffee consumption and pancreatic cancer disappeared [6, 7].

Prospective cohort studies are also susceptible to the effects of confounding variables. This is because the observational nature of prospective cohort studies makes it impossible to randomly assign patients to the exposed or unexposed portions of the cohort.

Minimizing the potential bias introduced by confounders in a prospective cohort study can be done through a variety of ways at both the research design phase (randomization, restriction, matching) and the data analysis phase (stratification, regression modeling, propensity score matching), but these strategies are beyond the scope of this chapter [8].

## 22.7 Pearls and Pitfalls of Conducting Prospective Cohort Studies

While prospective cohort studies provide vital information for optimizing clinical care, they can easily fail without the appropriate support, which can vary considerably depending on the study design. If there is a single-center cohort study with patient-reported outcomes only and no physical exam or in-person follow-up required, then a research assistant would be helpful but not required. If physical examinations are required for the study, then a research assistant should be employed to ensure that the study runs smoothly.

When adding imaging or biomarkers to the single-center cohort study, some more experience is typically required for the principal investigator (PI) and a dedicated research coordinator is needed. When a multi-center cohort study is constructed, the PI should have moderate to extensive experience, and a team of research coordinators and biostatistical support should be assembled.

Obtaining follow-up is a second major challenge for prospective studies. For publication, it is often required that the authors have achieved 80% follow-up at 2 years post-intervention. To obtain this follow-up, passive forms of collection such as scheduled email can be employed, but often that method is not able to achieve responses from 80% of patients. Therefore, active follow-up such as patient calls by research assistants, research coordinators, resident physicians, or attending physicians can be helpful and required [9].

## 22.8 Prospective Cohort Studies Versus Randomized Controlled Trials

Prospective cohort studies and randomized controlled trials (RCTs) have both strengths and weaknesses, and they can work in concert to augment one another. An RCT works optimally for determining whether a new intervention or technology is effective in a population as a whole or for evaluating potential major shift in clinical practice. It compares the mean effect of treatment against a control or clinically standard treatment. An RCT that shows effect is demonstrating that the "average" experimental intervention is better than the "average" control or clinical standard. Within the overall study population, the RCT is not able to identify the individual patients who are at the highest likelihood of benefiting from an intervention. This was recently recognized by the medical community and spurred the PATH publication in the Annals of Internal Medicine which stated that RCTs should publish risk stratified results to be able to best apply the findings at the patient level. However, while this is feasible in the large RCTs typically conducted in the medicine specialties, orthopedic, and other subspecialty surgery RCTs are often smaller in size and so stratified results are not able to be obtained. Prospective cohort studies can provide this vital information.

One setting in which cohort studies are particularly important is post-market surveillance. After an intervention has been implemented, such as following an RCT that demonstrates clinical success, the medication or device should be evaluated after release for any beneficial or adverse effects not previously identified in the form of a post-market surveillance cohort study. The importance of this can be clearly seen in the example of Vioxx, where an approved medication was found to substantially increase the risk for cardiovascular events through a cohort study conducted post-market [10]. This ultimately led to the medication being pulled from the market for safety concerns.

## 22.9 Controversies Surrounding Reporting of Prospective Cohort Data

One area of controversy that has developed with the increasing popularity of cohort studies (related to the renewed understanding of their importance) is how to report data that is obtained through retrospective review of prospectively collected data. When data is initially collected in a prospective fashion, it is almost always collected with the aim of understanding one or more specific clinical questions (as outlined above). However, often the data collected can be analyzed to answer questions that the data was not initially designed to answer. Thus, the question has become whether these should be seen as level 2 evidence and reported as a prospective cohort study since the data was collected in that fashion or if they should be considered level 3 retrospective cohort studies as the question was identified after data collection and the data that was prospectively collected was retrospectively analyzed. There is not currently a clear answer to this question, and so authors in conjunction with the journal should discuss and come to an agreement on how to describe studies with this foundation of evidence.

## 22.10 Conclusion

A prospective cohort study is a powerful tool for clinical research that was helpful when developed in the time of King Nebuchadnezzar and that has only grown more important with time. A cohort study permits researchers to answer an a priori clinical question in a group of individuals without a control over a period of time with longitudinal data collection. With this data, there is the ability to make patient-level decisions through complex statistics designed to identify individual risk factors. When the study design accounts for confounding, a major risk for the conclusions drawn, by including a large sample size and many variables, valid conclusions can be drawn with more confidence. To ensure smooth completion of the study, using the appropriate team such as involving a research coordinator or biostatistics assistant is essential. In the future, while randomized controlled trials will provide important information on how the average result from an intervention performs against the average clinical standard or placebo, the decisions made at the individual patient level will continue to be informed by well-conducted prospective cohort studies.

## References


1. Beynnon BD, Vacek PM, Newell MK, Tourville TW, Smith HC, Shultz SJ, Slauterbeck JR, Johnson RJ. The effects of level of competition, sport, and sex on the incidence of first-time noncontact anterior cruciate ligament injury. Am J Sports Med. 2014;42:1806–12.
2. MARS Group, Brophy RH, Wright RW, Huston LJ, Haas AK, Allen CR, Anderson AF, Cooper DE, DeBerardino TM, Dunn WR, et al. Rate of infection following revision anterior cruciate ligament reconstruction and associated patient- and surgeon-dependent risk factors: retrospective results from MOON and MARS data collected from 2002 to 2011. J Orthop Res. 2021;39:274–80.
3. Brophy RH, Huston LJ, Briskin I, MOON Knee Group, Amendola A, Cox CL, Dunn WR, Flanigan DC, Jones MH, Kaeding CC, et al. Articular cartilage and meniscus predictors of patient-reported outcomes 10 years after anterior cruciate ligament reconstruction: a multicenter cohort study. Am J Sports Med. 2021;49:2878–88.
4. MOON Knee Group, Jones MH, Oak SR, Andrish JT, Brophy RH, Cox CL, Dunn WR, Flanigan DC, Fleming BC, Huston LJ, et al. Predictors of radiographic osteoarthritis 2 to 3 years after anterior cruciate ligament reconstruction: data from the MOON on-site nested cohort. Orthop J Sports Med. 2019;7:2325967119867085.
5. MOON Group, Everhart JS, Jones MH, Yalcin S, Reinke EK, Huston LJ, Andrish JT, Cox CL, Flanigan DC, Kaeding CC, et al. The clinical radiographic incidence of posttraumatic osteoarthritis 10 years after anterior cruciate ligament reconstruction: data from the MOON nested cohort. Am J Sports Med. 2021;49:1251–61.
6. MacMahon B, Yen S, Trichopoulos D, Warren K, Nardi G. Coffee and cancer of the pancreas. N Engl J Med. 1981;304:630–3.
7. Zhou CD, Kuan AS, Reeves GK, Green J, Floud S, Beral V, Yang TO. Million women study collaborators: coffee and pancreatic cancer risk among never-smokers in the UK prospective million women study. Int J Cancer. 2019;145:1484–92.
8. Braga LHP, Farrokhyar F, Bhandari M. Practical tips for surgical research. Can J Surg. 2012;55:132–8.
9. Cleveland O, Piuzzi NS, Strnad G, Brooks P, Hettrich CM, Higuera-Rueda C, Iannotti J, Kattan MW, Molloy R, Lynch TS, et al. Implementing a scientifically valid, cost-effective, and scalable data collection system at point of care: the Cleveland Clinic OME cohort. J Bone Joint Surg Am. 2019;101:458–64.
10. Krumholz HM, Ross JS, Presler AH, Egilman DS. What have we learnt from Vioxx? BMJ. 2007;334:120–3.

# 23 Surgical Registries

Jon Olav Drogset, Andreas Persson, and R. Kyle Martin

## 23.1 Introduction

Information from registry data can be used to guide management, help answer questions commonly encountered in clinical practice, and ultimately to improve patient care [1]. In medicine, a registry is a standardized database designed to prospectively collect information on a patient population with a common disease or intervention that is followed over time [2].

It is estimated that more than 234 million surgical procedures are performed each year worldwide and a further 134 million lack the possibility to get necessary surgical treatments [3, 4].

Optimization of surgical outcomes relies on constant evaluation of and improvement in surgical indications, devices, techniques, and perioperative care. The surgeons should receive feedback on their own outcomes, compared with population-based averages. This may enable the surgeon to recognize and seek to improve upon suboptimal outcomes. This goal of optimizing patient outcome represents the core mission of registries.

## 23.2 History

The first known medical registry was the National Leprosy Registry of Norway which was established in 1856 [5, 6]. More than a century later, the Swedish knee arthroplasty registry became the first national registry in orthopedic surgery in 1975 [7]. Finland (1980), Norway (1987), and Denmark (1995) followed with arthroplasty registers and were soon expanded to include all joint replacements. The primary objective of the first arthroplasty registers was the early detection of inferior results based on implant revision data. This proved successful in 1995 when two studies identified inferior implants at an early stage, a determination made possible through the arthroplasty registry [8–10].

J. O. Drogset (✉)
The Norwegian Knee Ligament Registry, Orthopedic Department, Haukeland University Hospital, Bergen, Norway

Department of Orthopaedic Surgery, Trondheim University Hospital, Trondheim, Norway

Norwegian University of Science and Technology, Trondheim, Norway
e-mail: jon.o.drogset@ntnu.no

A. Persson
The Norwegian Knee Ligament Registry, Orthopedic Department, Haukeland University Hospital, Bergen, Norway

Department of Orthopaedic Surgery, Oslo University Hospital, Oslo, Norway

OSTRC, The Norwegian School of Sports Sciences, Oslo, Norway

R. K. Martin
Department of Orthopedic Surgery, University of Minnesota, Minneapolis, MN, USA


S. Lyman et al. (eds.), *Introduction to Surgical Trials*,
https://doi.org/10.1007/978-3-031-77563-5_23

Today, the use of registries in the medical field has expanded to include many specialties and several national, regional, and local registries have been developed. Building on the early experience of the arthroplasty registers, important changes have also been made to the data collection and outcome measures that are captured. The first knee ligament surgical registry was created in Norway in 2004 (NKLR), followed in 2005 by Sweden and Denmark [11]. While revision surgery and conversion to total knee arthroplasty were determined to be important outcome measures, it was also recognized that inferior clinical outcome and graft failures may not always go on to further surgery and therefore may go undetected by the registry [8]. To account for this, the knee ligament registries also include patient reported outcome measures (PROMs), specifically the Knee injury and Osteoarthritis Outcome Score (KOOS) [12], pre-operatively and at standard post-operative time points. Thus, the ability to detect inferior results and early failures is improved without relying on subsequent surgery as the sole endpoint.

In 2014, the International Society of Arthroplasty Registries created a PROMs Working Group [13, 14]. The working group outlined the rationale for the inclusion of PROMs in the arthroplasty registries and noted that several have incorporated PROMs into their data collection [14]. They also made several recommendations regarding the use of these outcome measures in arthroplasty registers [13].

## 23.3 Importance of Registries

The goal of surgical registries is to improve health care delivery via prospective surveillance of surgical outcomes. Continuous feedback to hospitals and surgeons allows comparison to the population average and can help establish best clinical practices [8]. This, in turn, encourages improvement by setting and continually updating the standard of care [7, 15]. The detection of procedures and devices that result in early failure can be identified by following revision or reoperation rates and deterioration in patient reported outcome measures [11, 16]. Prognostic variables associated with positive and negative outcomes can be ascertained via large cohort studies performed on the registry data [8]. Epidemiological trends and the burden of disease can also be followed for changes over time.

One of the biggest advantages of registries is the ability to include a high volume of data over time. This creates a large database of short and long-term follow-ups from which cohort studies can be undertaken. This confers several important strengths:

1. There is little or no selection bias to influence these large datasets.
2. The data already exists at the onset of a study, making the analysis less time-consuming and more cost-effective.
3. When subsequent surgery on included patients is linked with a personal health identification number, there is minimal risk of attrition bias.
4. Data is collected independently of future research questions—there is no differential misclassification.
5. The high volume of data allows the assessment of several different endpoints and exposures at the same time.

While randomized control trials (RCT) are considered the gold standard research design for evaluating and comparing interventions, they are often not practical or possible to perform owing to ethical, financial, procedural, or other barriers. RCTs also often have stringent inclusion and exclusion criteria which limit the external validity and the generalizability of the results to patients seen in clinical practice. In contrast, well-designed observational studies from registry data can offer similar results regarding treatment effects, while largely avoiding the hurdles faced by RCTs. These studies can be complementary to RCTs by assessing real-world applicability of the experimental findings and may serve to generate new ideas for future RCTs [17–22].

Registries also have limitations. Non-randomized cohort studies are subject to bias from confounding variables which must be corrected for; either by selection of homogeneous subgroups or through multiple regression analysis [23]. Even if risk factors are considered in a regression model, there is always a risk of unmeasured confounding in observational studies due to variables that are either not considered in the model or not yet recognized or collected. Compliance is essential for an effective registry database and can be difficult to achieve, especially in the initial stages if no prior database existed. Furthermore, the need for a high response rate can conflict with the goal of optimizing the amount of useful data that is to be collected. To encourage form completion by the surgeons and patients, details regarding demographics, diagnosis, surgical procedure, and implants, along with objective and subjective outcome measures must be streamlined to avoid survey-fatigue and non-compliance. Finding the optimal balance between details collected and, for example, the surgeon's precious time can prove to be difficult. Consequently, the relevance of every requested input must be carefully considered by the steering board members to keep compliance high.

## 23.4 Research Questions

When creating a registry, it is important to understand the research questions that can be answered through the database as this will influence what information should be recorded. Registries can be used to track epidemiology and provide quality assessment of treatment protocols, devices, and outcomes for a defined patient population. Regional variations within a country can also be identified.

The NKLR provides an example of how registry data can be used to provide quality control. Epidemiological data gives an actual number of anterior cruciate ligament (ACL) and posterior cruciate ligament (PCL) reconstructions and revision surgeries performed on an annual basis. Using this data, the NKLR established that a failure of a specific device is suspected if only 14 patients with this device are identified as having failed, based on recorded outcome measures [8]. This early warning system is ongoing, and problems may be identified long before they would have been uncovered by traditional methods such as RCTs. While causality of failure may not always be evident in these cases, it raises flags and directs further assessment and research.

Selecting which outcome measures and variables to record has been eluded to above. Revision surgery or subsequent conversion to arthroplasty are two end points that are clear and indisputable. In addition, patient reported outcome measures offer a subjective end point useful in identifying inferior results that may not proceed to further surgery. Selection of patient-based subjective outcome measures to include should take several variables into consideration. These include validation for use given the target population, availability in multiple languages, cost, and completion should be self-explanatory and fast (ideally less than 10 min) [8, 13].

Data recorded by, for example, the surgeon should be minimal and necessary, generally limited to a one-page reporting system. As it can be beneficial to compare data between registries, it is also important to use a core minimum data set that is in use across several different registries. In the development of the NKLR, this data was chosen based on the following three criteria [8]:

1. Can the question addressed be clearly specified and justified?
2. Is the question clinically relevant?
3. Can the item be completed post operatively while dictating the surgery notes, not needing to seek information from other sources?

Finally, as medical practice is dynamic and ever-changing, variables should be re-evaluated on a regular basis and changes made according to current practice and evolving literature.

The Single Assessment Numeric Evaluation (SANE) is a patient rating from 0 to 100. Patients rate their current illness score in relation to their pre-injury baseline. SANE scores are most used by orthopedic sports specialist surgeons, and usually for the shoulder and the knee. Current best evidence demonstrating good correlation of shorter and more general measures with longer and more specific measures suggests even a single simple question (SANE) could be sufficient [24–30].

The minimal clinically important difference (MCID) is the smallest change in a treatment outcome that an individual patient would identify as important and which would indicate a change in the patient's management [31, 32].

Patient Acceptable Symptom State (PASS) has been defined as the highest level of symptom beyond which patients consider themselves well. The most widely used anchoring question to identify PASS cut-off points is, "Taking into account all the activities you have during your daily life, your level of pain, and your functional impairment, do you consider that your current state is satisfactory?". The response options are "yes" or "no." Studies have also addressed the robustness of the PASS cut-off points. It appears that PASS cut-off points are stable over time [33].

## 23.5 Structure of a Registry

The registry collects prospective information on all patients in a defined population. Patient consent to participate may or may not be required, based on the specific national privacy legislation. In general, if the data is to be used in future research studies, patients should be made aware and informed consent should be obtained when they are initially enrolled. In surgical patients, information is obtained from the patient and from the surgeon at pre-specified time points. In general, baseline subjective data is obtained from the patient pre-operatively and repeated at defined intervals post-operatively. Information related to the diagnosis, surgical findings, procedure(s), implants, and complications is recorded by the surgeon immediately following the surgery [8]. Bar-code stickers from implanted devices can often be scanned or included with the report form to ensure accurate tracking [8, 23]. Some registries also include clinical and/or radiological follow-up data at subsequent post-operative visits [34, 35].

All documents are sent, either electronically or on paper, to a central location to be checked for completeness and stored in the registry database. Incomplete forms are returned to the sender for completion to assure data quality and completeness. A copy of the form is also retained in the patient's hospital chart. In Norway, for example, a small staff is responsible for the day-to-day operations of the NKLR, overseen by an advisory board. This includes a secretary, a computer engineer, and an administrative head of the registry. Each participating hospital employs secretarial assistance and the NKLR also has access to experienced statisticians for registry studies [8]. In 2017, the operating budget for the central NKLR office was 1,800,000 NOK (approximately $218,000 USD) and includes the salary of additional staff involved in NKLR-based research projects.

Orthopedic registries are most often publicly financed either through direct funding or grants. For example, the Norwegian, Swedish, and Danish knee ligament registries are financed through the national public health system. Similarly, the Canadian Joint Replacement Registry receives funding from Federal and Provincial government sources, via the Canadian Institutes for Health Information [3]. Privately owned and financed registries also exist, for example, in New Zealand. Collaboration with the local and national Orthopedic Association is important in all cases to advocate for continued financing and support ongoing activities of the registry. In general, it is advisable for registries to avoid industry sponsorship to maintain objectivity and avoid bias which may affect research and clinical practice.

## 23.6 Data Reporting

Data contained in the registry can be released for evaluation via annual reports, hospital specific data requests, or more extensive research projects. Annual reports present descriptive information including compliance rates and are often broken down into regional subsets for comparison to the national and historical data. Tables and figures are used to present overall and regional epidemiology, survivorship curves, complications, and other information (Figs. 23.1 and 23.2). These reports are frequently published online for public viewing.

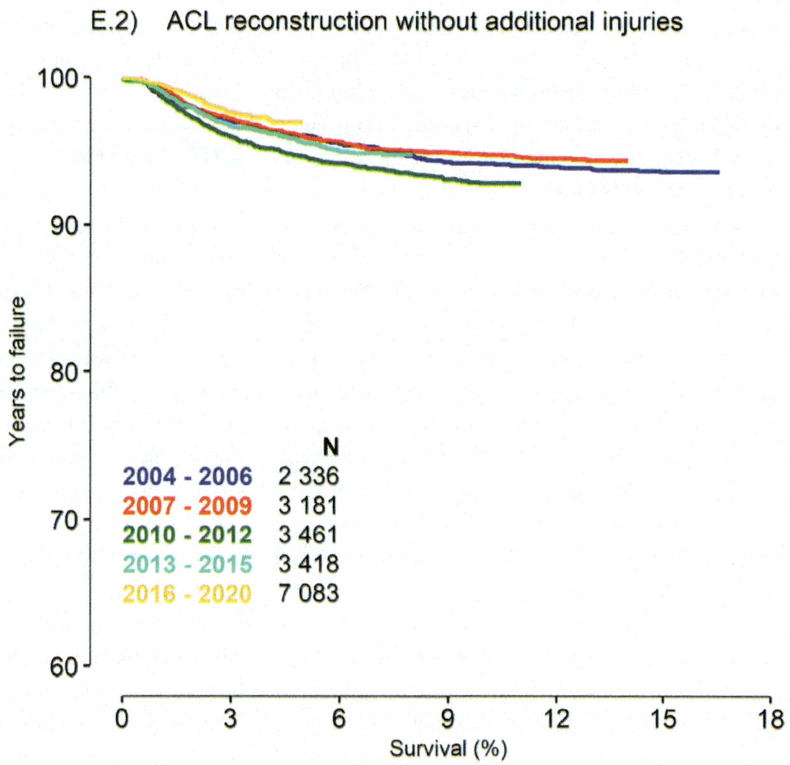


**Fig. 23.1** Kaplan-Meier survivorship curve of primary ACL reconstruction from the Norwegian National Knee Ligament Registry 2017 annual report

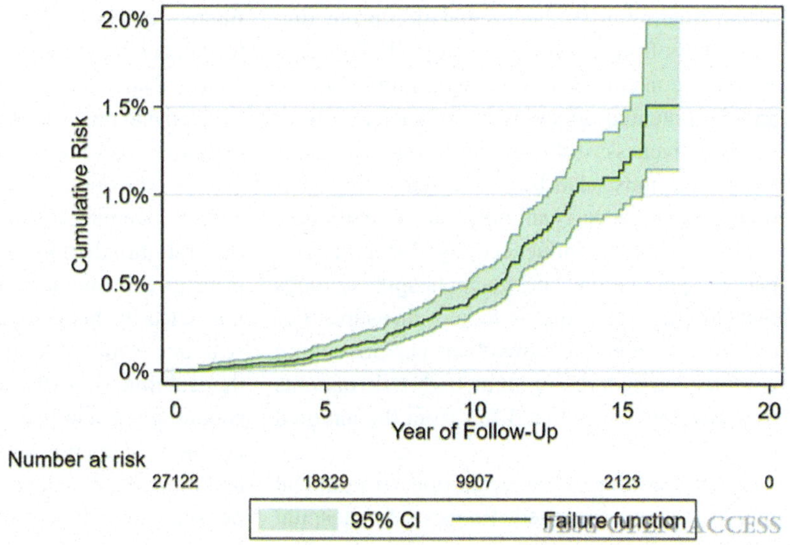


**Fig. 23.2** Cumulative risk of knee arthroplasty following ACL reconstruction

Since attaining and maintaining a high compliance rate is paramount to the success of a registry, it follows that accurate determination of this rate is of equal importance. Hospital, regional, or national databases that capture information related to the number of procedures performed are often used as the denominator in determining the compliance rate of registries. For example, in Norway, hospitals track their procedures and send the information to the central office for reimbursement according to the Diagnosis-Related Groups schedule. This data is then compared with the information received by the registry over the same time to determine the compliance rate. Any discrepancies are included in the annual report as hospital specific compliance rates. In Norway, it is mandatory for the surgeons to report to the NKLR.

Registries may report only national and regional data, keeping surgeons unidentified, or they may use the information to produce surgeon specific reports [36]. In one Canadian province, annual surgeon specific reports are generated for all hip and knee arthroplasties, hip fractures, rotator cuff repairs, and knee meniscectomies. These report cards allow hospitals and individual surgeons to compare their data with that of their peers. Furthermore, the regional Standards and Quality Committee also reviews the reports and notifies surgeons that fall below the regional averages. If outcomes remain below the average for 2 or more years, the committee meets with the surgeon to review the data and to develop a plan to correct the identified issues. This initiative is possible owing to the mandatory nature of regional registry participation, strong leadership of the steering group, and legislation protecting the reports from court subpoena [37]. Concerns over surgeon confidentiality, legal ramifications, and the potential effect on compliance rate limit the effectiveness of this model in other jurisdictions. One must also be aware that using endpoints in a register as an indicator of health care quality might be influenced by differences in patient populations between hospitals/clinics that might affect the outcome measure. For example, surgical centres that perform more complex procedures or treat high-risk patients may have outcomes that differ from the national average.

Access to information in addition to the annual report is also encouraged. Requests for hospital specific data often requires approval by the advisory board and are made by the official hospital contact person. This potentially patient- and surgeon-identifiable information can be used by the hospital for evaluation and local quality improvement projects. More extensive requests for information to be used in research projects can be applied for in writing to the governing body and additional Health Research Ethics Board approval may also be required [36].

## 23.7 Pearls

The strength of a registry lies in the completeness and accuracy of the data [38], and therefore compliance is crucial. This can be difficult to achieve for several reasons that have been described previously. Some ways to improve compliance include the way in which data is collected, rules and laws governing its collection, and perception regarding the importance and uses of the registry.

Whether paper-based or electronic forms are used, they should be user-friendly and not time-consuming. Only the necessary data should be included and if possible, as much of the data should be recorded in advance (i.e., operating room nurses can enter the operative information and scan the implant bar-codes during the surgery [37]). Missing data should be flagged immediately, and a notice sent to the surgeon to address the deficiency before too much time has passed after the surgery. In the future, machine learning/artificial intelligence techniques may drastically improve the ability to collect data while minimizing the burden on the surgeon and this concept is discussed further in the discussion on future directions.

The collection of personal information is and always should be an important discussion. Several jurisdictions require informed consent prior to enrollment in a registry while others do not. Clearly this can play a role in compliance, with one National Registry reporting that 31% of the submitted forms were missing the corresponding consent [39]. Strict adherence to confidentiality standards including secure data storage and limited authorized access may bridge the gap between privacy concerns and data collection. Decisions related to the necessity of obtaining consent must ultimately involve regional Heath Research Ethics Boards and established legislation.

Legislation can influence compliance with national registries in other ways. In Denmark, the hospitals do not receive reimbursement for cruciate ligament surgeries that have not been reported to their national knee ligament registry. Creating a user-friendly data submission environment for the surgeon and introducing policy mandating compliance is a powerful way to maintain a high rate of data completion on a national level.

Perception of the registry in the eyes of the public and the orthopedic community also plays a role in compliance. This begins on the first encounter with each patient which should include a discussion on the importance of the registry and an overview of their contribution. It is also an opportunity to build a good report that may influence their future compliance. The regular publication of reports highlighting trends and important findings, both positive and negative, provides constant reminder that the data is being collected for a purpose. Major publications that may change clinical practice further reinforce the importance of participation in the registry. Finally, data should be used to foster best medical practice, rather than seeking to identify and punish individual surgeons who may fall below this current standard. A supportive community approach to the registry should be sought to ensure that all surgeons feel comfortable participating and remain open to the feedback it provides.

## 23.8 Future Directions

Moving forward, registries will continue to play an important role in medicine. As more national registries are established, there is a vision to create a common international knee ligament registry in Europe. The development of a common software program to collect and store the data is an additional goal that could be used by those nations who will not join an international database for legal or other reasons. Standardizing data collection across several nations would have several benefits including increased power for large studies and the ability to directly compare data from one part of the world with another. There is also an ongoing effort to expand registries to include the non-operative management of orthopedic conditions such as ACL deficiency which are not currently captured in most databases [40].

## 23.9 Register-Based RCT

The classic RCT remedies confounding bias by randomly allocating patients to each treatment ensuring equal distribution of measured and, importantly, unmeasured characteristics. However, RCTs often have strict inclusion and exclusion criteria leading to diminished generalization to the general population. One may ask what good are RCTs if they can answer questions regarding only a fraction of the population. They are often expensive and time-consuming, limiting the possible number of patients included. Recently, as an answer to these limitations, the implementation of randomization into registers has been proposed, and termed "the register-based RCT" (R-RCT). The promise of this approach has been highlighted in high-ranking journals as the "next disruptive technology in clinical research" [41]. Simply put, patients are included in a quality register, and the treatment is randomized. The outcome data is collected automatically through the register, cutting the costs, and simplifying the follow-up. Analysis of the subsequent register data can conclude on effect estimates between treatments with the same level of evidence as those from regular RCTs, only with a greater external validity [42]. The feasibility R-RCTs has been shown mainly in trials relating to interventions in cardiology and has only very recently been used in orthopedic trauma surgery [41] . However, linking an R-RCT to a national quality register represents a novel innovation.

Recruitment problems have been highlighted as a challenge in a previous RCT on ACL treatment. The R-RCT mediates this by facilitating multi-center collaboration to ensure rapid inclusion of patients in the proposed trials [28].

## 23.10 Machine Learning

One way registries have started to evolve is using machine learning. Machine learning is a branch of artificial intelligence and represents a set of advanced statistical techniques. These techniques enable the processing of large volumes of data to identify complex relationships within the dataset that may not be feasible through more traditional statistical approaches. Going one step further, deep learning and neural networks allow interpretation of highly complex and unprocessed data. Within healthcare, machine learning is primarily used for pattern identification and outcome prediction. This may take the form of clinical calculators capable of predicting the patient's diagnosis or prognosis, software that can automatically interpret imaging modalities, and tools for text-based data extraction from clinical notes and electronic medical records.

National orthopedic registries have been prospectively collecting large volumes of data for decades and machine learning analysis has the potential to yield clinically relevant algorithms capable of predicting patient-specific outcome. Early clinical models to estimate a patient's risk of experiencing a revision surgery or inferior clinical outcome following ACL reconstruction have recently been developed [43, 44]. These algorithms were based on analysis of the Norwegian knee ligament register and demonstrated moderate prediction accuracy. The revision model has also been externally validated using the Danish knee ligament registry [45]. Similar analysis of the Danish Hip Arthroscopy Registry led to a prediction model of limited clinical utility, however, emphasizing the need for improvement in both the quality and quantity of the data being collected [45].

Accuracy of registry-based clinical prediction models is presently capped by the subset of variables being recorded. Accuracy of subsequent models may be improved through the inclusion of additional variables that are likely to be associated with the outcomes of interest. Machine learning techniques such as computer vision (automatic image interpretation) and natural language processing (interpreting text such as operative and clinical notes to extract additional variables) are tools that enable registries to collect additional variables without increasing the burden on those typically responsible for the data collection. For example, natural language processing can be trained to extract details from the operative report and computer vision can interpret imaging for automatic documentation of radiographic parameters such as posterior tibial slope. These methods can vastly increase the range of variables being collected while simultaneously minimizing the manual inputs currently required by the surgeons. These innovations could also be applied retrospectively to capture data from past clinical notes and images to improve the existing databases. Finally, these machine learning techniques could also be deployed to create *new* registries for institutions, regions, or nations based on retrospective data.

## References


1. Ivers N, et al. Audit and feedback: effects on professional practice and healthcare outcomes. Cochrane Database Syst Rev. 2012;(6):CD000259.
2. Drolet BC, Johnson KB. Categorizing the world of registries. J Biomed Inform. 2008;41(6):1009–20.
3. Weiser TG, et al. An estimation of the global volume of surgery: a modelling strategy based on available data. Lancet. 2008;372(9633):139–44.
4. Meara JG, et al. Global surgery 2030: evidence and solutions for achieving health, welfare, and economic development. Lancet. 2015;386(9993):569–624.
5. Irgens LM. The origin of registry-based medical research and care. Acta Neurol Scand Suppl. 2012;195:4–6.
6. Irgens LM, Bjerkedal T. Epidemiology of leprosy in Norway: the history of the National Leprosy Registry of Norway from 1856 until today. Int J Epidemiol. 1973;2(1):81–9.
7. Knutson K, et al. The Swedish knee arthroplasty register. A nation-wide study of 30,003 knees 1976-1992. Acta Orthop Scand. 1994;65(4):375–86.
8. Granan LP, et al. Development of a national cruciate ligament surgery registry: the Norwegian National Knee Ligament Registry. Am J Sports Med. 2008;36(2):308–15.
9. Havelin LI, et al. The effect of the type of cement on early revision of Charnley total hip prostheses. A review of eight thousand five hundred and seventy-nine primary arthroplasties from the Norwegian arthroplasty register. J Bone Joint Surg Am. 1995;77(10):1543–50.
10. Havelin LI, et al. Early aseptic loosening of uncemented femoral components in primary total hip replacement. A review based on the Norwegian arthroplasty register. J Bone Joint Surg Br. 1995;77(1):11–7.
11. Granan LP, et al. The Scandinavian ACL registries 2004-2007: baseline epidemiology. Acta Orthop. 2009;80(5):563–7.
12. Roos EM, et al. Knee Injury and Osteoarthritis Outcome Score (KOOS)—development of a

self-administered outcome measure. J Orthop Sports Phys Ther. 1998;28(2):88–96.
13. Rolfson O, et al. Patient-reported outcome measures in arthroplasty registries report of the patient-reported outcome measures working Group of the International Society of arthroplasty registries part II. Recommendations for selection, administration, and analysis. Acta Orthop. 2016;87(Suppl 1):9–23.
14. Rolfson O, et al. Patient-reported outcome measures in arthroplasty registries. Acta Orthop. 2016;87(Suppl 1):3–8.
15. Maloney WJ. National Joint Replacement Registries: has the time come? J Bone Joint Surg Am. 2001;83(10):1582–5.
16. de Steiger RN, et al. Joint registry approach for identification of outlier prostheses. Acta Orthop. 2013;84(4):348–52.
17. Benson K, Hartz AJ. A comparison of observational studies and randomized, controlled trials. N Engl J Med. 2000;342(25):1878–86.
18. Comber H, Perry IJ. Observational studies for intervention assessment. Lancet. 2001;357(9274):2141–2.
19. Concato J, Shah N, Horwitz RI. Randomized, controlled trials, observational studies, and the hierarchy of research designs. N Engl J Med. 2000;342(25):1887–92.
20. Horan FT. Judging the evidence. J Bone Joint Surg Br. 2005;87(12):1589–90.
21. Naylor CD, Guyatt GH. Users' guides to the medical literature. X. How to use an article reporting variations in the outcomes of health services. The evidence-based medicine working group. JAMA. 1996;275(7):554–8.
22. Pocock SJ, Elbourne DR. Randomized trials or observational tribulations? N Engl J Med. 2000;342(25):1907–9.
23. Havelin LI, et al. The Norwegian arthroplasty register: 11 years and 73,000 arthroplasties. Acta Orthop Scand. 2000;71(4):337–53.
24. Winterstein AP, et al. Comparison of IKDC and SANE outcome measures following knee injury in active female patients. Sports Health. 2013;5(6):523–9.
25. Williams GN, et al. Comparison of the single assessment numeric evaluation method and two shoulder rating scales. Outcomes measures after shoulder surgery. Am J Sports Med. 1999;27(2):214–21.
26. Schmidt S, et al. Evaluation of shoulder-specific patient-reported outcome measures: a systematic and standardized comparison of available evidence. J Shoulder Elbow Surg. 2014;23(3):434–44.
27. Williams GN, et al. Comparison of the single assessment numeric evaluation method and the Lysholm score. Clin Orthop Relat Res. 2000;373:184–92.
28. Bradbury M, et al. Relationship between scores from the knee outcome survey and a single assessment numerical rating in patients with patellofemoral pain. Physiother Theory Pract. 2013;29(7):531–5.
29. Taylor DC, et al. Isolated tears of the anterior cruciate ligament: over 30-year follow-up of patients treated with arthrotomy and primary repair. Am J Sports Med. 2009;37(1):65–71.
30. Edmonds EW, et al. The pediatric/adolescent shoulder survey (PASS): a reliable youth questionnaire with discriminant validity and responsiveness to change. Orthop J Sports Med. 2017;5(3):2325967117698466.
31. Schunemann HJ, Guyatt GH. Commentary—goodbye M(C)ID! Hello MID, where do you come from? Health Serv Res. 2005;40(2):593–7.
32. Wright A, et al. Clinimetrics corner: a closer look at the minimal clinically important difference (MCID). J Man Manip Ther. 2012;20(3):160–6.
33. Kvien TK, Heiberg T, Hagen KB. Minimal clinically important improvement/difference (MCII/MCID) and patient acceptable symptom state (PASS): what do these concepts mean? Ann Rheum Dis. 2007;66 Suppl 3(Suppl 3):iii40–1.
34. Lind M, Menhert F, Pedersen AB. The first results from the Danish ACL reconstruction registry: epidemiologic and 2 year follow-up results from 5,818 knee ligament reconstructions. Knee Surg Sports Traumatol Arthrosc. 2009;17(2):117–24.
35. Mygind-Klavsen B, et al. Danish hip arthroscopy registry: an epidemiologic and perioperative description of the first 2000 procedures. J Hip Preserv Surg. 2016;3(2):138–45.
36. Granan L, et al. Development of a national cruciate ligament surgery registry: the Norwegian National Knee Ligament Registry. Am J Sports Med. 2008;36(2):308–15.
37. Singh J, et al. Trends in revision hip and knee arthroplasty observations after implementation of a regional joint replacement registry. Can J Surg. 2016;59(5):304–10.
38. Robertsson O. Knee arthroplasty registers. J Bone Joint Surg Br. 2007;89(1):1–4.
39. Bohm ER, Dunbar MJ, Bourne R. The Canadian joint replacement registry-what have we learned? Acta Orthop. 2010;81(1):119–21.
40. Engebretsen L, Forssblad M, Lind M. Why registries analysing cruciate ligament surgery are important. Br J Sports Med. 2015;49(10):636–8.
41. Lauer MS, D'Agostino RB Sr. The randomized registry trial—the next disruptive technology in clinical research? N Engl J Med. 2013;369(17):1579–81.
42. Mathes T, et al. Registry-based randomized controlled trials merged the strength of randomized controlled trails and observational studies and give rise to more pragmatic trials. J Clin Epidemiol. 2018;93:120–7.
43. Martin RK, et al. Predicting anterior cruciate ligament reconstruction revision: a machine learning analysis utilizing the Norwegian knee ligament register. J Bone Joint Surg Am. 2022;104(2):145–53.
44. Martin RK, et al. Machine learning in sports medicine: need for improvement. J ISAKOS. 2021;6(1):1–2.
45. Martin RK, et al. Limited clinical utility of a machine learning revision prediction model based on a national hip arthroscopy registry. Knee Surg Sports Traumatol Arthrosc. 2022;31:2079.

# The Future of Trials

# 24

Bálint Zsidai, Alexandra Horvath,
Eric Hamrin Senorski, and Jón Karlsson

## 24.1 Introduction

The increasing complexity of surgical research provides new and exciting challenges to be overcome in the design of future trials. The aim of this chapter is to provide a bird's-eye view of the emerging trends in orthopedic surgical trials with the aid of a handful of examples. These trends include the recognition of the importance of pragmatic trial design and harnessing the use of prospectively collected registry data and international research networks. Moreover, multicenter trials generating statistically robust and generalizable trial data and artificial intelligence-based (AI) tools promise a potential new frontier in orthopedic and sports medicine trials.

**Fact Box 24.1**

Key ideas in the future of trials:

1. Pragmatic trial design.
2. Implementation of international research networks and registry data.
3. Trials with multicenter collaboration.
4. Adoption and evaluation of artificial intelligence and machine learning technologies in clinical trials.

## 24.2 A Shift Toward Pragmatic Surgical Trials

Randomized controlled trials (RCTs) have historically been considered the gold-standard of evaluating devices, pharmaceuticals, and surgi-

B. Zsidai
Department of Orthopaedics, Institute of Clinical Sciences, Sahlgrenska Academy, University of Gothenburg, Gothenburg, Sweden

Sahlgrenska Sports Medicine Center, Gothenburg, Sweden

A. Horvath
Sahlgrenska Sports Medicine Center, Gothenburg, Sweden

Department of Internal Medicine and Clinical Nutrition, Institute of Medicine, Sahlgrenska Academy, University of Gothenburg, Gothenburg, Sweden

E. H. Senorski
Sahlgrenska Sports Medicine Center, Gothenburg, Sweden

Department of Health and Rehabilitation, Institute of Neuroscience and Physiology, Sahlgrenska Academy, University of Gothenburg, Gothenburg, Sweden

J. Karlsson (✉)
Department of Orthopaedics, Sahlgrenska University Hospital, Sahlgrenska Academy, Gothenburg University, Göteborg, Sweden
e-mail: jon.karlsson@telia.com; jon.karlsson@vgregion.se


S. Lyman et al. (eds.), *Introduction to Surgical Trials*,
https://doi.org/10.1007/978-3-031-77563-5_24

cal interventions in medicine. The strength of RCTs stem from the methods they employ in order to reduce the impact of assessor- and participant-related bias on the outcomes of any study. These methods include various randomization techniques, allocation concealment, carefully selected control groups and blinding, each of which safeguards clinical trials from bias at different stages of the investigation. Traditional RCTs are explanatory in nature and typically investigate the efficacy of interventions under ideal conditions with strict eligibility criteria applied to the patient populations involved in the study. While the application of rigorous inclusion and exclusion criteria to a study population may limit the effect of confounding variables and biases, such groups are unlikely to be a true representation of patients treated for a specific orthopedic pathology in everyday clinical practice. A meticulously controlled study environment and blinding of the patient, operating physician, and outcome assessor is often unattainable or unfavorable in surgical trial design, warranting the investigation of treatment effectiveness under conditions closely resembling the average clinical setting. Consequently, surgical trials in orthopedic surgery have shifted toward a more pragmatic trial design in order to collect evidence supporting the best-practices in surgical interventions, in a manner that is applicable to a diverse population [1]. Consequently, it is not possible to adequately assess the efficacy and effectiveness of a treatment under the same experimental conditions. While efficacy trials investigate a causal relationship between a treatment and outcomes under ideal experimental conditions, effectiveness trials aim to evaluate how well different treatments perform under the everyday clinical conditions, where they would be applied [2]. It is generally accepted that all trials fall somewhere on a continuum between explanatory and pragmatic trials.

The Pragmatic-Explanatory Continuum Indicator-2 (PRECIS-2) tool [2] and updated Consolidated Standards of Reporting Trials (CONSORT) checklist [3] have been developed in order to clearly define the characteristics of pragmatic studies with respect to several important dimensions. According to these guidelines, the extent of pragmatism of a surgical trial can be determined based on features such as;

1. Eligibility criteria and recruitment method of patients' representative of a disease group in a usual clinical setting,
2. Organization of the intervention and flexibility of delivery and adherence to the given therapy,
3. Quality and intensity of the follow-up compared with everyday clinical practice and
4. The assessment of relevant and high-quality outcome measures and data analysis [4].

While future surgical trials are likely to benefit from the generalizability of results derived from a pragmatic study design, their main objectives should be to collect high-quality evidence capable of shaping everyday clinical practice, rather than strict adherence to pragmatic criteria. However, it is worth considering that while explanatory RCTs aim to generate consistent results with high reproducibility, pragmatic trials confer the advantage of yielding consistent and valid results by accurately assessing relevant outcome measures under generalizable conditions. Several recent surgical trials serve as good examples with various degrees of explanatory and pragmatic features. The Meniscal Tear in Osteoarthritis Research (METEOR) trial [5] aims to evaluate the efficacy of arthroscopic partial meniscectomy versus a standardized physical therapy protocol in symptomatic meniscus tear patients. The Treatment of Meniscal Tear in Osteoarthritis (TeMPO) trial [6] focuses on assessing the differences between four different non-operative regimens in reducing pain and improving function in patients with meniscal tear and osteoarthritis. Finally, the STABILITY

**Fact Box 24.2**

According to the PRECIS-2 tool and updated CONSORT checklist, the extent of pragmatism in an RCT depends on:

1. Patient recruitment and eligibility representative of the disease group in the everyday clinical scenario.

2. Organization of the intervention and flexibility in terms of delivery and adherence to the treatment.
3. Quality and intensity of the follow-up compared with everyday clinical practice.
4. Evaluation of relevant and high-quality outcome measures and data analysis.

trial [7] compares outcomes between patients undergoing anterior cruciate ligament (ACL) reconstruction with those undergoing lateral extraarticular tenodesis (LET) in conjunction with anterior cruciate ligament reconstruction (ACL-R).

## 24.3 International Research Networks and Registries

The use of data recorded in registries enables researchers to explore the epidemiology and evaluate the quality and outcomes of a variety of treatment methods available for a patient population with a given disease. A large volume of prospectively collected registry data on patient- and intervention-related variables, along with the collection of outcome measurements over time, enables the investigation of trends in terms of surgical techniques, factors impacting surgical and patient-reported outcomes, and the current standard of care on a nationwide or international scale [8, 9]. Simultaneously, registry-based studies may also serve as substitutes for RCTs, where they are unfeasible and generate hypotheses to be investigated by future RCTs [10]. One recent editorial discussing the lessons learnt from 15 years of research on the Scandinavian knee ligament registries proposed three key ideas to guide the future use of registry data [11]. According to this report, surgical registries should be encouraged to recruit patients undergoing non-operative treatment for a specific injury in order to avoid selection bias against this patient group and to gain a deeper understanding of how operative and non-operative treatments truly compare in terms of functional outcomes. Moreover, conducting registry-based RCTs have the potential to provide a low-cost alternative compared with conventional RCTs, as previously collected prospective data is readily available and patient recruitment can be completed relatively quickly. Lastly, international collaboration involving multiple national registries enable recruitment of large cohorts for a particular study, improving generalizability of its results and the ability to investigate subpopulations of the treatment groups. However, several challenges must be overcome in order to implement these strategies, such as consistency and standardization of data collection across registries, methods to assure data security and obtaining consent from participating patients and healthcare centers. Most importantly, studies conducted on registry data are only as strong as the completeness and reliability of the data they contain [12]. Future strategies should therefore be aimed at finding ways to facilitate and increase patient compliance with the reporting of outcome measures, which can result in more accurate assessment of patient populations and higher reliability of the subsequent studies performed.

Small studies conducted by individual institutions are unlikely to lead to any major new clinical evidence that can be published in high-impact journals, let alone breakthroughs with a worldwide impact on the practice of the orthopedic society. In the future, establishment of national and international collaborative research networks will enable researchers to answer questions of a study by accumulating data from large patient populations recruited across geographically separated surgical sites. The robustness of data collected in this manner will enhance the reliability of the conclusions drawn from a particular trial and influence patient management and care. Operation of an international research network requires:

1. A motivated and well-organized leadership committee comprised of investigators from individual institutions with sufficient expertise in designing and implementing study protocols,

2. Interdisciplinary teams consisting of trial experts, statisticians, and senior surgeons with academic backgrounds and.
3. Trainees, including medical students mentored by senior physicians responsible for recruiting patients and data collection [13]. Formalizing of such trial networks is advantageous from the perspective of standardizing research methodology and data management and protection through a centralized repository as well as from an economic standpoint.

**Fact Box 24.3**

The key ideas guiding the future use of registry data:

1. Inclusion of patients treated non-operatively.
2. Performing registry-based RCTs.
3. International collaboration between national registries.

## 24.4 The Role of Multicenter Trials

Over the last decade, multicenter trials have been at the forefront of answering important research questions that provide high-quality evidence in the field of orthopedic surgery. One of the many challenges of surgical trials is the collection of large datasets with sufficient statistical robustness and power, obtained from patient groups with generalizable characteristics. Multicenter surgical trials address this particular challenge by recruiting patients for a study from several surgical centers, often located across different countries or continents. An inherent advantage of this type of study design is the inclusion of heterogeneous patient populations with a wide variety of ethnicities and demographic parameters. Development of a well-framed common research goal, often initiated by the leader of an institution at which previous efforts have been made to study the given subject, is followed by the creation of a leadership committee, consisting of researchers tasked with supervising the trial at their home institution and coordinating between different centers. The STABILITY trial [7] is a good example of a successful multicenter, randomized, pragmatic surgical trial performed on parallel groups of young (14–25 years old) patients undergoing ACL-R. Patients recruited from seven Canadian and two European centers were randomly allocated into one of two groups, one in which patients undergo single-bundle, hamstring tendon autograft ACL-R alone and another, with patients undergoing the same technique of ACL-R augmented by LET. Randomization of eligible patients was conducted in a 1:1 ratio using telephone or web-based services stratified according to factors such as sex, surgeon, and concomitant meniscus repair in order to eliminate bias across the patient groups. A critical component of multicenter trials is the selection of appropriate, validated clinical outcome measures for answering the proposed research questions. In the STABILITY trial, patients were evaluated at 3, 6, 12, and 24 months, respectively, following operative treatment [7]. Primary outcome measures included ACL-R clinical failure consisting of composite measures of rotatory laxity, pivot shift grade, and graft rupture, while secondary outcome measures comprised an array of patient-reported outcome measures including but not limited to the International Knee Documentation Committee (IKDC) score, ACL Quality of Life Questionnaire (ACL-QOL), and Knee Injury and Osteoarthritis Outcome Score (KOOS) [7]. Ensuring that the appropriate number of patients is recruited in order to answer the proposed research question is one of the central components of multicenter trials. A recent review of the orthopedic literature has, in fact, shown that 28% of negative RCTs are underpowered [14]. Partnering with a statistician is always recommended in order to facilitate the process of performing power calculations, adjusting for correction of patient dropout during the follow-up period. In the STABILITY trial 300 patients per group (600 in total) were determined to provide sufficient power to detect a significant decrease in the relative risk of ACL-R failure following either of the two procedures. Findings of the study showed that augmentation of ACL-R with LET resulted in a statistically significant reduction of ACL-R clinical failure rate compared to ACL-R alone (25% vs. 40%, respectively; relative risk reduction = 0.38; 95% CI = 0.21–0.52; $P < 0.0001$) [15]. The Femoroacetabular Impingement Randomized Controlled Trial (FIRST) [16] is another multicenter RCT that has demonstrated the successful application of power calculations in order to provide reliable answers to the research questions proposed in the study. In order to achieve 80% statistical power for the detection of the minimum clinically important improvement in primary and secondary outcome measures, accounting for loss to follow-up, a total of 220 patients were recruited. The RCT identified that osteochondroplasty was superior compared to lavage with or without repair of the labrum in the hip joint in terms of reoperation rate within 2 years for the surgical correction of femoroacetabular impingement. Both treatment groups displayed a similar rate of 1-year improvement in hip function and pain [16].

In the future, multicenter trials should aim to address several pitfalls and complicating factors in order to improve communication, transparency, and efficiency of the research process between the participating institutions. Importantly, guidelines have been developed for centralization of data repositories and protocols submitted for institutional review board (IRB) approval, which may expedite study initiation across the involved surgical sites and provide a more streamlined platform for subsequent data management and analysis [17]. Perhaps one of the most important goals of multicenter trials in the future should be the implementation of novel ways to maintain communication and coordination between dedicated investigators who are often geographically separated. Finally, surgical trials involving research groups from different countries encourage multinational collaboration, which has the potential of creating long-standing partnerships between institutions capable of undertaking future large-scale research projects together.

## 24.5 Validation of Artificial Intelligence and Machine Learning Models

Over the last decade, the emerging role of artificial Intelligence (AI) and machine learning (ML) have been observed across a wide variety of industries, including healthcare and medical practice. While fields like radiology, oncology, and pathology have already started to permit the adoption of AI, practical applications in orthopedic surgery are also being demonstrated. Clinicians face the everyday challenge of making decisions in terms of diagnostic and therapeutic interventions with long-lasting implications on patient quality of life. While they may be supported by long years of clinical training, these decisions are subject to errors in human cognition and judgment [18]. Rapid advances in the field of AI have paved the way for novel research efforts to investigate the possibility of shared diagnostic and therapeutic decision-making using ML models trained on robust datasets. A recent review of ML applications in orthopedic surgical outcome prediction identified spinal surgery, arthroplasty, and trauma as the subspecialties in context of which ML algorithms have most frequently been studied [19]. The same study reported medical management, survival, complications, and patient-reported outcome measures to be the most frequently studied outcome domains using this method [19].

In the field of orthopedic sports, medicine prediction of injury risk, automatic interpretation of medical images, evaluation of patient-reported outcome measures predictive of certain clinical outcomes, and optimization of value-based care and decision-making are some areas that may benefit from novel, innovative approaches made possible by the use of AI [20, 21]. An example of a proof-of-concept study conducted using this technique is a recent model developed to predict functional outcomes in patients following primary hip arthroscopy based on the most relevant variables identified by ML algorithms applied to patient data [22]. In this study, the best performing ML algorithm identified eight factors that were able to reliably predict the minimal clinically important difference in 2-year postoperative Hip Outcome Score—Activities of Daily Living scores with an 84% success rate (Table 24.1). While this study demonstrates an internally validated example of a ML application, external validation of such algorithms in the context of RCTs will be essential in order to evaluate the generalizability and justify the future use of ML models in clinical decision-making. However, as we

**Table 24.1** The most important features contributing to achieving clinically significant improvement on the Hip Outcome Score—Activities of Daily Living (HOS-ADL) subscale determined by random forest feature elimination [22]

| |
|---|
| 1. Baseline HOS-ADL score |
| 2. Body mass index |
| 3. Baseline visual analog scale (VAS) pain score |
| 4. Age |
| 5. Sex (male/female) |
| 6. Tönnis grade (0 or 1) |
| 7. Preoperative symptom duration (greater or less than 2 years) |
| 8. Drug allergies (presence of 1 or more) |

*HOS-ADL* Hip Outcome Score Activities of Daily Living, *VAS* visual analog scale

acknowledge the excellent predictive abilities of AI, recently performed studies applying ML algorithms to the diagnosis of meniscus and ACL injuries [23, 24] highlight that current models still do not outperform clinicians and should therefore be regarded as a tool for augmenting diagnostic accuracy and outcome prediction rather than a substitute for human expertise. In the future, the everyday use of such AI-based predictive models will facilitate surgical decision-making and help individualize treatment based on patient characteristics.

## 24.6 Conclusion

At the conclusion of this overview of some of the trends at the forefront of future trial design, it is important to mention that the benefit of a well-executed surgical trial will not be limited to answering of the primary research question. Instead, surgical trials embracing pragmatic approaches, the use of multinational registries, collaboration across surgical sites and new technological tools are likely to generate further important research questions to explore and new approaches to evaluate these questions with. Ultimately, these trends will facilitate the emergence of new partnerships and international collaboration essential for the future investigation of new and existing surgical interventions.

## References

1. Schwartz D, Lellouch J. Explanatory and pragmatic attitudes in therapeutical trials. J Clin Epidemiol. 2009;62(5):499–505. https://doi.org/10.1016/j.jclinepi.2009.01.012.
2. Loudon K, Treweek S, Sullivan F, Donnan P, Thorpe KE, Zwarenstein M. The PRECIS-2 tool: designing trials that are fit for purpose. BMJ. 2015;350:h2147. https://doi.org/10.1136/bmj.h2147.
3. Zwarenstein M, Treweek S, Gagnier JJ, Altman DG, Tunis S, Haynes B, et al. Improving the reporting of pragmatic trials: an extension of the CONSORT statement. BMJ. 2008;337:a2390. https://doi.org/10.1136/bmj.a2390.
4. Ford I, Norrie J. Pragmatic trials. N Engl J Med. 2016;375(5):454–63. https://doi.org/10.1056/NEJMra1510059.
5. Katz JN, Brophy RH, Chaisson CE, de Chaves L, Cole BJ, Dahm DL, et al. Surgery versus physical therapy for a meniscal tear and osteoarthritis. N Engl J Med. 2013;368(18):1675–84. https://doi.org/10.1056/NEJMoa1301408.
6. Sullivan JK, Irrgang JJ, Losina E, Safran-Norton C, Collins J, Shrestha S, et al. The TeMPO trial (treatment of meniscal tears in osteoarthritis): rationale and design features for a four arm randomized controlled clinical trial. BMC Musculoskelet Disord. 2018;19(1):429. https://doi.org/10.1186/s12891-018-2327-9.
7. Getgood A, Bryant D, Firth A, Stability G. The Stability study: a protocol for a multicenter randomized clinical trial comparing anterior cruciate ligament reconstruction with and without lateral extra-articular Tenodesis in individuals who are at high risk of graft failure. BMC Musculoskelet Disord. 2019;20(1):216. https://doi.org/10.1186/s12891-019-2589-x.
8. Granan LP, Bahr R, Steindal K, Furnes O, Engebretsen L. Development of a national cruciate ligament surgery registry: the Norwegian National Knee Ligament Registry. Am J Sports Med. 2008;36(2):308–15. https://doi.org/10.1177/0363546507308939.
9. Ahlden M, Samuelsson K, Sernert N, Forssblad M, Karlsson J, Kartus J. The Swedish National Anterior Cruciate Ligament Register: a report on baseline variables and outcomes of surgery for almost 18,000 patients. Am J Sports Med. 2012;40(10):2230–5. https://doi.org/10.1177/0363546512457348.
10. Benson K, Hartz AJ. A comparison of observational studies and randomized, controlled trials. N Engl J Med. 2000;342(25):1878–86. https://doi.org/10.1056/NEJM200006223422506.
11. Hamrin Senorski E, Svantesson E, Engebretsen L, Lind M, Forssblad M, Karlsson J, et al. 15 years of the Scandinavian knee ligament registries: lessons, limitations and likely prospects. Br J Sports

Med. 2019;53(20):1259–60. https://doi.org/10.1136/bjsports-2018-100024.
12. Ueland TE, Carreira DS, Martin RL. Substantial loss to follow-up and missing data in National Arthroscopy Registries: a systematic review. Arthroscopy. 2021;37(2):761–70e3. https://doi.org/10.1016/j.arthro.2020.08.007.
13. Pawlik TM, Sosa JA. Clinical trials. In: Success in academic surgery. 2nd ed. Cham: Springer; 2020.
14. Abdullah L, Davis DE, Fabricant PD, Baldwin K, Namdari S. Is there truly "no significant difference"? Underpowered randomized controlled trials in the orthopaedic literature. J Bone Joint Surg Am. 2015;97(24):2068–73. https://doi.org/10.2106/JBJS.O.00012.
15. Getgood AMJ, Bryant DM, Litchfield R, Heard M, McCormack RG, Rezansoff A, et al. Lateral extra-articular Tenodesis reduces failure of hamstring tendon autograft anterior cruciate ligament reconstruction: 2-year outcomes from the STABILITY study randomized clinical trial. Am J Sports Med. 2020;48(2):285–97. https://doi.org/10.1177/0363546519896333.
16. Femoroacetabular Impingement Randomized Controlled Trial I, Ayeni OR, Karlsson J, Heels-Ansdell D, Thabane L, Musahl V, et al. Osteochondroplasty and labral repair for the treatment of young adults with Femoroacetabular impingement: a randomized controlled trial. Am J Sports Med. 2021;49(1):25–34. https://doi.org/10.1177/0363546520952804.
17. Flynn KE, Hahn CL, Kramer JM, Check DK, Dombeck CB, Bang S, et al. Using central IRBs for multicenter clinical trials in the United States. PLoS One. 2013;8(1):e54999. https://doi.org/10.1371/journal.pone.0054999.
18. Loftus TJ, Filiberto AC, Li Y, Balch J, Cook AC, Tighe PJ, et al. Decision analysis and reinforcement learning in surgical decision-making. Surgery. 2020;168(2):253–66. https://doi.org/10.1016/j.surg.2020.04.049.
19. Ogink PT, Groot OQ, Karhade AV, Bongers MER, Oner FC, Verlaan JJ, et al. Wide range of applications for machine-learning prediction models in orthopedic surgical outcome: a systematic review. Acta Orthop. 2021;92(5):526–31. https://doi.org/10.1080/17453674.2021.1932928.
20. Ramkumar PN, Kunze KN, Haeberle HS, Karnuta JM, Luu BC, Nwachukwu BU, et al. Clinical and research medical applications of artificial intelligence. Arthroscopy. 2021;37(5):1694–7. https://doi.org/10.1016/j.arthro.2020.08.009.
21. Ramkumar PN, Luu BC, Haeberle HS, Karnuta JM, Nwachukwu BU, Williams RJ. Sports medicine and artificial intelligence: a primer. Am J Sports Med. 2021;50:3635465211008648. https://doi.org/10.1177/03635465211008648.
22. Kunze KN, Polce EM, Nwachukwu BU, Chahla J, Nho SJ. Development and internal validation of supervised machine learning algorithms for predicting clinically significant functional improvement in a mixed population of primary hip arthroscopy. Arthroscopy. 2021;37(5):1488–97. https://doi.org/10.1016/j.arthro.2021.01.005.
23. Kunze KN, Rossi DM, White GM, Karhade AV, Deng J, Williams BT, et al. Diagnostic performance of artificial intelligence for detection of anterior cruciate ligament and meniscus tears: a systematic review. Arthroscopy. 2021;37(2):771–81. https://doi.org/10.1016/j.arthro.2020.09.012.
24. Fritz B, Marbach G, Civardi F, Fucentese SF, Pfirrmann CWA. Deep convolutional neural network-based detection of meniscus tears: comparison with radiologists and surgery as standard of reference. Skeletal Radiol. 2020;49(8):1207–17. https://doi.org/10.1007/s00256-020-03410-2.

The manufacturer's authorised representative in the EU is Springer Nature Customer Service Centre GmbH, Europaplatz 3, 69115 Heidelberg, Germany. If you have any concerns regarding our products, please contact ProductSafety@springernature.com

Printed and bound by CPI Group (UK) Ltd, Croydon, CR0 4YY
30/09/2026
02225594-0007